LEGENDS AND LEGACIES
Pacesetters in the Profession of Dietetics

Connie E. Vickery
Nancy Cotugna

University of Delaware

KENDALL/HUNT PUBLISHING COMPANY
2460 Kerper Boulevard P.O. Box 539 Dubuque, Iowa 52004-0539

Dedication

To my parents—Joe and Jennie Cotugna—who are the wind beneath my wings.

and

To my folks—Vic and Laomi Vickery—who must now go forth and move this book.

Contents

Preface

A profession is shaped and molded by dynamic and dedicated individuals whose careers have made a difference. Women and men who have given unselfishly are the legends; their expertise, time, and talent, are the legacies described in *Legends and Legacies*. Thirty-five outstanding leaders in nutrition and dietetics accepted our invitation to contribute their professional autobiographical sketches by sharing their careers that have taken a path for which they are well known.

As dietetic educators, we are always searching for ways to stimulate and excite students about the field and instill a sense of professional pride. Our fellow educators who are frequently asked "What can I do in dietetics?" will find this book to be a jewel of a resource. *Legends and Legacies* is intended to interest prospective students, motivate and help current students shape their career paths, and inspire professionals to examine their careers for continued growth and development.

Each story is impressive! We have been both stimulated and moved by their stories which graciously describe successes and failures, joys and sorrows, risks and adventures. Some stories will bring a tear to your eye, some will call forth a laugh, some may even make you angry, but none will leave you untouched. We have read each story over and over and never fail to extract something inspirational. We are confident that our readers, be they students, professional, or interested friend, will find the same inspiration on these pages.

To be sure, the list of contributors is by no means all-inclusive, but rather selective from legends in our own minds! From an initial list, we solicited the advice of three distinguished professionals. Our "blue ribbon panel," two past presidents of The American Dietetic Association and a presenter of the annual Lenna Frances Cooper Memorial lecture, reviewed the names and offered suggestions. Fifty professionals were invited to participate in the project. Several who could not contribute for various reasons offered encouragement and wished us success in what they thought sounded like an exciting and much-needed venture.

We wish to express our deepest appreciation and sincere thanks to each of the thirty-five contributors who, during the year 1989, generously shared his or her personal insights for the benefit of others. We have made a concerted effort in editing manuscripts to preserve each writer's style and personality. Many contributors wrote us more than once to ask, "Why me?" Most credit others for their success. Several contributors will learn that while they were writing about their mentors, they themselves were identified as mentors. A portion of the revenue from sales of *Legends and Legacies* will be contributed to The American Dietetic Association Foundation as a tribute to the professional excellence and dedication demonstrated by these individuals.

We would also like to take this opportunity to recognize our own mentors who have made a significant and lasting impact on our careers. Nancy credits Major Eleanor Mathewson, whose World War II escapades and Hospital Ship HOPE stories made dietetics come alive in the classroom for her and whose continued support and encouragement have meant so much over the years. Connie acknowledges the memory of Louise Hatch, who impressed her with high standards of ethics and professional responsibility and who seemed to thrive on making those around her look good and feel a sense of pride in their accomplishments.

With all the time and effort provided by the contributors, *Legends and Legacies* should be flawless. To the extent that it is not, we accept full responsibility.

Mary Ruth Bedford

Mary Ruth Bedford, PhD, RD, LD
is a Consulting Dietitian in El Paso, Texas

What resulted in a lifelong dedication to the field of dietetics did not begin with that as a clearly defined goal. But once Mary Ruth Bedford made the decision to commit her education, skills, and energy to dietetics, she became immersed in the profession. Her career includes experiences in clinical dietetics, food service management, administrative dietetics, public health nutrition, and dietetic education. Mary Ruth Bedford has always been involved with local and state dietetic association activities from Colorado to Iowa; Nebraska to North Carolina; Kansas to Virginia; Massachusetts to Texas. Time and interest devoted to these activities have not attenuated time and energy devoted to the national Association. She has served as ADA Liaison to the American Home Economics Association, Chairman of the Council on Education, and member of the Quality Assurance Committee—just to name a few!

Mary Ruth Bedford

Getting into the field of dietetics was not a clearly defined goal in my life. My parents did not discuss with my brother and myself whether we should go to college, the assumption was that we would. Beyond that we did not have specific direction from them. They had both been teachers and somehow I was certain that this was one thing I did not want to do.

But after two years attending a liberal arts college while living at home, the time had come to make a decision as to what I was going to do. These were the years of World War II, money was very tight in our family so choices were limited. Because I was interested in foods and had talked with the lady responsible for the foodservice at the college, I investigated dietetics. Madison College, now James Madison University, was the institution in Virginia which offered this option. To get in the required courses meant attending two years and two summer school sessions. I liked the option although I found the science courses most difficult. I felt I was most fortunate that I could intern at the University of Colorado Medical Center in Denver beginning that next January. We had many relatives in Colorado (both my mother's and father's families), my brother had graduated in electrical engineering from the University of Colorado (and I envied him that), and besides I have always loved Colorado.

I can remember a few highlights about those internship days. Six of us lived in a private home about 1/4 mile from the hospital, but we ate most of our meals at the hospital. We worked long and hard, studied at night in one of the dining rooms at the hospital. We had some of our experiences in a private hospital, St. Luke's, which had a Swiss chef in charge of the kitchen and at Children's Hospital where I did my staff relief experience. When I learned of a vacancy on the staff of Presbyterian Hospital, I wanted that job so much that I told the chief dietitian that I was the one that they wanted to hire permanently and not temporarily. She agreed, and I spent the next two and a half years working split shifts, weekends, did both clinical and administrative tasks and enjoyed the people and the opportunities.

Then I decided it was time to move on. Another dietitian whom I had known at Children's Hospital, Denver who was now at the Children's Hospital at the University of Iowa Hospitals told me of a vacancy on the staff in the Therapeutic Department. So, for the next five years I had many valuable opportunities to interact with and learn from many capable people. This was a 1000 bed hospital with outpatient clinics, with some of the best physicians in the country, with Dr. Kate Daum and other competent dietetic practitioners as well as dietetic interns who came because of the hospital and most often because of Dr. Daum. Dr. Daum, not the greatest administrator, was renowned as a scientist who loved her laboratory. Interns as well as her staff were in awe not only of her knowledge but also the respect and the relationship she had with the doctors who often consulted her about the patients. She received the Borden Award one year and her staff and interns shared in that celebration. Evelyn Brandt, the Chief Therapeutic Dietitian with whom I worked, was one of the most capable, effective dietitians I have

2

known. She had overall responsibilities for preparation and delivery of all modified diets and instructions related to them. I supervised the kitchen that prepared all the modified diets and delivered them and assisted her as needed including assuming all responsibilities when she was not on duty. Research diets served from our kitchen were usually prepared by the interns conducting that part of the study.

Next I left for a position at Nebraska State Teachers College, where I managed the college food service and the snack shop for a year. I was excited when I could move back to Denver where I was the dietitian at a home for mentally retarded for two and a half years. I learned to be patient with the "children" as we called those who assisted the small staff which I had. I did lots of negotiating and spent time trying to convince, not the administrator, but a non-professional individual who exercised authority over much of the institution, that I did know how to manage the foodservice. The situation was unreconcilable and I was glad to move on to the Veterans Administration hospital in southeastern Colorado where I was the Assistant Chief. It was great experience and I would probably have stayed with the VA, which would have changed the rest of my life. But I had the opportunity to return to Presbyterian Medical Center in Denver and be the Chief of Dietetics. It was a rough beginning but the administrator gave me tremendous support. My greatest joys included working with the total hospital staff, including the Auxiliary, hiring many young dietitians, and being highly involved with the team to renovate the foodservice. We moved the kitchen into what was to become the dining room while the "old kitchen" was rebuilt. Service to the patients which had been decentralized was changed to a centralized trayline. We opened a coffee shop which serviced the public as well as the staff who chose to eat there rather than in the cafeteria. I stayed long enough to enjoy the rewards of the agonizing days of construction and reorganization of the department. I was convinced that administrative dietetics was where I wanted to be even though I kept in touch with the clinical work of the dietitians.

Again, I sought a new experience. Since I had been challenged in designing a foodservice, including the selection of the type of system and the equipment, I pursued the opportunity of full-time employment with a foodservice consultant. This was not the time, although I continued to consider this as a future opportunity for another career move. Another friend, Marjorie Morrison Donnelly, a public health nutritionist and dietitian whom I had known in Denver had married a physician who was with the North Carolina State Board of Health and living in Raleigh. In fact, she has served in many elected positions in The American Dietetic Association (ADA) including its President as well as President of The American Dietetic Association Foundation (ADAF). She has been a true contributor to dietetics as a practitioner and in the Association. So, I made a big decision to leave Denver and take a position as the consulting dietitian with the Nursing Home Section in the North Carolina State Board of Health. What a change in pace and responsibilities. I travelled the state and worked with personnel in over a hundred nursing homes. I believe that I accomplished many good things and recruited dietitians back to the workplace as consultants to some of the facilities. Through my networking, I learned that Indiana State University was looking for a person to teach the management components of the dietetic program. I wanted to use my dietetic experiences in yet another way so I accepted this opportunity to teach and share them. I worked day and night to prepare classes. Not only did I teach management, layout and design, quantity food production, but I taught a beginning foods class as well as meal management. This opportunity was available because I was recommended by peers who recognized that my many years of excellent work experiences in dietetics were an asset.

But I realized that if I wanted to teach at the college level I would have to have at least a master's degree. I took classes at the University of Iowa in nutrition but I never completed the necessary work for the degree. Since it had been years since I had taken a college course for credit, I took classes during the summer. With some confidence I found that I could discipline myself and I did have the ability to go back to college and be successful. I did not have a good undergraduate record so I have much empathy for students whose grades have not been outstanding but are good at applying what they have learned.

I sought a program where I felt I could get the desired course work and be in an environment and would nurture my interests and abilities. Grace Shugart, then President of The American Dietetic Association and head of the Institutional Management Department at Kansas State University (KSU) was supportive of my efforts. So, off I went to Kansas determined to earn the masters in a calendar year, which I did. Course work completed, research defended, I headed back to my teaching responsibilities in Indiana. But before I left, Richard Vaden, who had been one of my instructors and had become a friend as had his wife, Allene who had completed her doctoral work and was teaching at KSU, encouraged me to stay and continue my studies. I was pleased with myself that I had earned the masters but the savings were gone. Most importantly, I was not prepared to accept such an enormous task at that time. However, I soon decided to return and was delighted to be offered an assistantship in which I would teach and supervise juniors in the coordinated dietetic program. Those were busy yet enjoyable years but I was glad to be back job hunting *with* a doctoral degree.

Again, because of my professional contacts, I was headed back east to plan the coordinated dietetic program at Virginia Polytechnic Institute and State University with strong support from Dean Laura Jane Harper. What a busy few months. We submitted the self-study and we soon accepted our first class. Once established I could begin to do some graduate teaching and supervising of research studies along with my other responsibilities. I was well into University activities when the chance came to go to Boston to teach and work with masters students. My greatest reward at Virginia Tech, and later in Boston, was students who graduated and became excellent practitioners and involved in professional activities and were happy with the choice they have made.

One of the highlights of those days just before departing for Boston was the surprise luncheon the students/graduates planned with assistance from the faculty and administrators. The plaque which I received ''in recognition and grateful appreciation for caring, sharing, and guiding'' along with the one I was presented ''for tireless efforts meeting the needs of patients and staff'' from Presbyterian Medical Center are among my prized possessions.

At the MGH Institute of Health Professions, classes were small but the students were bright and eager to learn. As always, I learned along with my students when we discussed the current environment and its problems as well as the management of food-service systems. This ended too soon when the program was cut from the budget of the Dietetics Program even though we had a good record of graduating our students and in spite of the need for a graduate program in foodservice systems management.

Job opportunities for which I was prepared and in which I was interested did not occur during the next months. I decided if I could not be challenged by a position as I had been with every job in the past, I would look at my alternatives. Since living in Boston was expensive, the situation forced me to move to El Paso, Texas where my brother lived. I settled in and have continued to be involved by doing volunteer work for The American Dietetic Association. Other opportunities have been proposed but this independence has made it possible for me to make choices as to how my time and energies will be spent.

During my career I have always been involved with local and state dietetic association activities. Because of my interests I have been active in the Dietetic Practice Group called DPG #41, ADA Members with Management Responsibilities in Health Care Delivery Systems and with the Foodservice Systems Management Education Council. Serving as Chair of both of these groups was truly rewarding and exciting to see the important work and influence they have had.

My current involvements with The American Dietetic Association are because of my previous activities and considered expertise. I have been a site visitor for dietetic education programs since 1980 except for the time I served on the now Council on Education, including its Chair. Because of my experiences as a site visitor, as a dietetic education program director, as a member of the hospital staff with an internship, I was appointed to serve for three years on the Review Panel for Accreditation/Approval of Dietetic Education Programs for the Council on Education. Also, I have been a member of the Knowledge Requirements Committee for the Role Delineation Study. I like these types of commitments not only because of the value to the profession and the Association but because I find them challenging, stimulating and rewarding.

Because of my involvements with the Council on Education I worked on the Committees for the Standards of Practice and Educational Standards Committee. It has been pleasing to see these Standards finally accepted and implemented and to follow their utilization. In my study of the background for the development of the Standards of Education I read extensively about guidelines for our educational programs from the beginning of the profession. We can be proud that we have had well articulated goals which have evolved over the years through the growth of the profession and through the quality of those dietitians involved with preparing future practitioners.

Being on the Board of Editors for the Journal of The American Dietetic Association is certainly a challenge and one which requires that I do thoughtful review of the manuscripts that are submitted for publication. My areas include dietetic education and adult education as well as foodservice management and its wide range of areas. Reading about the most recent research being conducted and having the opportunity to preview the findings is exciting. More practitioners need to write about the studies they conduct and not leave most of the reporting to the educators-researchers and their graduate students.

When I left Boston, I gave most of my professional library to the National Center for Nutrition and Dietetics (NCND) but I did share some of my books and materials with two former doctoral students from Virginia Tech who are now teaching in universities. Since my interest in books was well known by the staff of The American Dietetic Association Foundation, I was asked to Chair the Library Committee for the NCND which is well underway. As usual, I wanted to see more action but the staff and the Board have moved very carefully and thoughtfully in the planning of the NCND. Advice has been sought from those with expertise needed for such as undertaking. The financial support needed to implement and continue this project is enormous but a most worthwhile investment for our contributions of time, ideas and monies.

During my career in dietetics, I have been challenged and inspired by those with whom I have had contact and by those situations in which I have found myself. At times I have envied those who have had different talents and who have attained certain accomplishments that I would have liked to have achieved or achieved at their levels. But generally, rather than envy these persons, I have learned to enjoy sharing their accomplishments while admiring their unique abilities.

I have been a teacher in many different situations: in the academic environment with both undergraduate and graduate students, with those in nursing homes as a consultant, in the hospitals as one who helped teach dietetic interns as well as hired many dietitians in their first positions. I have tried to discern abilities as well as ambitions of these individuals and help them to learn and most importantly, to develop themselves.

It is very important that we attain satisfaction from whatever work we choose. In dietetics I have found this satisfaction because it has always provided opportunities for new challenges. For me, these challenges have been in different working environments, in many different positions in organizations, with individuals from a wide range of socioeconomic, cultural, educational backgrounds and in many geographic locations.

Occasionally I have looked at those who have worked within one organization for most of their careers and have continued to be stimulated by their work and environment and their profession. Such a situation has its advantages and rewards. However, I am sure that I would make the same decisions about my career changes having the same opportunities again. Without a well-defined plan I focused on increasing responsibilities of authority, which included planning new or more complicated programs, more involvement in the parent organization.

My own interests have been reflected in my studies and activities and have opened up doors not only in my employment but in my professional activities. Also, mobility has provided an abundance of opportunities to meet dietitians from many different

6

working environments, who had different philosophies associated with their professional as well as personal lives. Some of these individuals have affected my own thinking and behavior and I can identify that I have tried to emulate some of their characteristics.

And then there were others whose actions I have not looked upon favorably and I do not consider to be an asset to our profession. Working with many individuals on committees, I have observed the dedication of the charge of the committee by some while others are looking for recognition and personal advancement which could lead to exposure and recognition for them so seeking to be more influential among their Association members. At times, their behavior has not strengthened the purpose of our organization and has had negative affects on our work.

A concern which I continue to have is that some dietitians are functioning at a level below that for which they have been prepared and seem satisfied with their responsibilities as well as remuneration for their work. Our profession does not benefit from these individuals, so the dilemma continues as to what can be done about them. But we also have some members who are moving very fast into new areas and sometimes with little forethought of what they do want for themselves and their profession that will stand the test of time.

From the time I joined The American Dietetic Association until 1988, the membership increased from about 15,000 to over 50,000. The size of the budget has changed, the structure of the Association as well as headquarters have changed, the demands of our members and the environment including our clients have changed. The problems may not be any more complex or demanding than in the earlier years of ADA, they just seem so. We have made giant strides in a profession that has changed and continues to change. Through the years, the needs for all dietitians to have proficiency in managerial skills has become increasingly important and well documented. Regardless, of the area of practice each dietitian needs to have problem analysis, decision making skills, as well as an appreciation of the organization/system in which employed as well as the macro-environment. Because of the importance of affective behaviors of dietitians those associated with attitudes, beliefs and values, my dissertation research will probably be the most valuable contribution I have made to the dietetic profession.

We must not only continue to stress the importance of quality practice but we must be thoughtful in making our decisions about the direction that will be the most beneficial to the Association, its individual members as well as those for whom we provide our many diverse services.

Besides my family—my parents and my brother, I have been influenced by those dietitians whom I have admired because of their strengths of character, their professionalism, and their professional capabilities. I have also been influenced by both my academic preparation and professional practitioner experiences as well as by the environments in which I have worked and have visited in my travels. Travelling has certainly expanded my mind and my vision. I have read about each of the countries where I have toured. Then I have visited churches, museums, shops and markets, and other sites of importance to the various locales. Also, I have found by taking pictures and studying the foods and eating habits of the people I have been enriched while learning much about Hawaii, Mexico, Iran, Nigeria, and some of the countries of Europe as well as the Indians in the Southwest. I had hoped to participate in some educational programs in other countries but my timing has not been so that I could negotiate with the appropriate parties to do this.

Recently I have been studying and taking some of the examinations required to be an amateur radio operator. This opens up another area for contacts with people in the States and around the world. I find myself spending more time with this new found interest and other "hams" fascinated by this avocation. Because of my love of books and fascination for searching the literature on many different topics, I will be spending more and more time in libraries as a volunteer and pursuing my interest in genealogy.

Beatrice Donaldson David

Beatrice Donaldson David, PhD is Emeritus Professor
Food Administration, Department of Food Science
University of Wisconsin—Madison

Beatrice Donaldson David credits her successful career in dietetics to her mentors, those professional role models who supported her efforts and were willing to take a risk on the talent they perceived in her. Educated during the Great Depression and joining ADA in 1934, her career spanned 45 years in food service management and academia. From 1952 until her retirement in 1978, Beatrice Donaldson David was a faculty member at the University of Wisconsin where she wrote more than 75 articles reporting research in food administration and related topics. She served ADA as Food Administration Section Chairman and Chairman of the Editorial Board of the journal. She was the recipient of the Copher Award, the highest tribute awarded by ADA to a member. In 1989, she received one of two College of Home Economics Outstanding Alumni Awards from the University of Nebraska where she earned her undergraduate degree.

Beatrice Donaldson David

In the business world it is said that every one who makes it has a mentor; that is, an older person in the profession who encourages and supports the career progress of emerging colleagues. They are risk takers who bet on perceived talent in a young person and risk emotional involvement in working closely with that protege. I would like to acknowledge my mentors who, at various stages of my career, have helped me "make it."

They were: Kate Daum, University of Iowa Hospitals, who continually challenged me to move out of a routine, secure position and into the far from routine and secure world of graduate study and research; Mary de Garmo Bryan, Teachers College of Columbia University, who enthusiastically encouraged my decision to teach; Fern Gleiser, Iowa State University, who, during my first years of teaching, gave me a variety of emergency assignments and was always so sure that I could achieve her expected standards of performance; Grace Augustine, Iowa State University, who delegated to me responsibilities for curriculum planning and teaching, always with the commensurate authority to make major decisions when necessary; and Hester Chadderdon, Iowa State University, who made me aware of the discipline necessary for developing, conducting, and reporting research. I thank my mentors; they were wise advisers and loyal friends.

This then is the story of how these and other mentors, influenced the conception and development of my professional career.

How It All Began

Having a brother at the University of Nebraska while I was in high school was a major factor in helping choose a career in Dietetics and Institution Management. Textiles and clothing had been a major interest but one had to think of job opportunities during the depression. My brother talked with faculty and students and, knowing that I liked science courses and math, was certain that Dietetics would interest me. He was told there would be many positions available. There was concern about taking another year for an internship, but it seemed wise since I would be only 20 when I graduated and obviously needed some added maturity. So from the first year in high school, there was that determination to be a dietitian. There is no recollection that I ever questioned my ability to qualify.

University of Nebraska 1931–33

My professional career mentors were acknowledged in the introduction. But in recalling college years, others come to mind. Transferring to the University after two years in a small junior college was a traumatic experience. There were no special orientation days and although I had my basic sciences and general education courses, planning a schedule was difficult. Classes with freshman who were all new and had been in group orientation, left me feeling alone. In sophomore and junior classes, I was a stranger among groups of students who knew each other from previous years. But always, as it was through my education years and professional career, there seemed to be the right person there for me when I needed guidance. My brother's roommate had a sister in Home Economics who took me under her wing involving me in professional and social activities. Such participation was the first opportunity for me to become aware of ability for assuming responsibilities for leadership and enjoying it. My contribution to the various organizations was recognized by election into membership in Phi Upsilon Omicron, national Home Economics fraternity. Becoming a member of Kappa Delta social sorority extended the range of activities and friendships in the University.

Courses in Institution Management during the senior year and an excellent teacher in the area, Martha Park, were factors influencing my interest then and during my entire career, in the management aspects of dietetics. I loved those courses and the instructor.

Michael Reese Hospital 1933–34

A young graduate assistant wanted someone from Nebraska to have an internship at Michael Reese Hospital and suggested me. I was interested. In 1933 internships were few and dietetic students were increasing in numbers; appointments were not easy to get. This person, by visiting the hospital dietary department, influenced my selection and in July I was there. Another mentor influencing my educational career.

My mother always said that during that year in Chicago "Bea grew up." We new interns really didn't know what to expect but became so involved that soon were believing that the hospital could not get along without us. There were many low points but we learned to accept responsibility and be accountable. At times we felt that we were always being shifted from one service to another or substituting for someone before we learned much about what was going on. This being able to adapt to different situations, and working with personnel and patients with varying levels of education, and of different race and religion, was more of a social education than technical training. Adapting to a new position was less difficult following that concentrated year of learning.

Observing and working with Katherine Mitchell Johnson, the director of dietetics, continued to influence my interest in and concern for the management and administrative aspects of dietetics. And through all the years I remember her telling me that one never assumes something has been done—"You find out!" It was also there that I learned to enjoy working with children in the hospital.

On August 15, 1934 receiving my internship diploma and becoming a member of The American Dietetic Association was achievement of a long sought goal. And I also remained a registered dietitian from the time of its inception until after my retirement.

First Position—Nebraska FERA 1934–35

After completing the internship, anything but hospital dietetics was my major criterion for that first position. So off I went to Blair, Nebraska to accept, with confidence, a position as County Nutritionist for the Federal Emergency Relief Administration. Had that position been offered me ten years later, I would never have felt qualified

11

to be responsible for planning food and clothing budgets for clients, supervising and promoting use of government commodities by demonstrating food preparation and writing newspaper articles, and managing a community canning center. For the cooperation and support of the county nurse and social workers, I was grateful.

After a year in this position, the urge to become a hospital dietitian returned. And when an offer came for a position in my native state of Iowa and not far from my home, accepting was easy.

University of Iowa Hospitals 1935–37

Only a few days before my twenty-third birthday, I felt that my goals and ambitions were finally achieved. I was an administrative dietitian in the Children's Hospital of the University of Iowa Hospitals. Working in this dietary department under Dr. Kate Daum was a different but challenging experience. It was a fun time in my life participating in campus social activities and working with the many students associated with the hospital; having 25 working in the department for their meals really kept me on my toes. Dr. Daum was exciting, rigid, and at times difficult to work with; but she was a kind and caring person. Department and staff were held in high esteem by others in the hospital, especially the medical staff. Learning from her to perform required assignments ''now'' was an important step in alleviating my existing habit of procrastination. Dr. Daum also introduced me to Iowa Dietetic Association meetings.

These were two happy, satisfying years. Personnel during that time of economic depression always came to work and on time. For every position there were at least ten applicants waiting and willing to take time to learn the job without pay until there was a vacancy.

Change came after these years of content routine, by Dr. Daum suggesting that I was wasting my time and should think of moving on to a position with greater opportunities for advancement as well as for graduate study. Graduate study was not one of my priorities at that time; and I had never believed that I qualified. Dr. Daum's faith in my ability supported me through all subsequent advanced study. Her last words to me ten years later, indicating her pleasure in seeing me starting a doctoral program were ''I always knew you could do it.''

Accepting a position in New York City was an agonizing decision to make but the opportunity for working in another children's hospital, the anticipation of eventually studying with Mary de Garmo Bryan, as well as the excitement of living in New York over-ruled other opportunities.

Babies Hospital—Columbia-Presbyterian Medical Center 1937–42

After being promoted to Head Dietitian, concentrating my time on developing a much needed diet manual, planning children's menus, supervising personnel in setting up and distributing trays and keeping the formula room in good order, my interest in and concern for the management and administrative aspects of food service systems strengthened. It was time for me to consider beginning graduate study at Teachers College of Columbia University.

Participating in activities of the New York Dietetic Association was an opportunity to become acquainted with well-known dietitians; persons whom we had read about, whose books we had used in classes. We younger dietitians were impressed because these experienced professionals made us feel welcome and important to the profession. At a busy ADA meeting, Lenna Cooper took the time to ask me what I was doing professionally and what were my goals. She enthusiastically supported my decision for graduate study with Dr. Bryan.

Studying at Teachers College was entirely different from what I had experienced before. The personal contact with faculty and their interest and belief in a student's potential was unbelievable in such a large university. Students were encouraged to do as much as they wanted in projects usually related to their profession. The MA degree was awarded after two years of part-time study while having a full time position. During discussions with Dr. Bryan, concerning the apparent lack of emphasis on management in undergraduate programs of dietetic interns, my thoughts turned to the possibility of a career in higher education teaching what was then called Institution Management. There was an opportunity for me to become an instructor at Iowa State University and to be near home and family once again.

Iowa State University 1942–52

Assisting in managing the student operated "Tea Room," helping Lenore Sullivan teach catering classes, assisting the dietitian and being responsible for food cost accounting in the cooperative residence hall, and counseling freshman and sophomore students were all experiences I later realized to be important in finally having the opportunity to teach Quantity Food Preparation, Equipment Planning, and Organization and Management. And to be promoted to Assistant Professor. All this with guidance from Fern Gleiser.

When Grace Augustine became chairman of the department, her major focus was on developing a graduate program. Recognizing that to advance in higher education, this was an opportune time for me to be the first doctoral candidate in the department. I was not the first to graduate. It took me seven years of taking one course a quarter while working full time and going to summer school. Was I ever discouraged? Yes. Just before prelims and after being told by a counsellor in the graduate school office that some experimental tests indicated a possible lack of aptitude for planning, conducting and reporting research. There were other times, too. But encouragement from friends, advisors, and co-workers was supporting. Invitations from Phi Kappa Phi, Omicron Nu and Psi Chi, all national honor societies were rewarding. My thesis, "Management Aspects and Educational Criteria for School Lunch Programs in Iowa," was accepted and a Ph.D. in Institution Management with a co-major in Education and a minor in Food Science was granted. Recognizing through this research, that many factors affecting quality of food and time planning were major problems in Food Service Systems, ideas began to develop for future research.

Opportunities for research and teaching in universities were available to me. When discussing concerns about ability to direct programs of study and research for graduate students, Dr. Chadderdon helped me realize that my role would be changing. Now I would be the mentor; and she and others of my mentors would feel their time and efforts with me fulfilled.

University of Wisconsin–Madison 1952–78

Accepting an appointment as an Associate Professor in the Department of Foods and Nutrition of the School of Home Economics involved organization and management of the new student operated "Tea Room," re-organizing and teaching Institution Management courses, developing a graduate program and initiating research projects. Continued support and encouragement from administration, faculty and personnel of food service facilities on the campus made much of this possible. Promotion to Professor was achieved. And an invitation to Sigma Delta Epsilon, a professional honor society for graduate women in science was appreciated.

The opportunity to be a chairman of a committee to develop a program for Regional Research project was a challenge and the beginning of the North Central Region Project #120 which continues to function and includes research on various aspects of food service system administration.

A six month sabbatical in 1968–69 gave impetus to on-going research on factors affecting labor time in hospital food service systems. Convincing faculty and researchers in Industrial Engineering and Business Administration at the University of Michigan that their courses and research methods could contribute to the methodology and analysis of my research was not an easy task. Continued research in activity sampling was possible because of their assistance and eventual understanding of problems in providing quality food and service.

While attending a meeting in Chicago, I met Carl David. We had fun times when I was there for meetings and shopping. He was doing temporary work following retirement from extensive traveling for Hearst Newspapers. When we decided to marry in 1971, it was his decision to move to Madison to work at his hobby in retail selling so that I could retain my position until retirement. He loved Chicago and it took some adjustment to life in Madison often called the "mad city."

Retirement 1978

Since retiring as Emeritus Professor in the Food Science Department at the University of Wisconsin–Madison, life has been active and rewarding. Until my husband passed away in 1987, most of my time was involved with care for him following two severe strokes. Although extensive travel as we had planned was limited, we enjoyed short trips to visit friends and relatives. Currently church activities, volunteer responsibilities in a nursing home, participation in social and professional organizations fill my time. Gardening in the summer and reading and sewing in the winter provide relaxation. Travels include visiting relatives and friends in Iowa and Nebraska.

After 45 years in a professional career, I looked forward to retirement. Things seemed to become more complicated and not as exciting. Or perhaps I was just tired of working. I do miss the contact with professional co-workers and other friends. Retirement can be exciting and rewarding and was for me upon receiving these honors:

> September 25, 1978 Selected as the Sixteenth Lenna F. Cooper Lecturer at the 61st Annual Meeting of The American Dietetic Association, New Orleans.

> September 13, 1983 Presented with the Marjorie Hulsizer Copher Award at the 66th Annual Meeting of The American Dietetic Association, Anaheim, California.

> April 29, 1989 Recipient of the 1989 College of Home Economics Outstanding Alumni Award at the University of Nebraska Lincoln.

Professional Motivators

In retrospect, faith of mentors, activities in professional organizations, association with students, and a supportive family—all were effective in motivating me to achieve professional goals. Recognizing that mentors had objectives and standards, for my performance, which at times seemed to be beyond my potential, was a major incentive.

Interaction and cooperation with professional colleagues not only stimulates personal and professional growth, but also the expansion and development of the profession itself. It has been a privilege for me to participate in the growth and development of The American Dietetic Association, the American Home Economics Association and others through a variety of activities. As a member, the benefits to me and my professional career have far exceeded the contributions I have made.

The experiences of being chairman of the Food Administration Section of The American Dietetic Association and of the Institution Management Section of the American Home Economics Association were both educational and motivating. And worth all the time and effort involved. Learning to know all the people who participated in a four year project for the ADA was satisfying. The results of their efforts were published in the Journal of The American Dietetic Association.

The AHEA and ADA sponsored the first Conference for College and University Faculties of Institution Management in 1962 when I was the AHEA Section chairman. This was an opportunity for us to meet and plan with those who were long-time members of both organizations. We were concerned about the development of guidelines for course content common to all curricula in Institution Management. The group continues to meet and discuss common problems. The name has been changed to "Food Service Systems Management Education Council."

Rather than list all the professional organizations of which I am a member and the activities involved, I would like to emphasize the importance of eventually arriving at a balance of activities in personal and professional life. There came a time in my career when, feeling overwhelmed with responsibilities, determining my priorities was necessary for satisfactory performance both at home and at work. Believing that it is wise to encourage younger professionals to take over more of the activities in professional organizations, I did not continue as active as I was in several. Focusing my career on the development of research programs and devoting most of my time to advising and directing graduate student programs, made living and working more satisfying and relaxing. So contact with undergraduate students and professional colleagues at other institutions was moved lower on the priority list; that was a difficult decision to make.

There is no greater incentive for doing things differently and better than being involved with students: undergraduate, interns or graduate students. This was evident in my first position and, thinking back on my career, the positions I was really interested in accepting were those where I could have contact with students. Extracurricular activities with student organizations were an enjoyable part of being a faculty member of two universities. For the most of that time, I served as advisor to students in Omicron Nu, Phi Upsilon Omicron, Home Economics Clubs and a social sorority.

Whenever I am commended for research projects developed and the content and the number of publications credited to my name, I always emphasize that little of that would have been possible without the intelligence, dedication, ingenuity and cooperation of nineteen Ph.D. and thirty-nine M.S. candidates. Students are super motivators.

There were times during much of my professional life, when the responsibilities of caring for my mother and my physically disabled husband might have limited my opportunities, activities and interests. The advantages were soon obvious to me. They were my greatest supporters—not always understanding what I was doing or why but believing I was *right* and always the *best*. This was a rare and effective kind of motivation for me. And I liked being "needed." And I shall always have a real understanding of and compassion for the elderly and the disabled. The "need to be needed" motivates my volunteer activities in a nursing home.

Reflections—A Pot-Pourri

What have been the effects of changes during these 45 years on the profession? With the growth of The American Dietetic Association the changes in focus and the many new and different positions made available, the profession thrives. The economic depression, World War II, the fabulous fifties, the Viet Nam War, the unrest of the sixties, minority problems, and the explosion of knowledge, all required adjustments in educational content and methods, management of human and physical resources and methods of achieving objectives in food service systems operations. There is evidence that the profession has, over those years, met these challenges.

What of the future? From 3000 members in 1934, when I joined, to more than 50,000 in 45 years is progress. Now reading about all the committees, activities, and areas of specialization in the Annual Reports of The American Dietetic Association, boggles my mind. But it is exciting to observe activities of young members and the variety of opportunities created by them through motivation, ingenuity, and initiative. However, to have adequate professionals to meet changing needs in the future, depends a great deal on the emphasis given to the *content* of educational programs as well as the *methods* used. The future looks great.

What has been my philosophy of personal and professional life? That is difficult for me to write. Most of it, I hope, has been woven throughout the story of my professional career. That it, along with goals and priorities, changed throughout the years is evident and reflects the influence of family, friends, professional colleagues, church, age and sociologic and economic events.

Just before retiring, a women's organization on the campus asked in a questionnaire, to what women's organizations or social movement did I attribute my rank, salary, research grants, equal rights with men, and general progress in my career. My answer was "none." I attributed progress in my career to having mentors there for me at the right time, a supportive family, a good educational background, an exciting and interesting profession, taking advantage of opportunities that came my way, and having lots of faith. Plus utilizing many hours of "good hard work" to achieve my personal and professional goals and taking one day at a time.

Judith L. Dodd

Judith L. Dodd, MS, RD
is a Nutrition Education Consultant with
the Dairy & Nutrition Council, as well as
Adjunct Assistant Professor of Clinical Dietetics/Nutrition,
University of Pittsburgh, PA

It is obvious after reading Judy Dodd's story that she has an unique ability to take advantage of opportunities whenever and wherever they present themselves. Although the theme appears to be "in the right place at the right time," colleagues and associates know better. She built upon early interests in people and food through a solid knowledge foundation. Her professional background is rich in experience. Judy Dodd purports that the traditional hospital role prepared her for some very non-traditional roles she has selected—something which is important for tomorrow's professional to consider today. Throughout her sketch, she subtly points out obstacles she faced as a woman trying to build a career and how she faced each as a challenge. Her commitment to the profession of dietetics is clear. In 1988, Judy Dodd was honored by the Pennsylvania Dietetic Association with the Distinguished Service Award.

Judith L. Dodd

As a senior Food and Nutrition major in a traditional Home Economics program, it was expected I would become a dietitian. I was resisting! The decision to enter a dietetic internship was the first of many career opportunities that put me on a path different from one I had envisioned. And, as with the internship decision, taking the new direction offered challenging and exhilarating experiences. As I relive my career choices, I realize that a certain amount of risk taking and the influence of several key mentors have brought me to this point. Through it all, the drive to make a difference has kept me on target.

My only recollection of a career choice, once I was past a short-lived goal of entering classical ballet, was to study something that combined food and people. I was surrounded by family members who prepared and enjoyed good, honest fare. My maternal grandmother was a "receipt" collector who shared with me a love of cookbooks. Even today I find great entertainment value in the narratives of regional cookbooks. From working in our family's retail business, I gained an appreciation of what it meant to work with people of all ages and backgrounds.

I entered Carnegie Institute of Technology, now Carnegie Mellon University, because of the reputation of the foods and nutrition program and because it was in my home town. To go to college meant commuting to enable me to continue to work in the family business. I realize now that the hectic pace I set for myself during these years prepared me for the schedule-juggling roles of managing family and multiple jobs.

Since I wanted more experience in my field, I maintained additional jobs during the summers in my junior and senior years of college. As the student dietitian in hospital and then in a commercial food service, I was put through the paces of both line and staff jobs. These summer experiences provided me with an "edge" in many ways. It was in these jobs that I learned the employee and customer side of food preparation and service. Although I had quantity food experience at Carnegie Mellon, my associates there were other students. As a paid employee, my peers were other employees who knew that someday I might be their supervisor. My people skills and my work management skills improved rapidly since I was expected to be a useful employee first and a learner second. It was an opportunity to observe people at work. Since food was involved, these experiences provided insights and experiences that I use daily in my current position. My advice to students is to choose at least one summer's job in a food-related position. Often the experience to be gained is in the observation rather than in the assigned tasks.

By my senior year, I was convinced my niche was consumer education. I had not applied for a dietetic internship. At that point I had no interest in being a part of a profession I believed was linked to hospital kitchens and starched whites. In addition, like so many college seniors, I was anxious to get on with earning a salary. This was the early sixties and I was headed for one of the popular and traditional positions of that era, a foods and nutrition specialist with a utility company. On the back burners were offers from a food company and a commercial food service operation.

In May it appeared a job with a utility company was mine with one hitch, I would have to relocate to a small town in another state for at least one year. It was time to stop and think! The advice being given to me was to continue my education since it appeared that jobs for dietitians would be more stable than those in home economics. As fate would have it, my college advisor knew that Pittsburgh's Shadyside Hospital had one more opening for an intern. Armed with a solid work background, excellent grades, and the support of my college advisor, Barbara Cross, I applied and was accepted the same day.

In the space of those next few weeks, several decisions not only shaped my career path but also tested my professionalism. A few days after my accepting the internship, three jobs I had originally sought, including another with a utility company, were offered to me. I found myself saying no because of a sense of responsibility to my original decision. In retrospect this was initiated from the values and strong work ethic that my family initiated. During my years at Carnegie Mellon, three dietitians continued to shape this foundation for my professional life. Melva Bakkie, who also served as the department head, my advisor Barbara Cross, any my quantity foods instructor, Margaret Alexander, reinforced the sense of commitment and developed the professional pride that has made decision making easier for me. I entered the internship because I was sure this direction had been made available to me for a reason.

The dietetic internship at Shadyside Hospital was directed by Irene Willson, one of the pioneers in dietetics. Miss Willson still commanded much respect in the hospital but actually had little to do with the six dietetic interns. The internship provided comfortable living quarters on the grounds, food, and a "salary" of about $35.00 a month (less the wage taxes). The required 12 white cotton uniforms with long sleeves were laundered for us. I still remember peeling the starched white sleeves apart in a uniform that surely could have stood upright in a corner. I was part of the white starched brigade!

At that point Shadyside, like so many internships of the era, was a "working" internship. Interns were expected to work weekends and holidays and all shifts. My recollections of split shifts starting at 6:00 A.M. and ending at 7:00 P.M. with a break after lunch and before dinner still brings chills. The clinical component of the internship was strong. Our instructors in this area were excellent role models who inspired us to be clinical dietitians. The department had the respect of the medical staff and interns were encouraged to consult on diet prescriptions.

Main kitchen was a learning experience not easily forgotten. Interns rotated through all the kitchen stations, something that was tedious for those who were aiming for clinical positions. Since all food was prepared from scratch we learned meat cutting and baking as well as special diet and formula preparation. Private room patients received special menu items and even a la carte attention. As interns we were expected to evaluate and enforce quality in all areas. To this day it is second nature for me to evaluate meals and service using the same critical eye I developed under Margaret Alexander at Carnegie Mellon and Ruth Reuning at Shadyside.

Early in the internship it was obvious that we were being "slotted" into clinical or management directions. I was one of the two interns obviously labeled *management*. My food service experience gave me an edge in the management end of the internship, but again I was resisting. In my mind I was still looking for ways to teach!

The concept of teamwork took on new meaning during this year. It was apparent early in the internship that our collective lives would be easier if every member of the group survived each rotation. For this reason, we developed strong support systems and literally bailed each other out when necessary. Our people skills were developed in part by our efforts to survive. We were exposed to 10 staff dietitians at Shadyside, each with a different personality and professional style. In addition there were two particular para-professionals who were poised ready to pounce on us when the professional staff wasn't looking. Since we affiliated with dietitians in three specialized hospitals, a health department, and a metabolic unit, we interacted with at least 10 other professional styles. As with any group of professionals, there were some conflicting styles that had to be "-scoped-out" and "adapted-to" in our rotations.

I realize now that our habit of sharing and discussion of observations contributed greatly to our developing personal styles. The internship residence was the site of many a "debriefing" session where we compared thoughts and plotted to change the future of dietetics. At the time our thoughts were not so global but were more oriented to graduation. Since two of the other interns, Joan Light Robertson and Sue Rau Gibbon had been classmates of mine at Carnegie Mellon, our college introduction to group problem solving moved into high gear. Even today I enjoy working with a group to solve common problems or to strategize.

Opportunity for intensified and varied role modeling is a factor I believe every educational system must offer today's student. Although the current coordinated programs support modeling, internships offer the maturity and knowledge base of the additional year. Affiliations with practicing dietitians offer students an opportunity to develop a personal style while being exposed to the various roles of a dietitian. In my opinion, more emphasis needs to be given to supporting the dietitians in these sites. Successful role modeling starts with quality practice but requires other skills that may need to be prompted. The ability to share ideas, to delegate appropriate responsibility, and to provide fair evaluation are some of these skills.

My own recollections of the affiliations I enjoyed and those I hated are still vivid enough to play a major role in shaping my attitude toward students and interns. After affiliations as interns, we would critique the positions and the people we had encountered. It was easy to spot the dietitians who enjoyed being a part of the educational processes and those who resented it. Experience has expanded the theories developed during my internship. It would seem that age, experience, or sex are not factors. The dietitians who offer the most support and who today offer my students similar support, appear to be those who enjoy their job and who bring enthusiasm. Those who are unhappy either with their position or with the profession often exhibit a certain complacency or frustration in their interactions.

These early observations have led me to deliberately evaluate my frustrations and change direction when necessary. In some cases this has meant a major career change. Upon graduation from the internship, I assumed the expected management position at Shadyside Hospital as an Assistant Administrative Dietitian with the promise of a move to the clinical area soon. After two years I found myself in a traditional dietetic box. My responsibilities had expanded to relief for the teaching dietitian and working with the interns, but it appeared to me I was locked into a slot. Marriage and a yen for more autonomy and less split shifts led me to a more lucrative job in commercial food service.

My responsibilities were to open a new facility. This included staff selection and training, recipe and menu development, and the management of the daily operations of a branch restaurant of a department store. This job met my need for new challenges for the first two years. By the third year I was in the routine phase and ready for a change. Again circumstances were in my favor since I was forced to make a decision. Pregnancy in the late sixties meant women were excluded from the work force. We were expecting our first child and that meant my job was terminated automatically by the fifth month. I left believing that I would follow tradition and return to work when my last child entered school.

The experience of being a "retired" professional is a phase of my life that was mercifully short-lived. Our daughter Wendy was followed three years later by the birth of our son Michael. During those years I became a professional volunteer for anything legal. Ask me about organizing church dinners, bazaars, and weddings. If there was food, I was the chairman.

It was during this time that I became active in the Pittsburgh Dietetic Association. Since I was one of the "grandfathers" in registration, I dug in to keep my continuing education hours intact. Since I was a willing volunteer, I soon found myself serving as the Chairman of what was then National Nutrition Week. Involvement with the Pennsylvania Dietetic Association followed quickly. Public Relations, National Nutrition Month, and Legislation fit my interests. The professional contacts I made during these years are ones that kept me active and sane.

It was during these combination baby and volunteer years that I found I could earn money as a consultant! Upon the recommendation of another dietitian, I worked as a writer and nutrition education consultant to a market research firm. One of the products was a weekly syndicated newspaper column called THE BUDGET MENU MINDER. The concept was simple, a daily menu with minor alterations to fit three budget levels. Recipes and nutrition tips were part of the package. For one year I researched my collection of cookbooks for ideas, priced the food on the local market, and developed the menus. Seeing the columns published was a joy. Simultaneously my husband found joy in seeking a paycheck come from my extensive cookbook collection.

Oh how I wish I had been able to tap with wisdom available today through the practice groups of The American Dietetic Association. I learned a great deal about the print media and about the lack of control one has over such a project. Since I was under contract to the firm, the columns could be used any number of times without any additional credit or financial support for me. Although the lead article featured my name, I was indeed the unknown dietitian with no byline. Of course, since the editor of any paper running the column had even more control, much of what I wrote was omitted. Even worse, the headlines for some of the columns bordered on the ridiculous. In fairness to copywriters I must admit it is hard to make news out of broiled chicken breasts! From this experience I learned the importance of clear objectives and understandable contracts. At the same time, I gained insights into my own need to seriously pursue a new direction for my career.

The opportunity for a full-time job in a new role came to me at a time when I was primed to move back full speed. Following the referral of another dietitian, I applied for a one year contract to be the Nutrition Education Specialist for the Pennsylvania Department of Education. It was a unique opportunity. Nutrition education was a new area in those early years of the seventies. The contract was to fulfill one of six pilot grants awarded by the USDA under Child Nutrition Funding.

On a personal note, I am still amazed that I had the courage to say yes to the job offer. Child care was a major concern since Wendy was entering first grade and Michael was three. Circumstances were in my favor when I located a former employee who had worked under me in my food service position. Catherine filled the need for child care for the next thirteen years. The need for other types of support was another matter! For the next few years I was a part of a group that knew open discrimination, the working mother! Potential employers asked how I was coping with childcare. Friends asked my husband if I was still cooking meals. Teachers scheduled me for the mid-morning appointments even when evening ones were available and requested. And some of our relatives were "waiting" for me to return to my senses and stay home.

My salvation was the fact that we needed an addition to our home and my paycheck could help pay for it. It was interesting to see how the "necessity" of gaining things made my working acceptable to those who couldn't accept my need to regain my professional life. Even in today's working woman environment, I see young professionals in the same dilemma. I can honestly say to them that they need to take a close look at their support systems. I could fight my friends and the school and organize the routine, but I could not have made it without the support of my husband and parents.

The job with the Pennsylvania Department of Education was a professional risk that set the stage for the future. The job fit the pattern I was now finding most attractive. Since it had never been done before, I had the opportunity to create and implement without the constraints of a past. It was short-term which limited my immediate risk, and it involved communication and education.

I remember during the interview being asked if I minded public speaking. Answering no, I squelched the urge to say yes thinking that I could ease my way back into facing groups. The term "baptism by fire" came to life when the first week of the new job I faced not one but two inservice programs for school food service staff and directors, each with over 150 people in the audience. That was the beginning of my new career path.

The end of the nutrition education grant led me to employment with the Allegheny County Health Department (ACHD) in 1974. My entry into public health was made easier by Dorothy Kolodner, the Chief Nutritionist of the Nutrition Services Section of ACHD. For the next thirteen years I was part of one of the most productive teams in public health. Dorothy was building a department and had sensed that my experience in nutrition education was important to the newly formed Women, Infants and Children Supplemental Food Program (W.I.C.). Nutrition Services operated by a team approach and this was an approach I enjoyed. Although my initial responsibilities were in the administration of the W.I.C. program, our accomplishments were indeed in total programming. We had a proven track record in meeting the nutrition consultation and education needs of both the public and other professionals.

During the seventies, two other people influenced my future. My approach to nutrition education followed the traditional lines of lecture/discussion with a touch of demonstration. Then one fall day I was an assigned hostess at a session at The American Dietetic Association meeting in Philadelphia. As I stood in a large auditorium in my serious senior suit, I was given instructions to "guard the ramp" that went from the back of an aisle to the podium. Suddenly, a blonde haired, leather jacketed motorcycle rider came up the ramp. Sarah Short of Syracuse University had made her entry. For the next hour she shared with the audience her approach to making nutrition live! Although I never have had the nerve to dress in a black light sensitive body suit painted with formulas, I have been known to dress in a housecoat and wear fuzzy slippers during a presentation on mid-life crisis nutrition needs. The message that Sarah Short burned in my brain was to meet the needs of the audience on their level. From that point on I have never apologized for teaching nutrition with games, role-playing, and fun! It is this philosophy that motivates me to continue as both a practitioner and as an educator. This same philosophy is a hallmark of my presentations to students and professionals who are trying to make a difference with nutrition education.

During this same period of my life, I was elected to the position of delegate for Pennsylvania to The American Dietetic Association. I had been asked to be on two national committees and had to choose between the Membership Committee of the House of Delegates or the Public Relations Committee. I was leaning to the role I enjoyed, public relations, when again circumstances made my decision easier for me. By chance on a shopping trip, I encountered Mary Ann Scialabba, then House of Delegates Coordinator for Area VI. Standing in the middle of a shopping mall, Mary Ann gave me advice that shaped my organizational future. On her advice I accepted the House of Delegates committee appointment, a decision that I will always remember as a major entry into leadership in The American Dietetic Association.

By 1980, following the advice of Mary Ann Scialabba and Dorothy Kolodner, I made the plunge into graduate education. I realized that an advanced degree was important to me, not for employment security, but for credibility. In addition, the urge to expand my formal background in administration and education led me back to formal education. I enrolled in the graduate program of the School of Health Related Professions at the University of Pittsburgh. For the next four years I tried to balance my many lives: personal, organizational, professional life, and student. My academic advisor and organizational mentor continued to be Mary Ann Scialabba. Under her guidance I was able to tailor my academic courses and integrate dietetics with a multi-discipline approach. I found that my experience and maturity made the coursework more meaningful than my undergraduate education. Since I knew where I was heading, selecting courses was more a process of elimination than a chore.

It was a time for self-evaluation and goal setting, something several of my professors advocated. I realized that it was also time to change my career directions during these years of balancing roles. To finish graduate school I would need a more flexible daylight schedule than a public health department schedule could allow. In 1982 I made the break from one full-time job to several part-time jobs. Continuing at the health department two days, I accepted a new job for a registered dietitian with the Dairy and Nutrition Council. The free day was used to finish my graduate teaching assignments and to free-lance in the community. As anyone who works part-time knows, there is no such role! However, I continued on this schedule until 1987 when I resigned my position as Public Health Administrator at the ACHD.

During those years I finished my degree and joined the faculty of the coordinated undergraduate program in Clinical Dietetics/Nutrition of the University of Pittsburgh. My private practice and my leadership roles in The American Dietetic Association continued to expand. At this point I am managing a unique community nutrition practice. As a Nutrition Education Consultant for the Dairy and Nutrition Council, I have the benefit of the team approach I find so important to my own professional survival. At the University of Pittsburgh I teach two courses to senior dietetic students, Principles of Nutrition Education and Professional Trends and Issues. The rest of my practice consists of such varied roles as teaching adult education fitness courses, collaborating on seminars and projects with my colleagues at the Allegheny County Health Department, appearing as a "regular" on a local television talk show, and teaching marketing for The American Dietetic Association.

The focus of my career is currently communication and education, but I would never say I am not open to changes in the future! I entered the profession reluctantly but looking for a way to make a difference. My involvement with the Pennsylvania and The American Dietetic Associations gave me the ability to be an active part of a changing, dynamic profession. The image of ladies in white starched uniforms is gone. As we work to attract males and minorities into the profession, stereotypes of dietitians should also change.

I realize now that each of my experiences was important in bringing me to this point. The traditional hospital role prepared me for the non-traditional role I have selected. I believe that food and feeding is the basis for everything we are, and I know that my background and interests in these areas of our practice strengthen my credibility.

By now it should be obvious to the reader that I believe that paramount to a strong profession is a responsive and strong professional organization. My years in the House of Delegates have provided me with background in leadership skills and professional issues. As I moved from delegate to Area VI Coordinator (with a year out as the President of the Pennsylvania Dietetic Association), I was appointed to several committee assignments. In addition to the Membership Committee, I served on the State Associations and the Bylaws Committees. Each of these assignments prepared me to better fulfill my role on the Board of Directors and as Speaker of the House of Delegates in 1988/1989.

As an association, I see The American Dietetic Association as a participatory organization of dedicated volunteers supported by an equally dedicated staff. Like so many delegates and members, I have learned that as a profession we are cautious and conscientious. During my years in the House of Delegates, the Association discussed, rediscussed, and finally supported several important Bylaws revisions, Advanced Practice Specialization, a major marketing effort, and State Licensure. I watched the House of Delegates vote against an advanced practice specialization proposal that passed several years later. Consistently it appears that timing, careful preparation, and consensus building is crucial if we are to make a difference!

In the twenty-five years I have been practicing, I have been a part of a profession in change. Safety nets have disappeared as increasing numbers of dietitians have made the move from illness to wellness and from institution to private practice. Specialization has become a critical part of the practice of peers in critical care and on health care teams. Communication and education skills are essential as we take our place in electronic and print mediums. The need for business and management skills and marketing is a permanent part of our practice. The public is demanding a new breed of dietitians and this new breed of dietitians is demanding support. It is an exciting time, a growing time, and one that fits my need to move forward.

Yes, there are still days when I would like to settle back and open a boutique. But, one call from a consumer or a student will usually bring me back to the reality that I enjoy being a part of a profession that deals with food, nutrition, and people.

Marjorie M. Donnelly

*Marjorie M. Donnelly, MS, RD is Professor Emeritus
Extension Home Economics, North Carolina State University*

A native Floridian, Marjorie Donnelly grew up as the daughter of a rural merchant from whom she learned basic management principles and business methods. This early training served her well as she went on to become treasurer and later the 46th President of ADA. During her presidency, the Association was in the throes of a "revolution" experiencing dire financial straits, in-fighting among members, and structural difficulties. Her adaptability, flexibility and problem solving skills helped steer the organization through turbulent times. Marjorie Donnelly has worked extensively in Public Health and with the Cooperative Extension Service. She represented ADA in the three White House Conferences. Among her many honors, she received the prestigious ADA Copher Award, the Member of the Year Award from the North Carolina Dietetic Association, and she has been listed in Who's Who of American Women. Since retiring, she has been traveling extensively and doing volunteer work for a variety of organizations, including the Shepherd's Table (a soup kitchen).

Marjorie M. Donnelly

A career in dietetics! That was the last thing I had in mind when I graduated from Florida State College for Women back in 1940. I left college with a double major in Vocational Home Economics and Textiles and Clothing. My plans were to teach for a year or two and then go on to the New York University School of Retailing. My career was to be in some area of textiles and clothing. George Bernard Shaw is credited with saying "Progress is impossible without change; and those who cannot change their minds cannot change anything." I changed my mind, and I hope that I helped bring about change in the lives of some of the people with whom I have worked.

My Career

I did teach home economics in Florida Public Schools for three years. I encountered many teenagers who were malnourished; many who came to school without breakfast. Though I had taken a minimum number of foods and nutrition courses in college, I began to appreciate them. I had disliked "rat studies" intensely, but I gritted my teeth, purchased white rats, and did a variety of demonstrations for the benefit of my students.

World War II was beginning at this time. Many young men were being rejected for military service because of their poor physical condition, and poor nutrition was the basic cause. Nutrition was beginning to be a very popular subject.

Three years led me to believe that although I enjoyed teaching, I did not like the confinement of the classroom. I decided, too, that I was no longer interested in pursuing a career in textiles and clothing. So, when the offer of a fellowship in Community Nutrition at the University of Tennessee arrived unexpectedly, I jumped at the opportunity even though I dreaded the thoughts of biochemistry. I shall always be grateful to Dr. Rex Todd Withers, Supervisor of Home Economics for the Florida Department of Public Instruction, who recommended me to Tennessee as a potential candidate for graduate work.

Studying with Dr. Ruth Huenemann and the late Dr. Florence MacLeod made nutrition come alive for me. The terms of my fellowship called for working in a mill area of Knoxville. Many of my experiences there are as vivid to me today as they were when they happened. I found that I could teach people in their homes, in schools, in grocery stores, in clinics, and in their places of work. Here I found the combination of the teaching I enjoyed and the variety I craved. I felt I had found my niche!

Following my graduation I joined the Maternal and Child Health Division of the Florida State Board of Health. It was a short stay, for some six months after I started to work there, the United States Public Health Service requested my release in order for me to participate in field studies being conducted to determine the nutritional status of various population groups throughout the country. I gladly joined the U.S. Public Health Service (USPHS) since the war was still on and I felt I was making some type of contribution. I enjoyed the travel, and I liked working as a member of a team. The late

Dr. Walter Wilkins was the first director of these studies; the late Harold Sandstead succeeded him. Both men had lots of knowledge to impart to a fledgling nutritionist. The individual in the central office in Washington who gave assistance with the dietary assessments was Helen Walsh. She was to become the forty-third president of The American Dietetic Association, and it was Helen who encouraged me to apply for membership in ADA.

While studying at Tennessee I met one Helen R. Stacey, Assistant Director of Nutrition Services for the Children's Bureau, Department of Health, Education and Welfare. When dietary assessments became a bit tiresome after 18 months, I contacted Miss Stacey for advice. She suggested that it would be good for me to learn more about the operation of voluntary agencies and to learn to work with a board of directors. I soon found myself serving as Director of the Nutrition Service Bureau of Springfield, Massachusetts—a Community Chest Agency. The Bureau received referrals from agencies such as the Visiting Nurse Association and Family Service Bureau. In addition to individual referrals, my assistant and I worked with community programs of all types and with industries.

A high point of the time spent in Springfield was being invited by the late Dr. Elda Robb to participate in the community nutrition course at Simmons College. Serving as guest lecturer there gave me a chance to experience teaching at a different level. I remain grateful to a generous Board of Directors who allowed me to do this because in those days, each trip to Boston to participate required a full day's absence from the office.

Family illness cut short my stay in Massachusetts, and I returned to Florida in October, 1948. Again, I joined the State Board of Health, but this time it was with the Division of Nutrition Investigations and Services headed by the late Dr. Walter Wilkins.

My parents were glad to see me back in Florida, but they were concerned about my rapid fire change of jobs. I had to agree with them that eventually it might not look good on a vita. I promised to stay at least five years to prove that I could hold a job, and in reality, I stayed ten.

As with any organization there were changes. Eventually I became the Chief Nutrition Consultant. It was my privilege to participate in developing regional nutrition positions, and finally to start some county programs. Nutrition Services in Florida did not grow as fast as in some other states, but the program continued to grow where some Southern states lost personnel almost as quickly as they had added them.

During my years in Florida, Helen Stacey served as a consultant to our state especially in the area of maternal and child health. On one occasion she said to me "What professional goals have you set for yourself?" I think it surprised both of us when I immediately said, One, I want to be a Children's Bureau Consultant like you; two, I want someday to be President of The American Dietetic Association." Of course, I had other shorter term goals, but these were major, and now that I had revealed them, I had to set about reaching them.

At the end of ten wonderful years in Florida, I had the opportunity to join the Children's Bureau staff in the Denver Regional Office. There were five states in the region—Colorado, Utah, Idaho, Montana, and Wyoming. There had been seven of us working in Florida and here I found only one nutritionist in the five states. Part of my job was to demonstrate the need for nutritional personnel. In order to do this, I did direct service as well as consultation. And, because of the shortage of personnel, the Children's Bureau and Public Health Service worked out an agreement that allowed me to work in all areas, not just with mothers and children. This was truly a growing experience because there were different cultural patterns to be learned; health departments were not always headed by a physician and this was a change; the distances between communities, especially in Montana and Wyoming, were hard to believe. Adjusting to the differences was a challenge and I enjoyed every minute of it. And, it was a thrill to see Utah, for example, hire its first nutritionist, though I don't claim credit to making this happen.

After two and a half years, I bid the West farewell and headed for North Carolina. My marriage to Dr. James F. Donnelly, a public health physician, was the reason for this change. During the years he lived following our marriage, I did not work on a full time basis. I found many offers for short term assignments coming my way, and I took advantage of most of them. They included consulting for the Head Start Program; planning and presenting a series of 30 nutrition classes on television; organizing teacher workshops in nutrition for three summers; teaching students of nursing at North Carolina Central University for one semester.

Following Jim's death, I decided to return to full time employment. The position I chose, since it would be similar to my work in public health in many ways, was that of Specialist-in-Charge, Foods and Nutrition, North Carolina Agricultural Extension Service located at North Carolina State University. I had been a 4-H'er many years before and so I was interested in working with the program in a different capacity.

The State staff was responsible for keeping Home Economics Agents in all 100 counties updated in nutrition, for preparing program materials for their use with both adults and 4-H'ers, and for participating in special programs upon request. Eventually, with the advent of the Expanded Foods and Nutrition Program, or EFNEP as it is commonly known, we shared the responsibility for training an additional 150 subprofessionals along with added supervisory personnel. I shall always be grateful to the staff who shared all this with me and who taught me so much. However, after 16 years I decided it was time to close the book on my professional career. I retired, feeling both joy and sorrow, on September 1, 1982, as Emeritus Professor of Extension Home Economics.

Professional Activities

Each of the agencies with whom I worked was most generous in allowing me time to pursue professional activities. Soon after I returned to Florida in 1948 I began serving the Florida Dietetic Association in various capacities. These included Career

Guidance Chairman, Bulletin Editor, Delegate, and President. (Through an odd set of circumstances I became President of the Florida Association without ever serving as Vice-President.)

In North Carolina I have been Public Relations Chairman and a Delegate and I have served on some committees. Responsibilities at the national level precluded my being too involved at the state level. Currently I am serving as Vice-Chairman of the N.C. Dietetic Association Foundation.

Activities in ADA began soon after I served as Delegate from Florida. These included Community Nutrition Section Chairman, Public Relations Chairman, Delegate-at-Large, Treasurer, President-elect, and President. I attended my first national meeting in Philadelphia in 1947; 24 years later I had the privilege of being President when we met in Philadelphia.

For three years following my presidency, I served as Advisory to the Hospital Institution, and Education Food Service Society, or HIEFSS as it was known then. (Currently, this is the Dietary Managers Association.) I had also been on the Board of The American Dietetic Association Foundation, and was its President in 1975.

I became Treasurer soon after joining the staff of the Extension Service. This office and the subsequent ones took a great deal of time—especially the Presidency. Fortunately for me, the Director of Extension Home Economics was Dr. Eloise Cofer, who as a nutritionist and an ADA member, gave unlimited support and understanding. This was true also of the specialists and secretaries in the Foods and Nutrition Department.

Reflections

Serving as President of The American Dietetic Association was perhaps the high point and the low point in my career. The turbulent sixties had not bypassed the Association, and the revolution came during my administration in 1970–71. A group known as "Concerned Dietitians" felt too much power was vested in the Executive Board. This was, perhaps, a valid complaint and we tried to expand the policy making group by including members of the Coordinating Cabinet. There already was a work group trying to develop a new structure for the organization, but they were not moving quickly enough. Financially speaking, our "cupboard was bare." A proposed dues increase led the Concerned Dietitians to take us to court in an effort to block a vote on it. The dues increase did not pass and then came the problem of cutting services without appearing to be punitive.

This group also threatened to disrupt the Annual Meeting of the Association. Fortunately, it did not happen. Since I was unaccustomed to working in a "we" vs "they" situation within an organization, it was hard to accept all the criticism that came my way. Luckily, I realized that the bitterness and dissatisfaction were not directed to me personally. And, with the help of a wonderful Executive Board consisting of Katherine E. Manchester, Isabelle A. Hallahan, Dorothy M. Rowe, Arlene Wilson, and the late Elsie Haff, I weathered the storm unscathed. Ruth Yakel, the Executive Director of

ADA, was always on hand to offer support and encouragement. I learned well, that in an age of dissent, it isn't easy to be a leader.

But there were bright spots in my tenure of office, and I prefer to think of them. It was an exciting time for ADA. A commission to study the profession was at work; the Journal was taking on a new look; computers were coming into use; innovative ways to meet the shortage of internships were being developed; a management team was working on office reorganization. These were but a few of the changes taking place.

As I look back over the years, I think ADA is moving ahead and, at the same time, going in cycles. New ideas and proposals are not always new—they may have been tried and failed. But timing is important, so this time may be the right time.

The Association has made progress, but I do not feel the minorities in our profession are given as many opportunities to serve at the national level as they deserve. This was one thing I worked for. Part of the problem, I believe, is that enough states do not elect minority members to office consistently enough to have them become well known at the national level. It is my hope that more states will begin grooming members, so to speak, for higher offices.

I admit to being politically naive. I was glad when we began legislative activity and I heartily endorse the recognition given each year to one or two congressmen who have supported our cause. I am sorry that we are pushing a PAC fund because I prefer selling ideas to buying votes, and this is what I feel PAC funds do.

I believe progress comes through being positive, patient, and persistent. It is important to deal in plain talk and hard facts. I am encouraged that dietitians are doing more documentation of their services and the costs of those services. This should help improve many work situations as well as move legislation forward at times.

I can see a bright future for ADA, and I am grateful to have been a part of its past. I was honored to be elected as an officer of the Association, and to represent the members at three different White House Conferences. Because of ADA activities, I was named North Carolina Dietitian of the year for 1969; I was invited to give a paper at the International Congress of Dietitians in Hannover, Germany. But, the greatest honor came when I received the prestigious Marjorie Hulsizer Copher Award in 1982. This came just six weeks after my retirement, so it was truly "the icing on the cake."

Somerset Maughan once said "One of the greatest differences between the amateur and the professional is that the latter has the capacity to progress." I like to think that I have been, and still am, a professional. My jobs and professional activities have been satisfying to me. They had led to numerous recognitions, but most of all, they have increased my understanding of human nature and made me a better person.

I like people and I like variety. In my career I was blessed with both. Though the career has ended, the opportunities to participate in a variety of activities continue. Many of the friendships I enjoy were made through ADA; the good health I enjoy is, I am sure, at least partially due to my trying to follow the principles of good nutrition. A career in dietetics—I couldn't have chosen a better one.

Johanna T. Dwyer

*Johanna T. Dwyer, DSc, RD is Professor of Medicine
and Community Health, Tufts Medical School; and
Director, Frances Stern Nutrition Center, Boston, MA*

Johanna T. Dwyer candidly admits that her choice of career focus is still incomplete and thus she improvises as she goes along. She most assuredly has the credentials and extensive experience to travel in any arena of nutrition and public health. She recounts how she selected schools to attend based on their excellence and then creatively worked to finance her education. She describes her own philosophy as "we are the happiest ourselves when we are doing things which are worthwhile to others." Johanna Dwyer believes that we must work together to enhance the career potential in the profession. Certainly her illustrious career is one which has brought needed recognition for the contributions made by professionals in nutrition and dietetics, and serves as a model for others.

Johanna T. Dwyer

I chose nutrition as a career and only secondarily became attracted to dietetics since it was the more practical and applied aspect of the field. I think it was the application ability and the ability to do good for people which made the dietetics aspect of the field of particular interest. What did not attract me was the rigid and rather inflexible undergraduate requirements and the overwhelming female dominance in the field. As a person who changed majors rather late in college it would have been virtually impossible to complete the requirements as they were laid out by the then required courses for internships. The notion of another year of unpaid training as an intern, which sounded to me like scut work also did not appeal.

My own professional path was via a home economics school, which was the way I could go away to school and still afford to go to university; since Cornell was a state school and I had a state scholarship I was just able to swing it with about $800 per year from my parents and summer jobs—otherwise I would have had to go to school in my home town, where the universities were not very good. Once I got to Cornell I majored in retailing but disliked it; it was really sewing and I didn't know how to sew. Therefore in my sophomore year I switched into food and nutrition, which seemed more interesting, more science oriented and like an overall more interesting way to go. I ended up majoring in that but not taking any more courses than I absolutely had to in it, since the requirements were already very rigorous to my mind, and I had many other interests. I did well in courses and didn't really feel I knew enough, not wanting to go into dietetics and needing to make some other career path, so I applied to graduate school. I ended up choosing the University of Wisconsin because I had read about all the vitamins which had been discovered there, and felt that with summer work before going there and the scholarships they offered along with a graduate assistantship I could make it financially. I ended up a little short for cash since waitressing through the summer prior to graduate school yielded very little money compared to what I needed. I was lucky because my family took their vacation to take me out to Wisconsin and so I saved on travel. I ended up in a boarding house there, which was all I could afford. I made many good and lasting friends at Wisconsin as well as learning a great deal of science. My only failure was that I continued to hate going to football games, which was a required Saturday activity in Wisconsin in those days. I stayed a second year at Wisconsin to finish my thesis on sterilized condensed milk, and started applying for jobs in the food industry. My interest in the food industry stemmed from a project I had done in a very interesting course I took on advertising in the Business School at Wisconsin. I applied to General Mills, Pillsbury, and Proctor and Gamble (P and G). P and G offered me a job first, although my preference was General Mills. By the time General Mills came through I had already accepted P and G. I moved to Cincinnati with P and G paying much of the bill and rented an apartment near the University there and began a two year stint at Proctor and Gamble in the test kitchens, where I really learned to cook. Advancement for women, in fact advancement for anyone, at P and G was a slow

36

process and I got bored and started applying to graduate schools. Also during that time I worked as a volunteer part time in Good Samaritan Hospital there to test my interests in clinical things, and liked it more than making cakes and pies.

Applying to graduate school, I applied to Cornell and also to Harvard, but Harvard demanded that I send my masters thesis to them and I didn't hear back after I sent it, so sort of forgot about it. In the meantime, Cornell had an opening in the Home Ec school teaching food chemistry labs since one of their instructors had resigned in mid semesters, so I took their job two thirds time and took courses the other third of a time at the School of Nutrition. The job was all right but there was a lot of personnel turmoil on the faculty and among the instructors so I was absolutely delighted when I finally heard from Harvard that if I wanted to come they had the money. I immediately quit for the following year, especially since they had doubled my teaching load at Cornell without doubling my salary. I then took a terrific 10 week vacation in Europe and ended up in Boston at the Harvard School of Public Health in the middle of August.

Public health nutrition held particular fascination to me since it seemed that I would be able to complete my doctorate in a field in which I could do some good and also fulfill my interests in science, while using my market related skills in the health arena. The School of Public Health was an extremely exciting place to be and that first year there, along with my first year in college, remain two of the best years of my life. I really enjoyed the public health and also the nutrition, although biochemistry courses at MIT were a terrible amount of work on top of a full load at the Harvard School of Public Health. Nevertheless I loved it all. The problem the next year was deciding who to do the doctorate with, and I finally settled on Dr. Jean Mayer, who was a brilliant teacher and a good scientist as well.

My professional path has had a couple of unique features. First, I have been able to enhance and use my interest in Spanish, which started at the University of Mexico in college when I studied there after several years of study in college. In the past twenty years, work has taken me to Guatemala, to Chile, and to Mexico, and in every case my ability to speak Spanish was invaluable. A second unique feature in my professional path was having to write a newspaper column for five years with Jean Mayer, every week. This was a syndicated column in about 100 papers nationwide. Two things resulted: a fair degree of visibility nationally, which led to me being invited to serve on a number of national level nutrition policy committees, such as the Office of Technology Assessment, the Institute of Medicine of the National Academy of Sciences' committees, and others, and chair of the 1980 Nutrition Education Conference sponsored by the Department of Health and Human Services, U.S. Department of Agriculture, and the Consumer Advisor to President Carter. The second thing resulting from the column was that I honed my writing skills which have stood me in good stead since then.

A second unusual aspect of my professional path is the year (1980–81) I spent as a Robert Wood Johnson Health Policy Fellow at the National Academy of Sciences, working for Senator Richard Lugar and now Senator, then Representative Barbara Mikulski. This really gave me a needed sabbatical and also permitted me to see a new world in terms of politics. I learned I wasn't a terrific politician but that I liked them and this has also served me well over the years.

A third unusual aspect of my professional path was my decision in 1981 to go back nights to get a certificate in management and administration at Harvard Extension. Again I learned a great deal which it was possible to apply in teaching and elsewhere. Also it opened some new vistas in terms of personnel and financial management. Also helpful has been a series of courses in epidemiology at Tufts Summer School, which have been absolutely first rate each year over the past three or four years. I believe if teachers don't continue to learn we are in big trouble.

People who shaped my professional life were several. First was my benign advisor in college, Dr. Jean Failing, who always said yes when I wanted to take oddball courses for broadness, like Spanish, for example, or literature. Dr. Maxine McDivitt at the University of Wisconsin was similarly benign. Then of course there were four key people at Harvard; Fred Stare, the then chair of the Department of Nutrition, who found me a fellowship; Jean Mayer, who served as my doctoral advisor and later as President of the University I later moved to; Dr. Mark Hegsted, a superb thinker and experimentalist; and Dr. Jack Feldman, a statistician and the man who really helped see me through all the various papers and analyses for my doctorate. At Tufts, the wisest of the wise has been Dr. Seymour Reichlin, who is and has been chair of Endocrinology for over two decades and a great support not only in obtaining a research career development award from NIH but in getting the Johnson Fellowship and many other good things. Also I must mention my parents, both fine health professionals, who always said I could do anything I decided I wanted to do, and made financial sacrifices to help me do it.

Many life events have had an impact on my career; perhaps most of all my interest in other countries which started when I was an exchange student to Germany as a teenager. I think my ability to write has also been helpful. I am also interested in a lot of things outside of my field, which has helped in relating to those in other fields.

My personal philosophies of life and work are difficult to put into words. Briefly I think we are the happiest ourselves when we are doing things which are worthwhile to others. Excessive work and lack of sense of humor cause nothing but trouble.

My professional motivators are the respect of people I respect, doing a job to the point I am vaguely pleased with it, and doing interesting things.

My beliefs about the profession are that it is important for dietitians to support each other as well as to seek their own advancement. I believe dietitians are often excessively timid and narrow in their outlooks, and tend to get walked on and passed over for advancement because of this.

I have learned and continue to learn a great deal about the practical aspects of the field from my peers, students, and colleagues in dietetics which I fail to see in the views of colleagues in nutritional sciences. Also invaluable has been the support and kindnesses of many individual dietitians.

My choice of career focus is still incomplete. I have never known exactly what I wanted to do with my life and have improvised as I have gone along. I continue interests in public health nutrition, political nutrition, and a side interest in international nutrition.

It is better to be male than female, even today, in the field of dietetics and also in the hospital field. However, there is less discrimination today than ever before, even though it still exists. I experienced wage discrimination in the 1960's and early 70's but not thereafter. So progress is being made.

Changes in the profession over time since I have observed the goings on have been a lesser attraction of young professionals to the field since so many other opportunities are available, making it hard for us to maintain high standards and good salaries. Thus the status of the profession has not risen nor have salaries as much as I would have like to see. On the other hand, in some states there are extremely bright and good people leading efforts within the dietetic associations to become more market oriented. Finally, many more dietitians have obtained doctoral degrees.

My personal perspective on my career is that I have been lucky to be involved in dietetics; it has given me some perspectives I otherwise would have lacked and I hope I have also made a contribution.

Risk taking is not exactly my forte. The biggest risk I guess was taking a year off to do a Robert Wood Johnson Fellowship in Congress. It set me back a year or more science wise but was well worth it. Similarly this past summer I took two months off in a time of budget crisis to go to the Far East and teach. Again this was an extraordinary growth experience. As to consequences, there is always a down side but we only go this way once, so we might as well enjoy ourselves.

If I knew then what I know now there are many good things I did which I would not have done so I am glad I did not have 20/20 foresight.

I don't know if I have a professional style so I cannot describe it.

My most important professional accomplishments are those that my peers gave me, such as the J. Harvey Wiley Award of the Society for Nutrition Education, and the Lenna F. Cooper award of The American Dietetic Association.

As to the future of the profession, the most urgent problems are status and money and recognition for the many contributions dietitians make. We must work, together, to increase the career potential of this field.

Susan Calvert Finn

Susan Calvert Finn, PhD, RD
is Director of Nutrition Services,
Ross Laboratories in Columbus, OH.

With a career that spans violence in the ghettos of Cleveland to visibility in the corporate boardroom, the professional life of Susan Calvert Finn has been a testimonial to her personal commitment to serving the public. Beginning as a home economist with a maternal and infant care project, she developed a deep concern for children and went on to conduct doctoral research on the nutritional habits of handicapped youngsters. Her career switch from the public to private sector raised some eyebrows, but she deftly maintained her crusading spirit and focused her efforts on hospital malnutrition and nutrition support. She has lectured extensively in Europe, the Far East, and the Soviet Union. Dr. Finn's mastery of marketing and networking have had a major impact on the profession of dietetics. She is an enthusiastic advocate of the Ambassador Program and continues to challenge dietitians to market themselves as the nutrition expert. Dr. Finn is Director of Nutrition Services for Ross Laboratories.

Susan Calvert Finn

Most careers—most lives—are a combination of design and chance. A childhood ambition, a fateful meeting with a person who exerts life-long influence, an experience which forever leaves its mark on your thinking. All may be factors which determine how and where we spend our professional days and years.

My own life is a testimonial to such turning points, events and plans. And today, at the chronological midpoint of my career, I have the perspective to review and analyze those landmark events which determined my professional life.

Childhood ambition was the starting point. Working in the ghettos of Cleveland during the 1960's was the influential experience. Entering private industry was the turning point.

The starting point: As a high school student in Berea, Ohio, my life was fairly typical of my times and my community. I was a cheerleader. Each Sunday I went to church with my family and out to dinner after services.

To help me decide on a career, my parents introduced me to people in a variety of careers—heads of personnel, executives, experts in what were regarded as suitable careers.

One of the people my parents arranged for me to meet was a dietitian in the Berea school system. She was one of the first in the series of many role models and mentors who have influenced my life and career.

As a student working toward a bachelor of science degree in nutrition at Bowling Green State University, still in my native Ohio, I thought I would teach home economics after graduation. When I shed my cap and gown to venture into the "real" world, that ambition began to pall.

And, like generation after generation of uncertain college graduates, I began studying the classified job ads hoping to find, if not inspiration, at least a clue.

I came across an ad for a person with food and nutrition background. I responded and was hired as a home economist with the Maternity and Infant Care Project, a Federal Program.

The year was 1967 and the Hough ghetto of Cleveland to which I was assigned was in turmoil. Violence was a daily occurrence.

I was part of a Metropolitan Hospital outreach program designed to reduce infant mortality. Our mission was to teach mothers, some as young as 12 and 13, about nutrition. I was then a young mother myself and I felt a strong affinity for these women—some still children, themselves—trying to deal with pregnancy or to take care of babies. I was especially interested in learning about the eating habits of pregnant women and their difficulties in obtaining good nutrition.

We made home visits and talked about prenatal care, breast feeding, empty calories—the entire range of maternal infant care. Often we would find people who just didn't have enough money to buy nourishing food.

As health care do-gooders do from the outside, we had to battle daily with the enemies of family life—unemployment, poverty, alcohol and drugs.

Women and children were fairly low priorities in the family hierarchy; the men took most of the food and the extras.

In the 1960's there was relatively little interest in nutrition and to accomplish anything, I had to develop "street smarts" and I needed to do it quickly.

I soon realized that hungry kids cannot learn. I observed that nutrition—good eating habits—makes a difference in people's lives. It can be one step in breaking the cycle of hopelessness which binds people to the ghetto. And, despite the overwhelming odds, research data demonstrated that these programs did produce results. They changed lives for the good.

The Cleveland ghetto experience was my lifelong influence. The lessons I learned there became a cornerstone of my life and career. The faces of the young mothers and their babies were permanently imprinted on my memory. Their plight and the desire to do more inspired my personal challenge—to design and help implement effective nutrition programs for women, children and the elderly.

The first step was to return to school to acquire an in-depth understanding of nutrition science and to complete the requirements for membership in The American Dietetic Association.

In pursuit of my goal, I applied for and received a United States Public Health Service grant from Case Western Reserve University in Cleveland where I completed a two-year program, earning a master of science degree in public health nutrition with a specialty in maternal and child health.

I then joined Project Head Start which, at the time, was the one of the favorite ventures of the Federal anti-poverty program. As a State Regional Training Officer, I served as a nutritionist in four Great Lakes States for one year, inspecting feeding programs, working with parent groups, developing nutrition education programs and ensuring that adequate meals were available for children.

Then, it was back to school for a doctorate. I began my Ph.D. program at The Ohio State University in Columbus, Ohio, intending to concentrate on education and public health.

However, at this point, another in my lifelong chain of mentors played a key role. She was Dr. Virginia Vivian, my advisor, who convinced me that in order to know "something," I needed more scientific training.

My doctoral work at Ohio State reinforced my love of teaching and communicating. And my concern for children was reflected in my dissertation which analyzed the nutritional habits of handicapped children—specifically those with Downs Syndrome. These youngsters tend to be overweight and I discovered the cause was parental overfeeding.

While completing my Ph.D. research, I travelled to California, where I taught full-time at Whittier College and, in the evening, at Cal State at Los Angeles. They were two totally different environments—Whittier with mostly white, middle-class enrollment and Cal State with working-class, older and mostly minority students. Each, I found, had its own challenges and rewards and this experience paved the way for much of what I do now—presenting educational programs to varied professional and lay audiences.

Subsequently, I returned to The Ohio State University where I was on the faculty at the College of Medicine in the Department of Medical Dietetics. I was teaching public health nutrition and pediatric nutrition to students affiliating at Children's Hospital. This assignment enabled me to keep my hand in both teaching and nutrition practice. Because I had access to public health agencies, children's hospitals and clinics and accompanied my students on field trips, I was broadening my own education.

What was, to date, the single most important turning point in my professional life, came shortly thereafter.

It had become increasingly apparent to me that my personal orientation was public health and children. So, when a good friend I knew through the American Public Health Association suggested I really belonged in private industry, where I would be more effective in accomplishing my long-term public service goals, I was somewhat skeptical.

However, because he was a friend, I accepted his invitation to visit the company he worked for, Ross Laboratories, the manufacturer of Similac infant formula. He wanted me to see how his Company approached public health and the marketplace. What began as a visit turned out to be an interview of sorts, with the offer of a job at Ross after this first meeting. It also brought home to me the importance of personal contacts and networking.

I was simultaneously flattered and intrigued by the opportunity. On the one hand, I thought hands-on experience with a company oriented toward children and nutrition would be valuable. On the other, was the concern, voiced by some of the University people, that I was "selling out."

Until the critical juncture, I was preoccupied with my challenge and I hadn't even considered the "private sector." It was 1974 and health care professionals hadn't begun to think about—or practice—marketing.

I accepted the offer and joined Ross' medical department where I was responsible for developing and monitoring medical clinical studies. I reported to the vice president of medical affairs, Dr. Henry Sauls, and with his support, I was free to expand my responsibilities in other areas.

Ross had just entered the medical nutritional market with "Ensure," the first total enteral nutrition formula providing completely balanced nutrition for those who can't get enough nutrients from food. It was a time when there were a number of studies indicating that malnutrition was not uncommon in hospitals and one of my early ventures was initiating the research program for medical nutritionals.

Drawing on my background in teaching and communicating, I worked with the Ross sales force, guiding them in the use of scientific data on medical nutritional products as both a sales tool and as background on how to provide better patient care.

The introduction of Ensure also widened the scope of my nutritional interests. To my abiding concern for the health and well-being of mothers and children, I added premium nutritional care for the elderly and hospitalized.

There is an ironic post script to this chapter. It is not unusual for our private and professional lives to intertwine. But it is not often in as dramatic a fashion as my experience with my own father five years ago.

Then 68 years old, he was brought to the emergency room of a Cleveland hospital with a bladder infection. As part of his treatment, he was catheterized. In the process, his bladder wall was perforated and the catheter went into his intestine—a complication I've since learned is not uncommon.

When I visited him, his six-foot frame carried only 118 pounds. The hospital staff had tried to feed him, but he couldn't tolerate the food and they seemed not to know what else to do.

I insisted they start him immediately on nutrition support. After overcoming several obstacles, including the staff's lack of nutritional knowledge, my father was given support. It took nearly three weeks, but he began to regain his weight and subsequently recovered.

My crusading instinct had been aroused by this experience and I learned my father's situation was all too typical. Many hospitals—and the situation still exists five years later—do not recognize the importance of nutrition support.

In fact, a recent private study conducted by the international public accounting firm of Arthur Andersen and Co. concluded that 55% of hospital patients were likely to be malnourished, but less than 5% received nutrition support prior to developing complications early in their hospitalization.

The opportunity to focus public attention on this problem and to work on nutrition awareness programs at Ross has been one of the most gratifying aspects of my experience in the private sector.

It wasn't long after I joined Ross that I also discovered what I felt was a compelling corporate need—the need to learn about dietitians and how to support them.

While it wasn't in my job description, I began to create a network of dietitians around the country. This network served a dual purpose: it would help me make my employer more successful in marketing its nutrition products and, not incidentally, it made this major company aware of the goals and needs of dietitians, benefiting the profession as well.

Not incidentally, my work with dietitians on behalf of Ross heightened my interest in the profession and I became more active in our professional organization, The American Dietetic Association.

That, in turn, provided the opportunity to be directly involved in a period of great growth and change for the ADA.

Through my dealings with dietitians across the country, I was aware of and concerned about the lack of visibility for our profession. I felt strongly that the dietitian should be the nutrition advocate and, as an active member of ADA, I could help effect this change. The best approach was a principle which was significant in my own career—marketing yourself.

So, I advocated—and continue to advocate—that dietitians learn all they can about marketing and sales. And then apply those principles to marketing themselves—and our profession.

Today, the ADA is 58,000 strong—and growing. And, although the battle is far from won, increasingly, our members are being recognized as equal partners on health care teams.

Registered dietitians currently hold positions in settings unimaginable 10 years ago, from wellness programs and food service management to life style improvement and personal nutrition counseling. Advancing our contemporaries and our discipline, and improving dietitians' status and career opportunities through the promotion of nutrition education are the result of the combined dedication and hard work of many people. Playing a role in this progress is among my proudest professional achievements.

One of the landmark accomplishments of ADA and its leaders during this period was the creation and expansion of the Ambassador Program.

The goal of the Ambassador Program is to create a positive environment for the profession and in just six years it has expanded to 83 spokespersons, with more than 20 functioning at the national level. In each state there are one or more Ambassadors who speak authoritatively in public on nutrition subjects.

In 1980 I made a media tour for Ross. The Company wanted to determine the level of public interest in nutrition support and, as part of that program, I spent a year-and-a-half speaking on malnutrition in hospitals and on the value of nutrition support—and listening to the feedback. There was extensive TV exposure, but no one to follow through in each city. The Ambassador Program was conceived as a way of delivering the good nutrition message to American on a continuing basis.

Another personal satisfaction is that I have been able to be an active participant in our profession's campaign to create public and legislative awareness of the nutritionally needy—low income families, women and children and the elderly. It has been particularly gratifying that Ross Laboratories has supported my efforts to help those very groups whose plight concerned me at the outset of my career.

My work on behalf of Ross and ADA also has contributed to my personal and professional growth. It provided me with the ongoing opportunity to do the two things I like best—communication and teach.

In those roles, I've been fortunate enough to regularly contribute to consumer magazines and professional publications and to appear on more than 400 radio and television programs. These media activities also have been educational; they've provided me with the opportunity to learn what journalists and the public think about nutrition and to utilize that information in my own work.

I've also been fortunate enough to travel and lecture to scientific organizations in Europe, the Far East and the Soviet Union.

In my visits to the Soviet Union—in 1982 and 1986—I spoke at the Institutes of Surgery and of Nutrition, updating them on nutritional research in this country.

It was a genuine educational experience for me as well. I discovered there are no dietitians in the Soviet Union so physicians were particularly interested in the subject. They still rely heavily on herbal medicine and cling to such outmoded therapies as starvation. But they were receptive to new ideas and eager for information. One of my talks lasted four hours because I was obliged to answer all questions before I left.

Although I have been practicing dietetics for quite some time, I regard myself as a young person. When I look backward, I realize how much I owe to so many. Few of us accomplish anything alone—we need the assistance and advice of many people. In my case, it has been unswerving love and support of my family, particularly my husband, Jim, and my son, John. The influence of role models and the guidance of mentors. And the encouragement of my colleagues in health care—especially in dietetics—and at Ross Laboratories.

When I look forward, I see so much work still to be done. And, I'd like to think I can continue to make a contribution to the crusade for nutrition, particular for the well-being of young mothers, children and the elderly.

Annie L. Galbraith

*Annie L. Galbraith, MPH, RD is Former Assistant
to the Provost for External Relations,
MGH Institute of Health Professions
and Director of the Dietary Department,
Massachusetts General Hospital, Boston, MA*

Annie Galbraith's childhood was filled with love from a family who taught her grace and respect for others through words and deeds. As is the case with most contributors to this book, she offers credit for many of her accomplishments to those around her. She is the epitome of a professional: commitment to the profession and service to her professional organizations. She has fully dedicated herself to dietetics because "halfway won't do!" Her focus on dietetic education has been steadfast. The pride she derives from the successes of dietetic interns and students of the Massachusetts General Hospital and MGH Institute of Health Professions with whom she has worked is revealed throughout her story. She candidly acknowledges, which may surprise those of us who thought it was a well-kept secret, that she, Louise Hatch, and Mae Dozier were known as "The Big Three." And yes, Miss Galbraith, it was a title of respect and admiration! Indeed, her career has inspired others to pattern their lives to also attain high levels of achievement.

Annie L. Galbraith

The third daughter, followed by two sons in a family where it was taken for granted that we would attend the University of Tennessee, I was destined for Home Economics. Mother (who had taught in elementary school) wanted at least one Home Economist and I was it! She wasn't really sure that dietetics was here to stay, so would I please also earn credentials for teaching in the Smith-Hughes Vocational Home Economics program? I did, and, in order not to require longer time for the double major, I carried at least one "extra" course per term throughout the upper division.

However, I need to step back before describing my college days and attempt to give readers an appreciation for the rich and special heritage I enjoyed as a child growing up in the heart of East Tennessee. When I was growing up, we lived with my Grandmother Galbraith who operated a resort hotel. The entire family helped with the operation which drew people from miles around to enjoy the splendor of the beautiful Appalachian Mountains. The hotel was celebrated for the medicinal qualities of its mineral springs and its wholesome food.

My father was more interested in farming than in resort management, and when the Tennessee Valley Authority needed the arable land of the tract which had been in the family since before 1800, he sold the hotel area also. We moved from Hawkins County to a Jefferson County farm. TVA's Cherokee Lake now covers the "homestead."

I credit my parents and grandmother with developing in me an early appreciation for social grace—and for scholarship. When I enrolled at the University of Tennessee-Knoxville my professional career really began!

While in college, I also worked in the University Cafeteria as a counterperson. In those days there was a large contingent of Air Force trainees on campus. The servicemen ate first, and later we served the resident students (all women). I observed then, and have not been convinced otherwise, that, as a group, men are far more cheerful and accepting of foodservice than women are.

Two professional role models emerged—Ruth Buckley, who not only chaired Foods and Institution Management in the Home Economics School, but was also the institution manager of women's residence halls. She operated a first-rate cafeteria (a popular dining-out spot for area residents) and oversaw housekeeping and staffing of resident halls. A veritable dynamo, she was my faculty advisor.

And then there was Jeannette Biggs. Miss Biggs was an enthusiastic teacher of lower division nutrition and child nutrition. She managed the nursery school's foodservice for 36 preschoolers (ages 2–4 1/2 years) plus assorted student and faculty teachers. Jeannette travelled extensively, was always elegantly dressed and impeccably groomed. I learned later that some independent income made some of those things possible for her.

Jessie W. Harris, Director of the School of Home Economics, professed to produce generalist home economists at the baccalaureate level. If one wanted to specialize, graduate work was essential. The School became a college and Jessie Harris a Dean a few years after I graduated.

I remember that on April 15th of my senior year Ruth Buckley and Florence Mac-Leod, Ph.D., Professor of Nutrition, together gave us our dietetic internship appointment letters. I asked for (and acted upon) their advice: "Since all hospital programs give essentially the same content, opt for the one farthest from home for the opportunities of cultural broadening." Sound advice for which I am ever grateful.

I was most pleased to receive an appointment to the Dietetic Internship of the Massachusetts General Hospital (the MGH). How well I remember writing at the beginning of that year, "At the end of these twelve months I shall not consider my education completed by any means, but I hope to be capable of doing my work so that others benefit from my labors." And certainly my formal education was not completed. In 1967 I received a Masters in Public Health from the University of Michigan in Ann Arbor.

As I look back on my professional career, I believe others have benefited from my labors. Following completion of the dietetic internship, I accepted my first staff appointment with Dr. Paul Dudley White's Hypertension Study Group at MGH—"The Rice Diet Project." Following that assignment and desiring to return to the beautiful Smoky Mountains, I began what was to be an 8 year association as a therapeutic dietitian at East Tennessee Baptist Hospital in Knoxville.

This newly constructed building was to house a newly organized general hospital. When I arrived, about 50 in-patient beds were occupied (of the capacity of about 300 when I left) and the Nursing School was about one year old.

Two "firsts" for that period. With the encouragement and assistance of the Knoxville Academy of Medicine, dietitians from St. Mary's, Fort Sanders, Knoxville General and Children's hospitals developed a city-wide diet manual. Geraldine Piper, then a faculty member at the University of Tennessee provided advice and guidance, and I chaired the committee.

We organized the Knoxville Area Dietetic Association. Organizational meetings were held in the living rooms of various members—one didn't dare miss a meeting! Soon we affiliated with the Tennessee Dietetic Association and right away hosted the state meeting in Gatlinburg.

Helen Hunscher, Ph.D., who was at the then Western Reserve University, was our ADA representative. I remember she advised us that committees should have co-chairs. "After all, dietitians are a bunch of tramps," and, if one left, the co-chair could carry on without lengthy start-up (or start over) time. It was my privilege to serve as first president of that newly organized district association, 1949–50.

As anyone who has ever affiliated with the MGH understands, bonds are strong. In 1956, a recommendation for dietary staff organization was made to the MGH Administrative Committee to meet the then-current needs for growth and enrichment. My college classmate (who had interned at Peter Bent Brigham Hospital in the July group) Edith Shipe Jones, Chief Dietitian, encouraged me to return to Boston to accept a senior staff appointment. In 1957, I assumed the position of Assistant Director, Department of Dietetics and began a 28 year history with MGH. Shortly after coming home to MGH, I was named Associate Director of the department.

As perhaps a more significant piece of the innovation in the MGH Dietary Department, Mae Dozier was invited to return at the same time. A report of a panel discussion presented at the 1958 ADA Annual Meeting describes this as follows:

> ". . . a new staff member has been added to the dietary department, a young woman graduate of the Management Training Program of Radcliffe College. As an administrative associate, her responsibilities include budget planning and follow-up with reports from the accounting department, job specifications, employee selection in cooperation with the personnel department, and in-service training for employees. Here is a fine working example of one way in which good business management practices and good nutritional practices can dovetail to the hospital's advantage." (1)

Former interns may recall "The Big Three" as Louise Hatch, Mae Dozier, and Annie Galbraith were—somewhat surreptitiously—called. Ours was a mutually rewarding and productive relationship since our talents and interests were complementary. There was quite enough responsibility to keep us all very involved. Two of Mae's mottoes bear repeating here. "Never underestimate the power of a personality" and "nothing is so infectious as example."

As I review my professional career, hopes, dreams, and accomplishments, I am proud of my continuing commitment to quality dietetic education. While a therapeutic dietitian at the East Tennessee Baptist Hospital, I also served as Instructor in Diet Therapy. At MGH I was deeply involved with the education of dietitians, ultimately serving as Director of the MGH Dietetic Internship.

During my tenure at MGH, I was to see the MGH Education Division, later to be renamed the MGH Institute of Health Professions, become a reality. Approval of amendments to the hospital's charter allowing it to award its own academic degrees—baccalaureate and masters' degrees in nursing and several allied health fields—was the result of more than 4 years of feasibility studies and planning within the hospital and a lengthy process of review by the Massachusetts Board of Higher Education and other state agencies. What an innovative and exciting concept! Several multidisciplinary committees cooperated in the planning of these programs from the outset. The Division's curriculum, administration, and faculty organization were intentionally designed to foster interdisciplinary exchange in the programs themselves. For example, the faculty functioned as a unitary rather than departmentalized group. Representatives from other disciplines served on each program's advisory committee. Many opportunities were made available for both formal and informal exchange and cooperation in teaching and learning, in conducting research, and in providing patient care. I was appointed Acting Faculty Representative for the Dietetics Program and elected Dean of Acting Faculty.

With the guidance of a distinguished Interim Steering Committee (serving as Board of Trustees might) and with the inspired leadership of Nancy T. Watts, Ph.D.,

R.P.T., Acting Provost, rudimentary organizational framework took shape, and Provost and Program Director faculty searches began.

It was an exciting time. One of its triumphs was when Mary A. Carey, Ph.D., R.D. accepted our invitation to become Professor and Director, Graduate Program in Dietetics. Mary's academic and experience credentials were impeccable—the bonus was that she had completed the dietetic internship and a tour of staff duty at MGH prior to graduate study at the Mayo Clinic and the University of Minnesota. The combinations which we sought—professional practice, research, doctoral degree and teaching experience are not easy to come by!

The first students in the Graduate Program in Dietetics, all registered dietitians, were accepted in the fall of 1981. The Master of Science Program in Dietetics offered experienced registered dietitians the opportunity to advance their careers through specialization in either clinical dietetics or foodservice systems management. Practicums designed to enhance individualized programs of study were to be conducted at MGH, its health centers, and affiliated institutions. Since the focus of the program was to prepare advanced practitioners, the faculty included individuals with academic credentials as well as practitioner experience in the health care setting. Two broad areas were incorporated into the program: the core in dietetics and the health professions core. In both areas, research, humanistic concerns and interdisciplinary approaches to health care were emphasized. The Graduate Program in Dietetics moved into full operation in the fall of 1982 as the 18-month Combined Dietetic Internship-Graduate Degree Program was offered for the first time. The internship component retained much of the traditional generalist internship with improvements, including a revised curriculum and evaluation strategy. Non-credit weekly classes in dietetics and classes with other Boston area dietetic internships continued. In addition, MGH dietetic interns completed 15 academic credits during the internship year.

Among changes made in the program when "real" faculty and students were aboard, was the decision to discontinue simultaneous enrollment in the dietetic internship in the hospital and degree candidacy in the Institute. Admission criteria for the dietetic internship continued to meet Institute requirements.

Following an active role over nearly a decade in the planning of the Institute before joining the administrative staff, I transferred from the Department of Dietetics and assumed the position of Assistant to the Provost for External Relations in January, 1983. The Provost I assisted was Julian Haynes, Ph.D. The Office of External Relations was responsible for many important links between the Institute and the rest of the world—other educational institutions, health care agencies, prospective students, and alumni.

My dedication to quality dietetic education and excellence in practice in our profession goes hand-in-hand with my commitment to and respect for our professional organization. Participation in professional activities provides opportunities for sharing expertise, interests, abilities, problems, solutions, and successes. I believe in being a builder; if you have the heart to criticize, have the will to work. I live by this precept and have kept myself busy and challenged with responsibilities in state and national dietetic associations and related professional organizations.

Elective offices have included service as Delegate and President of the Tennessee Dietetic Association; Secretary, President, and Delegate of the Massachusetts Dietetic Association; and Secretary of the Massachusetts Public Health Association. The membership of the Southeastern Hospital Conference of Dietitians elected me to serve as President, but I resigned with regret upon acceptance of the appointment at MGH. Additional memberships included the Society for Nutrition Education and the American Society of Allied Health Professions (ASAHP).

Contributions to The American Dietetic Association (ADA) have brought me more than I have ever given in terms of professional rewards and enduring friendships. I was a member of the Joint Committee, American Hospital Association. I have served as Chairman of both the Nominating Committee and the Diet Therapy Section. Committee memberships have also included the Academic Requirements Committee; Community Nutrition Sections Committee to Develop Guidelines for Community Diet Counseling Services; Journal Board Member; and Joint Committee, American Diabetes Association, U.S. Public Health Services, ADA. I represented ADA on the Advisory Group to the National Commission on Digestive Diseases Study for the National Institutes of Health. I was Speaker of the House of Delegates in 1972–73.

Surely one of the highlights of my career was the year (1975–76) I served as the 51st President of the Association. Truly a labor of love since ADA Executive Board members serve on a volunteer basis. I firmly believe the opportunity for a leadership role is a privilege and acceptance of the obligation must not be undertaken lightly. Case in point, during my year as President-elect, I recorded 75 days of ADA business, including trips to Chicago and to Washington, D.C., as well as to meetings in six states. That was excellent training, however. By mid-year of my Presidency, I had already logged 51,304 miles on my "Have Gavel, Will Travel" calendar—almost twice around the world!

The fact that my presidential year was the Bicentennial Year of the United States of America was especially memorable.

For several years in the mid-seventies, I participated in the national legislative initiatives of the ADA. I worked with Isabelle Hallahan, Betty Blouin, Jean Wilson Kruhm, Robert Barclay (our legislative counsel) and other member volunteers. We attempted interdisciplinary liaisons through representation on the National Nutrition Consortium, Inc. and the American Society of Allied Health Professions. For example, on December 2, 1975 I had the privilege of appearing before the U.S. House of Representatives' Subcommittee on Health of the Committee of Ways and Means. ADA was continuing its legislative thrust to promote preventive health care in legislation for national health insurance and amendments to Medicare. It was to this end that I directed my statement. On March 25, 1976 I appeared before the Agriculture Appropriations Subcommittee of the U.S. House of Representatives to testify on behalf of ADA regarding appropriations for legislated child nutrition programs, accompanied by Jean Sturdevant, ADA President-elect.

Although the ground work was laid earlier—by previous ADA Presidents—it was in my term that membership voted to expand membership categories. Isabelle Hallahan was the President who appointed the committee to revise the ADA Constitution (conversion to By-laws) which was chaired by Margaret L. Ross, Ph.D., herself a former ADA President.

Studies of the profession of dietetics in the seventies and eighties documented dissatisfaction on the part of some administrators and physicians as to the depth and adequacy of preparation of dietitians. This is due, in part I believe, to dietitians' efforts to be all things to all people. Current education programs no doubt are targeted to help students cope with the information and communication explosion.

I believe that I was a more effective diet counselor and supervisor at 21 because of exposures to "family life" education. One's own life experiences, which can enhance application of scientific knowledge to the needs of others, simply haven't been experienced at that age!

There were many fine role models at the Massachusetts General Hospital. I'll mention two. My first staff preceptor, and friend ever since, Shirley Wells, was the dietitian on MGH's Ward IV, renown metabolic research ward. She was so respected, so knowledgeable and so deft with quantitative techniques in those pre-electronic days!

And then there was Louise Hatch, then First Administrative Assistant to Miss Marion Floyd, the Chief Dietitian. Louise Hatch, also a lifelong friend, was an administrative dietitian par excellence, and yet she always had time for people—student dietitians included.

It was not always easy—I studied diligently and worked hard—as a student and as a practitioner. Dietetics is entirely too challenging a profession to undertake it if you don't love it—halfway won't do! Somehow I have never doubted that this profession is very worthwhile—essential to patient care—and that I was needed, necessary, wanted and even loved! Practice of the profession and the professional association provide so many opportunities!! The practice of a profession means continual growth, and that is the challenge and the reward.

As time passed, and the world became increasingly complex, dietitians-with-and-adjective became commonplace. Specialization is necessary—there is so much to know in order to practice effectively in management, clinical dietetics and education. I never really decided for what specialization to opt and think of myself as a generalist to this day.

In 1979 I was privileged and honored to be invited to deliver the 17th Lenna Frances Cooper Memorial Lecture at Annual Meeting (2). To me, this was a symbol of recognition which expressed personal admiration and acknowledged professional achievement. In my address I noted "there are precious hallmarks of excellence, talismans tried and tested, nuggets of gold." I named Lenna Cooper, Mary Swartz Rose, Mary de Garmo Bryan, Helen Hunscher, Charlotte M. Young, and Marjorie Hulsizer

Copher. In 1988, ADA bestowed on me its highest honor, the Marjorie Hulsizer Copher Award (3). Responding to this award afforded me the perfect opportunity to personally address former students and associates. "My greatest joy in this personal review is the realization that most of the individuals for whom I have been teacher or mentor exceed my accomplishments in knowledge, skills, creativity, and productivity. I am proud of them!"

I can only hope that my career reflects the intent of Dr. Glover Copher when he established this award in memory of his wife—that giving recognition to outstanding leaders of our profession would inspire other members to pattern their lives so that they, too, could attain high levels of achievement.

Notes

1. The challenge of today. J Am Diet Assoc 1959; 35(5):476.
2. Galbraith, A. Twenty-four-carat dietetic practice for the eighties. J Am Diet Assoc 1980; 77(5):529.
3. Annie L. Galbraith, M.P.H., R.D., receives 1988 Copher Memorial Award. J Am Diet Assoc 1988; 88(11):1449.

Joan Dye Gussow

Joan Dye Gussow, EdD
is the Mary Swartz Rose Professor
of Nutrition and Education,
Teachers College, Columbia University, NY

When you think of nutrition education, Joan Gussow's name invariably comes to mind. That is not surprising—she is widely published and much sought after as a speaker in that area. She has served on numerous committees, boards, panels, advisory groups, and tasks forces all the way up to the national level. What is really fascinating, inspiring, and perhaps a bit intimidating, is that she did not formally begin her career in nutrition until after the age of forty! She not only offers us a glimpse of how she came to be where she is and the origins of ideas that have shaped what she does, but she shares some basic lessons she has learned. Dr. Gussow is to be applauded for her support of her convictions. Her biographical sketch was accompanied by a note which she proudly identified as being penned on "directly recycled" paper.

Joan Dye Gussow

Because my career has been unconventional, I have been unable to devise a way to give a conventional description of its evolution. I am now the Mary Swartz Rose Professor of Nutrition and Education at Teachers College, Columbia University. From 1975 to 1985, I was the Chair of the Department in which I now teach. Now, mercifully, I am not.

In trying to create a narrative account of how I came to be where I am, I am going to start by talking about the origin of the ideas that have shaped what it is I actually *do*. Then I am going to describe, a bit more conventionally, what I did before I got to where I am, and finally, I will talk about some of what I think are the most valuable lessons I learned in the course of my odyssey.

I need to begin by confessing that there is a sense in which I am less interested than nutrition professionals are supposed to be in the actual food habits of my fellow eaters. That is, I care a lot about what our national eating habits are doing to the sustainability of global food systems, but if you choose to eat bacon and eggs in my presence, I will not lecture you. A couple of years ago, one of my Teachers College colleagues set down his plate across from me at a faculty luncheon. "Joan," he said, "I always worry when I sit across from you that you won't approve of what I'm eating." And because I was at that time nearly 60, and therefore risklessly fearless, I snapped back, "You know, Harry, I don't really care what you eat. I hoped you were afraid to sit across from me because of my ideas which—if you knew what they are—you might be." I was feeling fairly put out at the time about the way men had messed up the food supply and the environment, so he probably got hit harder than he deserved!

I went into the field of nutrition because I was upset about the American diet. I have two sons. When they were very young, I used to go to the market with them, and sometimes I let them watch television on Saturday morning. I hated what was being advertised to children; I thought much of what was in supermarkets was junk; and from everything I read, the nutrition profession seemed to be more worried about Adele Davis and faddism than about the sugared cereals, juiceless drinks, candy and other fads being marketed to our children. I don't know what I thought *I* could do, but I figured before I could do anything I needed to become informed—and that meant going back to school.

Actually, I wasn't at all sure I *could* go into nutrition. I had been a pre-med in college, but it was 20 years since I had taken organic chemistry, and I wasn't too certain that anything was left of my abilities in science. But I took my courage in hand, and in my 40th year, I went back to school.

I managed to get through biochemistry, and I began formally to learn nutrition. I took courses at Teachers College, and at Columbia's Institute of Human Nutrition, run at that time by public health nutrition pioneer Dr. Henry Sebrell. I learned a lot about intermediary metabolism, protein quality, nutritional needs, nutritional assessment, therapeutic diets, food science, current nutrition issues, educational techniques and so on, and on. I did well, actually, but I was also frustrated. Here was nutrition science, continually unearthing new information about nutrients and how they functioned in the body; but while all this knowledge-generation was going on, it seemed clear that our diets were getting worse, not better. I was old enough to remember when most of what people ate was actual food; now much of it seemed to represent the output of clever chemists. And next to faddism, the thing the profession seemed to worry most about was overweight, a topic that didn't interest me very much. I could not imagine myself devoting my life to telling people how to lose weight—not when there were, even in this country, people who didn't have enough to eat.

And that brings me to two major forces that strongly influenced what I *was* interested in. Before I formally entered the field of nutrition, I had gradually eased myself into work outside the house with a part-time job that led, over a three year period, to my writing a book with a psychologist-physician. The book (*Disadvantaged Children: Health, Nutrition and School Failure*) was about the ways in which the physical conditions of poverty affected the mental development of poor children. Some of the things I learned in the course of writing the book will come up later in this narrative. I bring the book up now because it dealt with poverty in America, and researching it pricked my already overdeveloped sense of responsibility and guilt (I had a Dutch reform mother!). A parallel influence was my husband's deepening involvement—and my own deep interest—in fighting for the survival of the global environment.

These underlying concerns were lying in wait on the day that Kendall King came to the Institute of Human Nutrition to give us students a lecture about the Mothercraft Centers he had helped set up in Haiti. The lecture was a revelatory experience. What I remember Dr. King saying was that the average peasant woman in Haiti had 12 children and raised about four of them to the age of five. The rest died, of something related to malnutrition, if not of outright starvation. I remember his telling us also that the amount of money such a mother had to feed her children was under 8 cents a day, and that he had tried to figure out what he could teach her to feed that would cost less than 8 cents a day.

I was deeply moved. I realized that I simply couldn't spend the rest of my life worrying about overweight Americans—or women who starved themselves down to a size one out of some desperate need to fit the bizarre norms of an indulgent culture. I listened to Dr. King and kept wondering what I *could* do. As he described the difficulties of getting the cooperation of the appropriately distrustful Haitian peasants, of finding local people who could be trained to help without losing their own credibility among the villagers, I counted up my liabilities. I couldn't run or even help run a Mothercraft Center because I wasn't Haitian. I couldn't take charge of the program because I wasn't a male M.D. I had a family so I wasn't really free to move (this was 1970, remember. Women's work was not what moved families—and what work was I talking about anyway?).

So what could I do? What I could do, I realized, was to try to wake Americans up to the meanings of their own wealth and the world's poverty. What I could do was to make people see, really *see*, the obscenity of a food supply that taught children to view food only as something fun, never as something scarce and special, and important. And so, little more than a year after I had started graduate school, I ended one of my term papers with a great cry of pain that says (with some allowances for the changes 20 years have wrought in me and in the food supply) essentially what I still believe:

> The growingly poor diets of many affluent Americans are—in the context of a
> world much more poorly fed in spite of itself—irrelevant, immaterial, and not
> worth worrying about were it not for the example we set to the world of what is an
> advisable end point of technological and material progress. Moreover, in a world
> context, the attitude of some American food manufacturers toward food—that it is
> just one more of the world's raw materials to be played with and manipulated for
> our amusement and for the greater delight of that 'consuming prince' the
> American—is immoral.

As my concern about poverty, food, hunger and the environment began to coalesce, I was given the opportunity to co-teach a course with Dr. Eleanor Williams who generously allowed me to inject into what had been her own course some of my ideas. Eventually that course became mine, and got the title "Nutritional Ecology." And the course led to a book *The Feeding Web: Issues in Nutritional Ecology*, which—thanks to my insanely loyal publisher—is still in print 11 years after it was first published. The course allowed me to discover that I loved teaching. The course, and the book, allowed me to discover that what I really wanted to teach people was how to make connections—between what we are and how we act and what that means for the food supply and the sustainability of the global systems that support food production.

All of which is intended to help explain what I actually *do*. What I do professionally these days falls into two major classifications:

1. I do all the things I am supposed to do—I teach nutritional ecology and other large classes every year. I teach seminars, attend staff meetings, committee meetings, college-wide meetings, I meet potential students, counsel current students, direct doctoral dissertations, correct papers, write papers, work on Food and Nutrition Board studies, write books, make speeches, talk with the press. . . .

2. AND I intellectually support all this activity by continually working to make a mesh of things—trying to figure out how the things that affect who has what to eat fit together. This means I read a lot, scan a lot, clip newspapers a lot, file a lot. One of our problems today is that we are overwhelmed with little bits of data. We have much less real information, even less knowledge, and very little wisdom at all. Under such circumstances, the temptation is to retreat into the narrowest space, seeking to know more and more about less and less. For reasons not entirely clear to me, I have opted to try to grasp some larger truths—which often leaves me feeling, probably accurately, that I know less and less about more and more. It is unsettling, but unavoidable.

60

Some of the larger truths I have tried to grab are laid out in *The Feeding Web*. Some of the more recent ones were presented to the Practice Group on Nutrition Education for the Public at ADA three years ago under the title "Women, Food and Power," a theme I continue to pursue.

That is some of what I do currently. I think and I teach—by a variety of routes and in a variety of fora—about the food supply and things that affect its sustainability, whether these are material threats or attitudes. What was my training for this? I smile at my own question, remembering Dr. Ruth Hueneman asking me that very question 18 years or so ago when she came to Teachers College for a site visit. I was a new (not young!) instructor, and I was, with all the enthusiasm of the novice, describing my course in nutritional ecology. Dr. Hueneman in her rich voice asked me solemnly, "And what was your preparation for this?" And I, unthinking, blurted out, "A highly developed sense of indignation."

Actually, I had somewhat more formal preparation than that. I was born in Southern California, one year before the Great Depression, in a small town surrounded—as were most small towns in Southern California at that time, by eucalyptus trees and orange groves. My father was an electrical engineer, who as a civil servant in the city of Los Angeles, did not find himself out of work during the crash. My mother was a beautiful, brilliant woman (though I don't think I recognized either quality at the time) who never was employed outside the home.

I went to public school, was ardently interested in science as a small child, and, at least 'til adolescence, had every intention of being an entomologist. Indeed, for my tenth birthday, my family (who always took their two daughters very seriously) bought me the textbook I wanted, Lutz's *Insects of Western North America*. I also read incessantly, a book a day during one particularly intense summer when we had just moved to North Hollywood and I was very lonely. I went to Pomona College as a pre-medical student. Why a pre-med? Asking myself that in retrospect, I have reluctantly recalled that it was for no reason more serious than that pre-med was "hard." I needed to prove something and I usually proved it by being very good in school. If pre-med was the hardest course of study, I would prove myself doing that.

So while my friends went skiing or to the beach (In spring you could do either within an hour's drive of Pomona), or spent the afternoon in an art studio enjoying every minute so they claimed, I dissected. (My God, was it really a fetal shark as I seem to remember?) I do recall the pickled cat that I and my laboratory partner dissected; when we slit it open it contained none of the expected organs, just a large undefined mass. As we cut deeper, we found, alas, pickled kittens—and sent a birth announcement on the lab's brown paper towels to our lab mates.

By the time I graduated, I was clear that I did not wish to go to medical school. This was 1950, at a time when few women went on to graduate or professional school. I had taken pre-med, as I said, because it was a challenge, not because I had ever really thought about being a physician. As graduation approached, and the men were applying to medical school, I didn't. How, I asked myself, could I justify taking a place in medical school when I really wanted to get married and have a family? This was the end of World War II. The class preceding mine was all veterans. Women were supposed to go home and leave the jobs for the men, and the model for combining a demanding career with wife and motherhood did not exist among mine or my mother's acquaintances.

But no one asked me to stay home! I was one of the minority who didn't get married right out of college. I came to New York, worked for 6 years as a *Time* researcher (wildly demanding, but viewed by me as a "job," not a life work) and ultimately quit to get married and have children at the advanced age of 28.

I had a son, moved to a big, run-down, inexpensive Victorian house in the country 20 miles north of New York City (where I still live) and had another son. When both boys were in school and I had lost all confidence in myself as anything other than a Mommy, I was rescued by a friend who suggested to one of her acquaintances that I might be able to do some writing and editing for him. He asked, I accepted, and through a succession of assignments (recorder and editor of several conference proceedings, abstracts editor for a new "information retrieval system"), I found myself working with Dr. Herbert Birch, a psychologist/physician on what ultimately became *Disadvantaged Children*.

In the summer of the year the book came out I was 40. I still did not know what my "own" work would be, but after three years of working with a male genius, I knew that wasn't it. I really wanted to write books on my own; to do that in the only way that would suit me—accurately—I had to become an expert. As I read galleys that summer, I asked myself over and over what I wanted to do when I grew up. One day it came to me—why had I not thought of nutrition? And my embarrassing reply to myself was: It doesn't seem to have much status. But—and here is another confession—I had been a reader of Adele Davis, whose book *Let's Have Healthy Children* was sent to me by my brother-in-law when I was pregnant with my first child. Old Adele had given me the confidence to go with that child—equipped with brewer's yeast—to an Island in Maine that had no telephones, no electricity and no doctor. Adam was only two months old at the time and he flourished, so I knew Adele wasn't all bad. On the other hand, I also knew, from my lengthy research for *Disadvantaged Children* that she was often wildly inaccurate, not someone you could confidently quote when your friends called to ask you for advice. And so, bolstered by the conviction that nutrition really was important, even if it carried a dull image, I spoke firmly to myself. If nutrition has a bad image, I told myself, that's a very silly reason not to do something *you* think is important—especially in your 40th year.

And so, as I said, I conquered (or at least made a truce with) biochemistry, and in my second year of graduate school, I met Robert Choate who had recently helped plan the 1969 White House Conference on Food, Nutrition and Health and was shortly to hit the front pages of newspapers across the country denouncing the poor quality of breakfast cereals. He gave a speech about the nutritional unworthiness of breakfast cereals to an audience in Brooklyn, and afterwards I went up and asked him whether he had ever watched the breakfast cereal commercials on TV. He said "no" and made a note.

Sometime later he called to ask whether my students and I would like to do a study of children's TV food commercials. I said we would; we did the study; and I, truly terrified, subsequently testified before Congress (which was what Choate had all along planned to do). My testimony was published in the *Journal of Nutrition Education*. Suddenly I was no longer an obscure graduate student; I was infamous.

I began to receive speaking requests—lots of them; and although I did not yet feel like an expert, I found myself being asked to act as one. I had been a *Time* researcher, responsible for putting a dot over *every word* in a story to show that I had checked its accuracy. I had spent three years arguing with Herb Birch over the exact interpretation of each research study cited in our book. I cared a lot about the truth; I had a big investment in accuracy; I wasn't sure I yet knew enough to speak. It was a stressful time.

I was helped out most by a new friend, Ruthe Eshleman, who had come to Teachers College to get her doctorate when I did and shared the anguish of biochemistry with me. She became not only an honorary member of our family, but my reality test. She had been in the field of nutrition for years. When I worked hard to understand the facts and the politics of the field, and reached a conclusion that seemed to challenge the majority view, Ruthe could disagree with me when necessary, and support my conclusions when they made sense—even if they were opposed by "experts." I don't think I would have continued graduate school without her support.

Much of the time between 1969, when I went to Teachers College to study, and 1975 when I received my doctorate, seemed a blur. I was often busy, often frightened, often over my head, often elated by teaching. I was suddenly thrust into a public speaking role that was entirely unexpected—and after the first year or so of doubts, surprisingly easy. (My husband who is a brilliant speaker, still gets tensed up before a speech. I never do—though I have no idea why).

On April 30, 1975, I passed my doctoral oral. On May 1, I made a speech on world hunger in Tennessee. Later that week, still an instructor, since my degree had not yet been formally awarded, I was appointed Principal Adviser (Chair) of the Program in Nutrition at Teachers College. I have never been more exhausted, frightened, anxious, or overwhelmed. You will need to ask Teachers College why they pressed me to take on a job I strenuously resisted taking. I felt unready, unable, and unwilling. My accepting had much to do, I think, with being pressured by two men, the President of the College and my husband, to take up the challenge. In retrospect, I'm astonishingly glad I did, but at the time I was truly depressed and terrified. Several months later, when the absolute panic had subsided and the reality of ADMINISTRATION had taken hold (Is *this* what I went to school for?), I was at a party where a woman whose clarity of thought I had long admired, asked me what I was doing. I told her, and added that it wasn't what I wanted to do at all. "What do you want to do?" she asked. "I went back to school in order to write books," I said. "Why do you want to write books?" she went on. That was harder to answer. "Well, I want my ideas to get out there so I can influence events." She smiled. "How do you know you won't better achieve that by doing what you're doing than by doing what you want to?'' There was a long pause. "That's a lousy question." I said. For of course, she was right.

For, of course, being a department chair (sometime in the 70s our "program" became a "department" and I became a Department Chair) is a bully pulpit in our profession. Of course it enabled my somewhat unconventional views to be more acceptable. And of course it gave me the chance to do things I would otherwise never have been asked to do. As far as my *job* is concerned I have in one sense been confined. I've stayed in one place. I've always taught. I've never worked in a hospital or health center, never worked as a diet counselor in any setting. I've never even taught many of the "straight nutrition" courses that are the bulk of many professors' careers.

But my *career* has been endlessly varied. It has taken me around the world to speak or participate in workshops in Uppsala (Sweden), Gran (Norway), Bangkok, Utrecht, Dar-es-Salaam, Budapest. It has taken me on a speaking tour of Australia and on repeated trips to one of my favorite cities, Montreal. This summer it will take me to Japan for a month of teaching, and this October to China where a former student is head of the Beijing Food Research Institute. I have spoken in almost every state in the Union, often to the state dietetic associations. I have testified to Congress, to the New York State Attorney General, before state assembly committees, and before a federal judge on behalf of the Federal Trade Commission on their proposal to regulate food advertising to children. With an intensity that has varied depending on who is in the White House, I have consulted on matters affecting the USDA, the FTC, and the FDA. I have been a consultant on a series of medical projects—from ABC's pro-social nutrition spots for children to the Children's Television Workshop health show "Feeling Good"—right up to the present when I am a member of the National Advisory Board of Project Lean. I have spent two busy terms as a member of the Board of Directors of the Society for Nutrition Education, serving as President 1979–80. I was the Chancellor's Distinguished Visiting Lecturer at U.C. Berkeley in 1980, have given memorial lectures in honor of Ellen Swallow Richards in North Carolina and of dietetics pioneers Violet Ryley and Helen Jeffs in Montreal. I have served as the only educator and the only woman on the three-year Diet, Nutrition and Cancer Panel of the National Academy of Sciences, and was subsequently appointed to the Food and Nutrition Board on which I am now serving my second term.

As I look at young women now, trying to balance a young marriage, young children and a young career, I realize that I have been exceptionally lucky. I worked at an exciting job (not every 22 year old gets to interview Marlon Brando at the height of his fame) for six years before I got married. I married a man who has always believed in me more than I believed in myself. I stayed home with my children, bored sometimes, but not anxious about my career. I picked the right profession at the right moment in history and was in the right place at the right time, so that—starting after 40—I was able to build a career that was exciting, satisfying and adventuresome beyond my wildest imaginings. It would therefore be presumptuous of me to give advice, to draw presumably generalizable lessons for those who might wish also to involve themselves as I have, in nutrition policy and philosophy. But I have learned some things, and come to value certain characteristics with which my parents appear to have endowed me and I want, in closing to share some of them.

1. It's important to do everything you have to do as well as you can, even if something seems "beneath" you, or boring, or both. When I was being given advice on going to interview for *Time*, fresh out of school, a wise counselor said to me "And for heaven's sake, don't say you want an 'interesting' job. Everyone wants an interesting job and most people have to spend some time stuffing envelopes." I've stuffed a lot of envelopes in my time and I've sometimes stuck things out longer than I should have, and I've often seemed to waste my time and energy working on things (like regulations controlling TV advertising to children!) that never saw the light of day. But since I always learned something in the process of doing the work, and since I usually impressed people with my seriousness along the way, payoffs often came later. A corollary rule is to do whatever seems important to do at the moment with all your heart, and not to hold back waiting to find *the one right thing* that will fully engage you.

2. Learn everything you can when you get the chance without worrying whether it is all relevant. Science and math especially should be learned early, first so you won't be entirely intimidated by it if you need to pick it up later. It's easier to escape than to grasp *de novo*. The second reason you need to understand science and math is so that you will understand what things they *cannot* deal with, so that you won't be intimidated out of your own common sense.

3. Care passionately about truth. Tell it, seek it, insist on it. Say what you believe to be true, even if it is unpopular, but always be willing to be taught. When someone attacks you and says (as they have said to me) "that's the most outrageous speech I have ever heard," don't be defensive. Ask them if they can be specific. Which statements are factually wrong. Always ask people if they will provide you with the information that you are missing, send you papers, give you citations, etc. You never learn by being sure you have all the right answers; you never win by assuming you don't have any of them.

4. I'm glad I was old enough when I went out into the world not to be intimidated by others' views of reality, and not to assume that truth was an absolute. I don't think I knew *that* until I had children! It is not a "loss of career time" to learn what Sara Ruddick calls *Maternal Thinking*. Subsistence knowledge, maintenance knowledge, cooking knowledge, gardening knowledge—all these are intensely valuable as we seek to make our profession relevant.

5. Sometime in your life you need to go into absurd detail in mastering something, though you will seldom have time to do that in regard to much of what you must do. Until you have once followed every single citation, talked to every single relevant person, to make sure you have covered every base, you have no benchmark for thoroughness and you do not know what—in real life, you can safely leave unexplored when time is short.

6. It's painful, but very useful, to be kicked out of the nest a few times, by being left on your own responsibility when you thought someone else was "the expert." In one of my husband's rare involvements in politics, he was appalled to realize that the people at the very top were working off the seat of their pants just as you and I. If you work with people every day, you are an expert on something. Act like it.

7. It's worth taking the time, even when you don't have it, to be a real friend to people, if only for the practical reason that if you do you will have friends when you need them.

Finally, I realize that I have always considered myself responsible for making the world a better place—a heritage from my parents, no doubt. That sense of responsibility has affected all my life choices. For someone who has had environmental concerns for more than 20 years, these last few years have produced confusing emotions. Last summer, as the midwestern drought once more cut into food reserves; as the nation began to wonder whether our industrialization had finally triggered a major upswing in the greenhouse effect; as even *Time*, my always conservative alma mater, acknowledged the need for government intervention to protect the global environment, I felt almost (almost) cheered by all the bad news. I would much rather have been wrong in the concerns I have been writing and talking about for almost 20 years. But short of having my anxieties proved baseless, nothing could have been more gratifying than to know that my anxieties were now mainstream concerns. It was nice to know you could begin to ask questions about the sustainability of our way of life without being considered a constitutional depressive! The other night in class, one of my students asked whether I thought I would win my battle to restore food, its home preparation, and its sharing to a place of importance in our society. "No," I said, "I probably really don't. But I sure intend to keep fighting and end up a fierce old lady."

Isabelle A. Hallahan

*Isabelle A. Hallahan, MA, RD, CHE served as a member
of the USDA Human Nutrition Board of Scientific Counselors
and as the 48th President of ADA*

When signing "R.D." after their name, dietitians have, in part, to thank Isabelle Hallahan who was on the original committee to explore registration for dietitians in the 1960s. Her countless hours of devoted effort helped make the registration credential a reality for the profession in 1969. An avid interest in legislation led her to play a key part in the development of the role of the Association in government affairs. She helped draft ADA's first legislative and public policy guidelines. Her early career was spent as a pioneer in school foodservice administration. She received the American School Food Service Association's Executive Director's Award for her service to children. Her concern for child nutrition also took her to Peru as a consultant for Operation Ninos, a U.S.A.I.D. program directed at increasing the nutritional status of children in Central and South America. Much of her later career was devoted to a 12 year tenure on the staff of ADA, including her position as coordinator of legislation and public policies.

Isabelle A. Hallahan

Writing one's personal saga of more than thirty years as a dietitian can be fraught with danger. First, one could be accused of being boastful if there be only a recording of successes and none of failures. Second, there is the pitfall of naming some who have contributed to the many projects and programs while unintentionally omitting others who deserve recognition.

Lest the reader go no further I hasten to say that it is my firm belief that individuals do not achieve success alone. Whether by chance or preordained circumstances, actions and decisions are influenced, promoted, deterred by the actions and reactions of others. Any and all named in this brief recollection I believe would agree that they too were influenced by others, directly at the time in which they are credited or by some previous experience while they tried to foresee and wisely influence the future.

According to Thomas Carlyle (1795–1881), "The history of the world is but the biography of great men." Perhaps that is what the organizers of this volume had in mind when they asked some of us to record our personal experiences and impressions over many years as practicing dietitians. Carlyle also said, "A well-written Life is almost as rare as a well-spent one."

Whether considered "great" or not seems scarcely as important as achieving the objective of presenting a well-written story that may possibly be of interest and value to history buffs.

My career began as a Home Economics teacher. At the time I started teaching many Boards of Education required that the Home Economics teacher manage the school lunchroom as a part of her responsibilities. This part of my work was a challenge and soon became a consuming interest. I knew, however, that I needed to know more about management and cost/accounting if I were to continue in foodservice.

I enrolled at Columbia University to pursue a master's degree with a major in Institution Management. Two of the professors made a lasting impression. Mary de Garmo Bryan, Ph.D., a founder and second President of The American Dietetic Association (1920–1922), was my major professor. Neva Henrietta Radell, Ph.D., taught food cost accounting. Each of these women brought a fund of knowledge and experience to her students. Each demanded no less than perfection in performance. Each was impeccable in her appearance and preparation for every class. They never compromised on quality and thus inspired this student and I am certain many others to try to emulate their behavior.

Having completed my master's degree and having experience under the supervision of members of The American Dietetic Association, I qualified for membership in The ADA but I did not immediately complete the application. It took a Public Health Nutritionist, a Kansas State graduate, Ruth Welton, to all but demand that I submit my application.

Ruth Welton was employed in Suffolk County on the eastern end of Long Island. I too lived and worked on Long Island where most dietitians found attending meetings in New York City was not convenient. Miss Welton was determined to establish a Long Island Dietetic Association (LIDL), but the requirement in the New York State Dietetic Association at that time was there must be 15 members of The ADA enrolled in a District before it could apply for State membership.

To this day I do not know who sent Ruth on my trail but I do know that she convinced me to attend the organization meeting of The Long Island Dietetic Association in the fall of 1951, at the Northport Veterans Administration Hospital. Miss Welton was elected the first president of the LIDA. By spring of 1952, my application had been filed with The ADA, and with Ruth's confidence and persuasion I agreed to consider the presidency of LIDA three years hence. Making us all potential officers was a maneuver to keep our interest. Three years before assuming the responsibilities of leadership gave me sufficient time to become a member of The ADA and to be relaxed about the whole affair.

Before the year passed the president-elect, for personal reasons, resigned. The president-elect, Ethel Tuman, was transferred by the Veterans Administration to Idaho. My application was still going through the review process when a telephone call from Ruth advised me that in the fall of 1952 I would be the LIDA president.

My first direct contact with both the New York State Dietetic Association and The American Dietetic Association began about 1959, when I became a Delegate. Shortly afterward The ADA Chairman of the Civil Defense-Emergency Feeding Committee, Dorothy Bovee, asked me to serve on the Committee. Dorothy was with the American Red Cross in Washington, D.C. At the end of three years of corresponding with Miss Bovee I became Chairman of the Committee. I was becoming more versed in the functioning of the Association. In 1961–62, I served as Secretary of the NYSDA; President-Elect in 1962–63 and President in 1963–64.

During this same time I continued to be employed in School Foodservice Administration and had observed the development of this program nationwide from small, single-unit operations to increasingly larger, sophisticated programs receiving considerable support through federal legislation.

In 1962–63, while on leave from my School Foodservice responsibilities, I was consultant to the U.S. Department of State, Agency for International Development for "Operation Ninos." This was a nutrition program directed toward improving the nutritional status of children in Central and South America. My service in Washington, D.C., and Peru afforded me the opportunity to become better acquainted with the operation of government, its sponsored programs and related legislative activities.

I was nominated in 1966, for the second time, to run for the office of Secretary of the Council of the House of Delegates. I probably would have declined if Charlotte Young, Ph.D., Professor of Medical Nutrition, Cornell University, had not urged me to do so. Charlotte had a long, distinguished career in the House, having served as a Delegate beginning in 1954; Speaker in 1963–64, and a Delegate at Large 1966–69. In urging me to stay active in Association affairs she said, "You know if it weren't for The ADA you and I probably never would have met and I would have missed our friendship." Charlotte thus expressed what dedication to the affairs of a professional association can mean. Her report to the House of Delegates 1968–69, in which she recommended changes that have come into fruition, is indicative of her deep concern and affection for her profession and colleagues.

The late 60's and the decade of the 70's found three major issues confronting both the profession and its Association: the structure of the Association, Certification vs Registration vs Licensure and participation of The American Dietetic Association in legislative activities. Education for the profession was an ever ongoing concern but I will leave that discussion to those more closely concerned with its history.

During the summer of 1967 a Committee of The ADA to explore Certification, Registration and Licensure for dietitians was appointed. I was honored to be asked to serve with Doris Johnson, Ph.D., as Chairman, Paul Damazo and Geraldine Piper.

Ruth Yakel, Executive Director of The ADA, on the advice of the Executive Board, had secured the services of an attorney, Frank Grad, a professor at Columbia University Law School, to guide the discussion and educate us in the fine distinction of each of the proposed qualifications as well as their privileges and restraints. Mr. Grad remained with this project as a consultant until legislation was achieved in 1969. Grace Shugart was Speaker of the House of Delegates, and at her invitation he appeared at the 1967 House of Delegates to speak to the members and respond to their questions on this vital issue.

In the fall of 1967, with Ethel Downey as chairman and the following committee members: Elsie Bakken, Marilyn Baker, Frances Fischer, Isabelle Hallahan, Jessie Obert, Sister Helen Marie Pellicer, Joan Sharp, Grace Shugart, Grace Stumpf, Charlotte Young, Mary Zahasky, Ex-officio Ruth Yakel, Consultant, Frank Grad, comprising the committee, there was a determined, organized effort to refine a proposal for registration, fully discuss it with the membership, put it to a full membership vote and develop a procedure to implement registration for dietitians.

Countless hours were devoted to this work. Memorable friendships were made. Tears and laughter intermingled as we met in Chicago to discuss, draft, re-draft, criticize until early morning and then agree to have a new draft ready when the committee reconvened the next day.

We all had assignments to be completed before the next formal meeting. The period between meetings seemed shorter than the meetings. One of my assignments was to draft a proposal for a system to enumerate continuing education hours with weighted values for the content and time expended. Needless to say, there were many drafts and revisions with full committee participation before any system was approved. In a moment of levity I referred to the hours as "Brownie points" and the term has never left my mind although the seriousness of the subject is indelibly entrenched.

A tentative proposal for Professional Registration was released on February 27, 1968, to the membership for review and response to the committee. To give more full detail of the numerous sessions and the "selling" of the concept would be a history in itself. Mary C. Zahasky was President of The ADA during this first year and continued on the committee until Registration was passed. Small in stature but a bundle of energy, dedicated to the cause, she kept the committee moving night and day, determined to bring this distinctive qualification into realization.

Members were wary of an additional requirement for practice even though they were well aware that more than membership in a professional association was needed to designate dietitians as health-care practitioners who were current in their knowledge and procedures. The requirement for continuing education to assure the public that dietitians were up to date was *avant garde* at the time and had been adopted by only a few groups.

Despite this apprehension the vote to accept the final Registration proposal was positive and dietitians were registered for the first time in 1969. By 1969–70 there was an appointed Interim Committee on Professional Registration with Grace Stumpf as Chairman. Those of us appointed to chair one of the five original panels served only until the Committee was fully elected by membership.

At the House of Delegates meeting in 1966, Massachusetts presented the following resolution which was adopted: that "The American Dietetic Association take such action as is necessary to insure the inclusion of nutrition and diet therapy services in all legislation concerning comprehensive medical care programs, and that . . . the Executive Board of The American Dietetic Association appoint a committee to recommend a policy and a plan of action to insure inclusion of the services of the dietetic profession in current and future medical legislation."

The support among members to become active in government affairs had been sparked by the passage of the Medicare legislation in which nutrition services were not designated for third party reimbursement.

Until 1966, the IRS tax classification for The ADA had prohibited the Association from becoming active in influencing legislation. With a change in this classification the Association could now implement this resolution. In November 1966, the Committee to Develop the Role of the Association in Legislation was appointed by the Executive Board. On June 26, 27, 1967, the Committee met for the first time in Washington, D.C. The members were Clare Forbes, Chairman; A. June Bricker, Ph.D.; Dolores Nyhus, and Isabelle Hallahan. Consultants were: Mary Egan, Helen Ger Olson, and Geraldine Piper. Miss Nyhus and Miss Egan did not attend this first meeting because of prior commitments.

The Committee had little precedent to follow but with the consultants employed in government there was a fund of knowledge on which to draw as the first guidelines for developing a program in legislation and public policy for The American Dietetic Association were written.

By 1968, the Committee's title had changed to Advisory Committee on Legislation and Public Policy, and two recommendations of the original Committee were adopted. First, Robert Barclay, a Legislative Consultant, was retained. Members of the Committee who held membership in American Public Health Association (APHA) knew Robert Barclay as a member of the firm of Swearingen and Barclay who were consultants to APHA. Mr. Barclay had previously served on the staff of Senator Lister Hill of Alabama, and was highly recommended. Second, even though finances were limited it seemed necessary that there be a staff member assigned the responsibility for acting as liaison between the Association and the Consultant as well as providing pertinent information to the membership.

Still employed in School Foodservice while representing The American Dietetic Association at the Southeastern Hospital Conference in 1968, I was awakened shortly after midnight to receive a telephone call from Clare Forbes and Mary Zahasky (They called collect. I still don't know why.). There were offering me the part-time job as Liaison.

We talked for quite some time. They knew of my avid interest in legislation; my experience in federally supported programs; my knowledge of ADA programs and goals. They were most persuasive and I agreed to give it a try for one year. Frances Fischer, Speaker of the House of Delegates, announced at the 1968 meeting in San Francisco that I had accepted the position. While my interest and support for all child nutrition programs has never diminished, my career as a School Foodservice Administrator came to an end.

My career in School Foodservice was most rewarding. There was satisfaction in being a Founder and later Chairman of the Nassau County School Foodservice Association on Long Island, Chairman of the Nassau Country Nutrition Council and a member of the American School Foodservice Association. In 1973 I was honored to receive the Executive Directors Award from the ASFSA for my "service to children." Later, I served as a member of the Child Nutrition Advisory Council, New York State Department of Education. As I reflect on this past, being a pioneer in School Foodservice had its problems but they were outweighed by the satisfactions.

The early years were a challenge. Clare Forbes and I gave our first reports to the House of Delegates in 1969. I operated from my home. The budget was tight. We started a Newsletter (the first release was June 10, 1969) and a page in the "Courier," which graduated to a page in the *Journal*. I audited the hearings of the Senate Select Committee on Nutrition and Human Needs and acted as Secretary to the Advisory Committee, as well as being the members' source of pertinent information. Trips to Washington were made as frequently as deemed necessary.

Mary Zahasky was the first Chairman of the Advisory Committee and brought her usual zeal to the assignment. Frances Fischer, President of The ADA 1969–70, was the first ADA representative under this new program to present testimony before a Congressional Committee. Jeanne Kruhm, a Washington resident-dietitian, became a part-time employee assisting in auditing hearings, arranging for meetings, and keeping current on legislation and regulations of concern to dietitians. Jeanne stayed with us until 1976, and following her resignation, Betty Blouin replaced her and soon became a full time employee.

Annual Meeting keynote speakers were selected from recommendations of the Advisory Committee as referred by the staff. Among those were Congresswomen Martha Griffiths of Michigan, the first woman to serve on the House Ways and Means Committee, and presently Lieutenant-Governor of Michigan; Lindy (Mrs. Hale) Boggs, Congresswoman from Louisiana; Senator Charles Percy of Illinois; and Senator George McGovern, Chairman of the Senate Select Committee on Nutrition and Human Needs, from which came the first "Dietary Goals for the United States" in January 1977.

In conjunction with the American Home Economics Association and the American Vocational Association, in 1971, we held six workshops across the country in an attempt to educate our members in the legislative process as well as to bring the Washington scene to those who had never observed it in action. Workshops have been held annually in Washington since then and in April 1975 a second workshop was also held in Salt Lake City.

The Legislative Network Coordinators, LNC's program was begun on October 21, 22, 1978, at the first ADA sponsored workshop for a representative from each of the fifty-two affiliated dietetic associations. Held in Alexandria, Virginia, all but one, the District of Columbia Association, had a "LNC" at this meeting. The program developed out of the need to create a network of dietitians charged with the responsibility of keeping their constituents alert to legislative activities and ready to respond as needed.

It also became apparent early in our efforts to speak before Congressional Committees that The ADA had to be prepared to take firm stands on issues within its expertise. Out of this need in 1970 the first "Position Paper on Position Papers" and the original guidelines for developing a Position Paper for the Association were written.

My relationship with The ADA took another turn in the 70's. I was elected Speaker of the House in 1970 and held that office in 1971–72. When I was elected President of The ADA for the term 1972–73, I resigned as Liaison for Legislation and Public Policy and did not return to the staff until January of 1974, when Arlene Wilson, then President, asked me to resume my responsibilities. My title then became Coordinator of Legislation and Public Policies. This too was on a part-time basis.

Our association with other groups of health care professionals grew in this decade. A Coalition of Independent Health Professions was formed in 1970, as a forum for major health professions to receive and share information on health policy and planning. It represented through its eleven member organizations nearly half a million health care professionals throughout the country. It was my privilege to be chairman of this group in 1976–77.

In 1973 The American Dietetic Association was one of the founding members of The National Nutrition Consortium, along with the American Society for Clinical Nutrition, the American Institute of Nutrition and the Institute of Food Technologists.

By joining forces the members of the "Consortium" hoped to develop a national nutrition policy by coordinating joint nutrition education activities for the public and by offering an opportunity to foster communication between organizations, thus providing greater visibility for the profession and the public. Mark Hegsted, Ph.D., of Harvard University was the first Chairman and some four years later it was my honor to be elected to head this group. In the early 80's Betty Blouin became the Executive Secretary for the Consortium and remained with the group until it dissolved in 1985.

The Nutrition Today Society was formed in 1978. Cortez F. Enloe, Jr., M.D., Editor and publisher at that time of *Nutrition Today*, was Executive Vice President. A long-time supporter of the capability of the dietitian to become a full partner in the health care of the public, Dr. Enloe founded the Society with the dedication to increase the dissemination of nutrition knowledge. Upon the recommendation of Grace Goldsmith, M.D., of Tulane University, I was invited to serve on the original Board of Trustees of the Society and later served as Chairman of the Board.

During this same decade the greater New York Dietetic Association invited me, in 1975, to present the Mary Swartz Rose Memorial Lecture.

Like a pebble tossed in a pool The ADA program in legislation and public policy created ripples every-widening as government intervention in health care grew rapidly in the 70's. Three outgrowths must be cited because they are ongoing and undoubtedly will continue to be a part of our history. Education and qualifications for health care practitioners, the costs and benefits of specific health care procedures, and quality assurance of health care all surfaced during this time as targets for government scrutiny.

The Coalition of Independent Health Professions received a grant to fund a workshop, April 2–5, 1974, to train members in the peer review process as a part of quality assurance. Each member organization was allowed to send representatives who would agree prior to their attendance that they would become teachers to go forth and train others in the process. Representing The ADA were: Mary de Marco, Farah Walters, Loyal Horton, Jack Bellick, Sara Crumley, Mary Lou South, Harriet Cloud, Kathryn Sheeler, Suzanne Hansen and Lois Good. Jean Kruhm and I attended as observers and members of the committee conducting the workshop. Our participants evolved into a committee that fanned out across the country, sharing their knowledge and training dietitians in the peer review process as an integral component in evaluating quality care.

In November 1977, 65 health and medical groups met in Miami, Florida and formed the National Commission for Health Certifying Agencies. The purpose of the Commission was to set tighter standards for testing and certifying the competence of the nation's more than three million health care practitioners. Original funding for the Commission came from the Department of HEW (now HSS) Division of Allied Health Manpower, Bureau of Health Manpower Education. Included in the convention were the AMA, the AHA, The ADA, Societies of physicians' assistants, dentists, dental hygienists, optometrists, nurse-midwives, physical and occupational therapists, and other technicians. One condition of membership in the new organization was that a profession must move toward some kind of periodic reassessment or evidence of continuing training of its members. Thus, from concern for the qualifications for health care providers had come a new organization. Annie Galbraith and Frances Fischer were The ADA delegates to the Constitutional Convention. It was my responsibility to be Arrangements Chairman for the Convention and later to serve on the Membership Committee where we reviewed the applications of organizations seeking membership in the newly formed National Commission for Health Certifying Agencies.

During this same time the government was seeking proof that provision of health care services was cost beneficial. As we lobbied to have nutrition services become a "covered" benefit we had to be able to document that they were cost beneficial in ambulatory nutritional care services. The ADA Washington staff requested that a committee be appointed to pursue this subject.

Marion Mason, Ph.D., was the chairman of the first committee given this charge. Serving with her was Patricia Mutch, Ph.D., Florence Smith, Eileen Buckley and Morissa White. The committee was specifically asked to develop a series of model research protocols that could be used in conducting cost/benefit analysis of nutrition counseling services provided in ambulatory care settings. Hundreds of documents were reviewed. My recollection as I worked with the committee is of a computer printout of sources that reached across the room.

In 1977–78 the Board of Directors of The ADA asked the committee to prepare a monograph which was entitled "Costs and Benefits of Nutritional Care—Phase I," which was published in 1979. Phase II was published in JADA 80:213, 1982.

At Dr. Mason's suggestion the cover of the monograph was a deep purple. Committee members rightly refer to this publication as the "Purple Passion" indicating their emotions over the hours spent in producing the monograph. From one who served mostly as a prod to the committee, desperately wanting the information to use for legislative purposes, I would suggest to the many who have referred to the monograph, you owe much to a few dedicated members of your profession.

With the publication in April 1989, of "Costs and Benefits of Nutrition Services—A Literature Review," again we should express our thanks to those who continue to see this as a vital issue.

The structure of The American Dietetic Association had been under review for several years before I assumed any leadership role. Membership was growing rapidly, members were asking for greater representation in the decision-making process. On the night before the 1972 Annual Business Meeting held in New Orleans I sought the advice of Marguerite Grumme, our parliamentarian who had served us for several years. She had been recommending that we revise our governing document, a Constitution, and adopt a set of bylaws as well. I asked how I might implement her recommendation. She replied, "As president you have the authority to announce the appointment of a committee to develop this approach for membership consideration." Courage in hand, I did so the next day. There was applause.

Margaret L. Ross, Ph.D., accepted the appointment as Chairman of the committee. It was truly an awesome task but Margaret had been ADA President, ADA Foundation President, a member of The ADA staff and a frequent spokesman for the Association. She was more than qualified for the responsibility. From the efforts of this committee whose work spanned most of three years, came a new Constitution, the first set of By-laws, and ultimately the basis for the present structure of the Association. Changes recommended were fully implemented in 1978.

Late in 1979 I felt it was time to do self-evaluation. My commitment for one year working for The ADA was stretching into twelve. My interest in Legislation and Public Policy was not diminished but it was time for a change. In February 1980 I told Clara Zempel, Executive Director of The ADA, that I would be leaving at the end of the year.

To conclude this narration without mentioning the influence, kindness and cooperation of The ADA Headquarters Staff would be a gross omission. To everyone who helped to achieve our goals my heartfelt thanks. In particular I owe much to co-workers who became fine friends: Ruth Yakel and Clara Zempel who were Executive Directors of The ADA while I was an officer and employee. Without their astute counsel I may not have enjoyed these many years; Dorothea Turner, Editor and Harriet E. Sankey, Managing Editor of The Journal of The American Dietetic Association, who were always ready to assist with publication; Dorothy Bates, Assistant Executive Director for Membership, who never failed to help me trace a member; Lorraine Thomas and Jewell Larkin who could take my scribbling and make it pristine.

Some who read this may question my points of emphasis. I have not forgotten the Study Commission Report of 1972; changes in Dietetic Internships; the proposal to move headquarters from Chicago, etc. I'm trusting that others will report these events. Much of all of these and what I have recorded can be found in the Journal of the ADA and *Annual Proceedings*.

Since leaving ADA employment I have taught at New York University and been a volunteer in a Head Start Program. From graduate students to four-year-olds is a quantum leap. Each has had its particular satisfactions. Serving as a member of the United States Department of Agriculture Human Nutrition Board of Scientific Counselors also had its rewards.

As I have written this I have thought often of the quote from Milton: "They also serve who only stand and wait." Leaders can only lead when and where members will follow. To the members who have had the faith to support the numerous activities in which I have been involved I pay my deepest respect and gratitude for affording me the opportunity to represent you. I continue to believe my remarks when you honored me with the Marjorie Hulsizer Copher Award in 1985. "To whom much is given, much is expected. I hope that I have lived up to your expectations."

The writer Willa Cather wrote: "The history of every country begins in the heart of a man or a woman." The history of Dietetics as a profession did indeed begin in the hearts of a few women. My hope is that the next 30 years will make me ever proud that the theme of my Cooper Lecture in 1976 will remain true—"Of The I Sing."

Laura Jane Harper

Laura Jane Harper, PhD, RD is Dean Emeritus,
College of Home Economics, Virginia Polytechnic Institute
and State University, Blacksburg, VA

Those who have worked or studied with Laura Jane Harper will attest that she is an individual who always credits others with good words and deeds, and her sketch exemplifies this. She uses such phrases as "never seen her equal," "placed students first," "one of the best teachers," and "a master of equitable and successful administration" to describe her teachers and colleagues yet these phrases most assuredly describe her as well. Who else would throw a "losers' party" for those who were unsuccessful candidates, herself among them, for an academic position and invite the successful individual to break the ice and pledge support? She believes that the professional should be well prepared through education, knowledge of the field, work habits, and purposive networking with others. One of her early lessons: "each individual with whom I came in contact was worthy of my best treatment and that excellent relationships with and on behalf of others were a premier achievement." She undoubtedly learned it well!

Laura Jane Harper

Reminiscing on My Career in Nutrition and Dietetics: Preparation and Practice

Since my first year in primary school I have wanted to be a teacher and by a circuitous route I arrived at human nutrition as the subject-matter interest. As a child I very much liked to get into the kitchen alone and experiment with food preparation and as a member of a 4-H Club I was fascinated by the food projects I attempted to perfect. I wondered why certain combinations of food components worked to the advantage of food products and others did not. I was puzzled as to why people developed different food habits, even in families where the same foods were served. In high school I excelled in mathematics, chemistry, and physics, subjects in which there were always unanswered questions. Probably that was the reason these subjects were my favorites. There were always additional questions to explore.

When I enrolled at Belhaven College, a liberal arts college in Jackson, Mississippi, I decided to major in mathematics and minor in natural science. However, in my sophomore year I elected a course in nutrition and, as a result, chose home economics with the idea of becoming a secondary-school teacher. Teaching positions at the high school level were scarce at that time so for a short period I was employed as a home economist for a utility company. In much of what I did, I constantly wanted to know more about food preparation procedures and eating practices. Thus, as quickly as I could I enrolled in graduate school at the University of Tennessee (UT) to work toward a master's degree in nutrition.

When I completed my work there I accepted a position at the Virginia Polytechnic Institute and State University (VPI) in Blacksburg, Virginia which involved both teaching and research in foods and nutrition. By that time the study of child nutrition had developed into a special interest for me. Thus I was particularly attracted to the VPI position due to the fact that the Department of Home Economics contained a nursery school that could be used as a laboratory for students wishing to learn more about the science of nutrition for early childhood. However, even before I completed work at Tennessee I knew I wanted to pursue further study in my chosen area, so I began to make plans for additional graduate study. This I did at Michigan State University where, on leave of absence from VPI, I received my Ph.D. in human nutrition in 1956. While there, I added supporting work in human physiology, physical chemistry, and anthropology. Along the way, prior to completing the doctorate, I added a few courses in statistics and industrial engineering at VPI and one summer at Cornell University studying human nutrition under Dr. Hazel Hauck.

Throughout my college years I worked to help defray expenses. These were valuable experiences. I should have paid for the opportunity! The first work-study grant I held at Belhaven was under the supervision of Mrs. Frances P. Mills, Dean of Students. I have never seen her equal in the way she helped students think through problems and reach solutions that were acceptable to them and their significant others. Even now, when a student comes to me with a problem, which is seldom now that I have retired from VPI, I often find myself considering how Mrs. Mills would approach a similar dilemma. During my senior year at Belhaven I assisted the librarian, Miss Mary Agnes Anderson. She, too, has been a continuing inspiration. I looked forward to each period of time that I worked with her, and I learned much from the library experience. I have often remarked that work in the library should be a required course for undergraduate students: it is by far the best laboratory a university has.

As a graduate student at the University of Tennessee, one of the first people I met was Miss Jessie Harris, Dean of Home Economics. Recognized by her peers as an outstanding home economics administrator, she became a special friend of mine and remained so throughout her long life, an authority whom many times I called on for advice and ideas. She sought me out to get to know me soon after I arrived at Tennessee, a tactic she used with graduate students whenever possible. She placed students and their needs and hopes for a better education first above any other group of constituents with whom she worked.

I was again lucky in having a work opportunity at the University of Tennessee to help with expenses: a teaching assistantship with Miss Jeannette Biggs, the professor who taught child nutrition. I helped with the courses she taught and supervised preparation and presentation of the food served in the nursery school (pre-school child development laboratories). Miss Biggs introduced me to excellent techniques in child nutrition as well as the theoretical concepts for their applications. In one of her classes I read a journal article written·by a recognized authority of that time in which she stated that young children dislike green and yellow vegetables and as they grow older this dislike usually becomes more pronounced. I questioned this statement and wanted to delve into it further, which I did periodically for years until I was certain this generalization is incorrect. There were so many unanswered questions, so much knowledge to pursue, so much to learn and teach that could help individuals and families develop better food habits. I knew for certain after my experiences with Miss Biggs and in the University of Tennessee Nursery School that I wanted to become a college teacher of human nutrition. The opportunity to pursue a better academic and practical understanding of the fields of foods and nutrition to pass on to students through teaching and experimentation became "my cup of tea."

Three years after coming to VPI I received a graduate fellowship from the Smith-Douglass Fertilizer Company, Norfolk, Virginia that helped me initiate study at Michigan State University (MSU). I also obtained several small fellowships granted through MSU. Again, I received a teaching assistantship which was maintained throughout the time I worked on my doctorate. Like the undergraduate, work-study program at Belhaven and my teaching assistantship at UT, this was a rich experience.

Upon arrival at MSU I asked my advisor, Dr. Margaret Ohlson, for permission to use my assistantship to teach under a different "master" teacher in the department each quarter. I wanted to learn as much as possible from many experts in the field. Thus, I put in extra hours learning about new courses and professors, but I gained from the experience. One of the masters I taught under was Fay Kinder, author of the text *Meal*

Management that has been used in many foods courses dealing with the subject. Another policy in force in the Foods and Nutrition Department at MSU was that each teaching/research assistant was usually assigned a desk in a professor's office. I benefited from this arrangement also, especially so from my contact with Dr. Dena Cederquist, recognized as one of the best teachers at MSU during her tenure there. I was lucky enough to share an office with Dena during the period she was working on an elementary course in general nutrition to be televised throughout Michigan. She helped me think through alternative methods for teaching and learning that can be used advantageously.

My ability to cope with a discipline more effectively and compete more confidently in the work place was strengthened, I believe, by drawing on several colleges for a body of knowledge. Such diverse situations provided additional opportunities to react to various frames of reference within a subject and to their applications; they also offered more opportunities to observe how others compete and succeed.

An important quality for a dietitian-nutritionist to develop is a capacity to solve problems satisfactorily. I don't know where or how I developed this quality, but most probably it came from experiences in my childhood and as an undergraduate at Belhaven College. Throughout my professional career, upon encountering unknown situations either alone or with a group, somehow I have found a way to work through most of them with some degree of success. Some individuals shy away from problem-containing situations; I enjoy them. I classify effective problem solving as one of the important competencies to develop as a nutritionist, whether one is engaged in higher education or in another aspect of the field.

During my last term of graduate study at MSU I was requested to return to VPI for a brief conference, at which time I was asked to chair a committee of nutrition researchers from the Agricultural Experiment Stations in eight southern states. This committee of researchers came together to plan for and later conduct a series of metabolic studies to establish nutrient requirements of pre-adolescent girls. The committee had already been assured funding for this research. Even though I had misgivings about my competence to handle this undertaking, I accepted the offer. I would try to succeed.

Dr. Harold Young was Director of the Virginia Agricultural Experiment Station at that time. The working relationships we developed during these experiments were the beginning of a long and highly beneficial professional association for me. The experiences I had in chairing and working in the pre-adolescent metabolism project were exciting and a research undertaking from which I benefited since the researchers came together in Blacksburg to help plan the study, collect the original samples and, in some instances, partially or completely analyze them there. These experiments continued in alternating years for several summers, the findings of which have been used in many parts of the world. To have adequate funding for such a venture and the combined scientific expertise of nutritional scientists from eight different locations was an opportunity-par-excellence for a nutritionist just out of graduate school. In addition, these studies provided thesis opportunities for graduate students with whom I was beginning to work.

We were a small department with a limited program at that time so one could not specialize in one's activities to any great extent. The faculty had to "cover the water front," so to speak. There were, of course, strengths and weaknesses in such a situation: on one hand there was an opportunity to coordinate and deal with many components and relationships within the subject-matter area; on the other, there was little time to treat each subject-matter component with as much depth as desirable. Having built-in research opportunities from the pre-adolescent metabolic experiments for my graduate students was helpful to the students and to me.

In 1958, the governing board of VPI recommended that the Department of Home Economics, than a part of the College of Agriculture, become a college in its own right, effective in 1960. The Board appointed an outside advisory committee to help the home economics faculty develop an organization plan for the unit. Two members of this committee were Miss Frances Zuill and Dr. Lela O'Toole, Deans of Home Economics at the University of Wisconsin and Oklahoma State University, respectively. I served as our faculty chair. Faculty and advisors provided excellent assistance in our developmental plans, as did Mr. L. B. Dietrich, Dean of Agriculture at VPI. Mr. Dietrich was a master at equitable and successful administration, a model for any young academician to try to follow.

During this time, Dr. Walter S. Newman, President of VPI, asked me to consider becoming the college dean, but I did not want to do so. "Why not?" he asked. At that point I had spent approximately half of my life preparing to become a nutritionist in higher education, a position I was just getting into and one that I enjoyed completely. I wanted to prove my competency and did not even wish to consider a diversion. For almost two years I resisted the idea, but finally Dr. Young, Miss Harris, Miss Zuill, and my closest faculty friends at VPI persuaded me that I should accept the president's offer. I continued to teach but the time I could devote to research grew less each year. My philosophy included the concepts that I should put home economics faculty and students and the general goals of VPI first in my planning and activities. My own specialization area of nutrition moved forward along with efforts on behalf of the total college, but I attempted in every way possible to see that foods and nutrition held no advantage over the other areas of study under my jurisdiction. When I joined the faculty at VPI, bachelor's and master's programs in foods and nutrition were already offered. In 1971 we received permission from the Virginia State Council for Higher Education to initiate a Ph.D. program in foods and nutrition and in 1976 The American Dietetic Association honored our request to include a Coordinated Undergraduate Program in Dietetics as part of our curricular offerings leading to a Bachelor of Science Degree in foods and nutrition. In both cases, these were the first such programs offered in Virginia.

I have long been a member of the American Home Economics Association and, after receiving the Ph.D., a member of The American Dietetic Association. I have been active in both of these associations at local, state, and national levels and at one time served as liaison between the two organizations at the national level. Whenever possible I have taken students to meetings, encouraged them to participate, and helped them organize and support student-member sections at VPI. My appointment as dean of home economics brought new avenues for development and opportunities for serve to my profession. One of these included membership, committee, and elected office assignments in the International Federation of Home Economics (IFHE) where I served on the Foods and Nutrition Committee and the Research Reporting Committee for the screening of research reports to be presented at international meetings. Altogether I have attended 14 IFHE Congress and Council meetings in eight countries. I cannot begin to count the ADA and AHEA meetings in which I have participated. Other organizations in which I served included the Home Economics Division, National Association of State Universities and Land Grant Colleges; the U.S. Association of Administrators of Home Economics for which I served as president for one term; committee appointments in government at district, state, and federal levels; and international advisory assignments in foods and nutrition in both developed and underdeveloped countries.

When I was a graduate student at the University of Tennessee and at Michigan State University I met and studied with students from many nations. This was a dividend to me. Once Miss Harris at Tennessee asked me to assist a student from Greece learn to use the university library, which of course I was glad to do. From time to time this student and I studied together and I found out first hand how difficult it is for an individual to learn how to study in a new culture. Many simple procedures that we take for granted are not handled in the same way in other countries. I'm not certain with the now-common-use of calculators whether long division continues to be taught in elementary school but I quite unexpectedly found out when I studied with my Greek friend that children in Greece, when they learn to divide, place the divisor where we place the dividend. This being the case, a simple chalk-board explanation by a professor who was working a chemistry problem for the class was utterly confusing to her. I learned the meaning of "It's all Greek to me."

At Michigan State University I studied with several students from India and the Orient and admired their facility to apply theoretical, abstract modes of thought so quickly and accurately, a process with which I still struggle. In addition to mutually increasing our subject-matter knowledge during these study periods, I used them to help overcome some of my lack of ability to quickly perceive the abstract basis of the topic.

In the early days of my employment at VPI, we always had a few undergraduate and graduate students enrolled from abroad, chiefly from Western Europe, China, India, and Latin America. In recent years we have received students from most of the developing world. Throughout this time, both early and recent, we have attempted in every way that we knew to help them develop programs of study for maximum benefit to them when they return home; and we encouraged them to return home rather than to find ways to remain in the United States. Later, we contacted them in their homeland and asked them to evaluate their programs of study in relation to how their "study-abroad" benefited them and, if they could again go through the experience, what they would like to change. We made a strong effort to use the information they shared with us in a positive manner. Through our contacts with expatriot students, both faculty and our U.S. students have been given broader cultural and environmental perspectives on nutrition.

During the time I was a graduate student at Michigan State University, President Hannah provided opportunities for large numbers of students from abroad to study there. In fact, in foods and nutrition more expatriot graduate students than patriots were enrolled. A prevailing emphasis throughout campus was on understanding international customs and needs and on education and research working together to help solve local inadequacies in all parts of the world.

Through my contacts with international students and from my affiliation with international organizations, I have had opportunities for travel and work with many people abroad. From these experiences I have accumulated a wealth of knowledge. As a result of these journeys the often obvious but sometimes hidden—yet always vital—relationships between food and culture and their impact on nutrition status have become one of my strongest academic concerns and one that I continue to pursue on an almost-full-time basis. Alumni of our program of study at VPI who have been employed by business firms of international interests express the same dilemma and encourage me to search further into this area. One of my former students, Maryellen Spencer, who was employed by a food-product-promotion firm that dealt with international contacts returned for a doctorate to research the subject and develop a framework for a systematic study of the topic. Due to her untimely death a few days after completing the Ph.D., she was not able to continue her study, but three articles relating to her dissertation have been presented and published with her name listed as co-author.

I do not wish to leave the impression that the majority of my former associates, including professional colleagues and students, are internationals. Through the years many of our students at VPI have come from Virginia but each year some have been admitted from other states. A look at alumni names and addresses from our undergraduate program of study shows that almost every state in the U.S. is represented, more from eastern than western states. Residential backgrounds of faculty and graduate students, from wherever they came, have been rewarding to all who associated with them. Our students have found professional appointments in many areas of work in a wide variety of locations. We have been gratified by their accomplishments, both professional and personal. I just hope that they learned as much from me as I did from them.

I and other members of our faculty worked constantly and democratically to move our programs of study forward and keep them "ahead of their time." In the mid-1960's we have the good fortune to receive funds for a new building which we occupied in January, 1968. That, of course, was a "red-letter" day for all of us. Faculty had not only worked on its scientific functions but also on the artistic environment it provided.

For the first two or three years after I became dean of the college I continued to take an active part in teaching nutrition courses and in advising both undergraduate and graduate students in foods and nutrition. However, I gave up these responsibilities as soon as a department head for foods and nutrition was employed. I continued to teach two general courses to all undergraduate home economics students: one to first-year students and another to third-quarter, third-year students. With two other home economics colleagues, Miss Oris Glisson and Dr. Shirley Farrier, in 1970 I helped develop a summer study-abroad program to Finland. In addition to serving as overall coordinator, my subject-matter responsibility for this endeavor was to assist in planning for the study of food and nutrition practices in Finland and some of the relationships between these practices and the health of Finnish populations. This study-abroad program continued through 1979.

My door was always open to talk to both faculty and students. I worked very closely with first-year students in an attempt to help each of them plan for a scholarly, profession-oriented program of study. I emphasize the "help-them" phase of this project, since each of them was expected to take responsibility for choices, in keeping with departmental and university requirements for completing a degree program.

In regard to my "open-door" policy, an undergraduate student once paid me what I consider the supreme compliment of my academic career: one day she came to ask my advice on a certain topic, at which time she commented that she didn't wish to bother me unduly; she stated, however, that the reason students liked to come to me for advice was that it didn't appear to upset me if—or when—they did not take it. I thanked her for the compliment, but her remarks "shook me up," so to speak. What if students took my remarks as "the Law of the Medes and the Persians"? If so, I would need to keep my big mouth shut! I was certainly not infallible; neither did I want to take responsibility for the decisions of others. The longer I considered this comment, the more pleased I became with the maturity of our students. They wished to take responsibility for their own decisions and actions.

In 1965, while a member of the Governor's Committee on the Status of Education for Women in Virginia, I learned of grants available through the U.S. Office of Education that could be used to help meet the special continuing education needs of professional women. I wrote a later-accepted grant proposal to develop and implement an off-campus graduate program for five centers across the state for study in the various subject-matter areas subsummed under home economics. This four-year grant was used to help meet the continuing education needs of Virginia's home economists. Thus, a wide-spread off-campus graduate program in several areas of home economics study was launched, an endeavor that continues to grow in northern Virginia. Numerous nutritionists and dietitians in Virginia have completed a Master of Science degree through this route; other's have up-graded undergraduate programs through continuing education.

I continue to keep in contact with many of my former colleagues and students. However, I closed the open-door policy I had maintained for faculty while I was dean at

VPI when I left that position in 1980. Two weeks after I moved out of my Wallace Hall office, I embarked on a Food and Agriculture Organization assignment in Southeast Asia to help develop plans for introducing the teaching of nutrition into the post-secondary education of agricultural students. The "new" dean of home economics at VPI was free to develop either similar or different programs of study and faculty/students relationships.

My professional path has not been unique but it has been personally gratifying all the way. If I had it to "walk-through" again, I don't know what I would do differently except for one thing: most people make their greatest contribution(s) to a position in the first ten to twelve years. I think I would have moved farther professionally if I had relocated in approximately that length of time instead of remaining in the same place for most of my professional life. But each time I was asked to consider an offer elsewhere, I looked at the faculty and students to whom I felt committed and decided to stay in place. By the time the College of Home Economics was "on it's feet," I felt that I was too old to be seriously considered for a move to a new position. In the final analysis, one's personal professional-development commitment is due more consideration than I gave to mine.

Almost all the professionals with whom I have had contact have made an impression on my activities as a nutritionist but no one individual has shaped my professional philosophy. Along with circumstances in which I found myself, I take responsibility for what I did and became. My parents began early to challenge me to do my best and opened many vistas to me, both interesting and challenging. They taught me to read early, beginning at age three; at the same time they began to help me develop an inquisitive nature. They expected me to achieve in whatever I undertook and never to accept mediocrity in my behavior or standards or conduct. They also helped me understand that I should not condemn myself when my expectations were greater than my accomplishments; that I should simply try again to excel, if not in the same activity, then in another one of equal importance to me. They impressed upon me that each individual with whom I came in contact was worthy of my best treatment and that excellent relationships with and on behalf of others were a premier achievement.

I have mentioned the names of some of the significant others, but certainly not all, who have influenced and supported me in career developments and activities. Administrators, faculty, other colleagues, and students have been influential in many ways.

Throughout this narration, some of my personal philosophies of life have been expressed. I have never compartmentalized my philosophy into "personal" and "professional." I don't think that way. What I subscribe to permeates my life in all its aspects. I believe that all professionals, of which I count myself one, should be well prepared through education, knowledge of the field, work habits, and constant contacts and interaction with colleagues and the general public with which the profession is concerned. I also believe that professionals have the responsibility to constantly improve their competencies and their subject-matter field through observation, continuing education, research, participation in professional societies, and interaction with colleagues and the general public. I believe that I should not take myself too seriously, that I should carefully think through assignments and what I plan to do. I hope to succeed most of the time but when I do not, I try to analyze what I did wrong and try again. I do not condemn myself for failure nor do I alibi; I only want to produce better results next time. I also agree with the adage that "All work and no play makes Jack a dull boy''; thus I have continually sought out activities and experiences unrelated to my profession. Although I cherish my professional colleagues, I also seek out additional activities not connected with my work. In a nutshell, my philosophy of life is to prepare for it well, plan democratically and thoughtfully, handle situations and analyze results expeditiously, never take myself so seriously that when things go wrong I condemn myself or others but instead to think through the problem and try again; I strive to choose and hold on to friends from many walks of life and enjoy each day's associations with them or alone.

A profession has been defined in several different ways. A description I used with students for many years is that a profession is an occupation established to help improve and subsequently assist in maintaining some aspect of the quality of life; for a profession: (a) minimum entrance and continuing intellectual and experiential study requirements have been established by active members of the profession and (b) careful monitoring of the acquisition of these requirements is carried out by the profession's associational society. In nutrition and dietetics our goal is to help improve the quality of human health through appropriate patterns of eating. Thus, as active members of the profession we are obligated to establish and keep up-to-date intellectual and experiential study programs of excellence, which on our behalf The American Dietetic Association must monitor continuously and thoroughly. If we accept this description of the profession, then our standards of professional preparation and performance will continue to improve. Such an outcome, however, depends on our personal commitments to and competencies in improving the quality of human health through appropriate dietary practices. The profession of nutrition/dietetics is a worthy one. I take pride in my membership in it.

To identify what I have learned from the profession is difficult—too difficult—since the profession encompasses so much of my life. I can, however, state that much of what I know, am, and do has come to me directly or indirectly from professional contacts: daily or frequent association with colleagues and students and attendance and participation in rewarding associational affairs and seminars at district, state, national, and international levels. Separating The American Dietetic Association and the American Home Economics Association into individual entities is difficult for me since I have been affiliated with and active in both organizations for so long. I not only find it hard to separate these two organizations, but to consider ''the profession'' outside of the two is impossible. Once in the early years of my career, for a short time I attempted inactivity in professional societies but that didn't work. Thus, I have been actively affiliated with both organizations for many years, at one time the liaison between the two organizations at the national level, and a member of AHEA's Food and Nutrition Section.

When I consider these factors in my relationships within and between these two organizations and their affiliates, the professional activities and opportunities they have mutually provided have been the spark for my professional dynamo.

In my career, I have encountered few minority struggles. If they were "struggles," they seldom seemed so to me; rather they appeared as conflicts of day-to-day living and working for which I should seek a higher plan of action. In fact, with my personality and behavioral mode, discriminating against me is not easily accomplished. I look at myself first as a human-being, after that as a woman and a nutritionist. Once a male colleague asked me to talk to one of our administrators about what he considered an incident of discrimination against a third party. I asked why he didn't talk to the administrator. His reply was that he thought I could get away with the discussion. Possibly I chose a "safe" occupation for women: home economics and nutrition-dietetics, but I have received opportunities for service that were open to women or men in local, university, state, national, and international affairs. I usually don't take affronts as personal. I am not a "flag-waver" but I have never minded speaking out for myself or others if I thought we were being unjustly treated or passed over. I have usually been able to accomplish the ends I sought by rethinking/reworking problems I or "we" faced. Presenting one's views in a low-key manner, positively, without bias, and with persistence helps. Even jest is sometimes effective.

I am not certain that I have taken any major risks in my career. I have never looked at new ventures as risks, rather as opportunities. The professional positions I have held were either offered to me without application or I was invited to apply for them. Thus, someone else took the risk. When anyone considers applying for a job, becoming a candidate for elective office, or entering some other competition or unknown endeavor, only two aspects of the venture need examination: (1) what will be done to carry through successfully if the offer comes through; and (2) what the anticipated endeavor will do to the individual if the offer is not received. When both eventualities are planned for, risk value of the enterprise does not exist. Let me explain how I handled what I consider one risk I took. The position of Vice-President for Academic Affairs was open on our campus and some of my colleagues who are women encouraged me to apply. I doubted if I had a chance to get the position but since I always urged them to try to move up the professional ladder, I did not feel I could treat their interest lightly. Thus I applied. The final group of persons considered for the position were three on-campus candidates of which I was one and one off-campus candidate who was later offered and accepted the job. Our president had a difficult time telling the on-campus candidates that we had lost and showed his embarrassment. To help relieve the tension, I had a "loser's party" to which I invited the local candidates, the president, and their wives, at the beginning of which we toasted the president and the vice-president-elect and pledged our support. We not only "broke the ice" but continued to work as a team.

Individuals and groups of people learn about professional opportunities in nutrition and dietetics much earlier than they did when I entered the profession. Today numerous students come to college aware of professional opportunities in the field that are open to them and with plans in place to choose one of them. Not only is there a wider range of professional opportunities available within the field but there is accompanying evidence of exerted efforts by practitioners to succeed in one of these new areas of work. Far more educational opportunities in the science of nutrition and in career escalation are available today to those who choose nutrition/dietetics as career options, either pre-baccalaureate or subsequent in-service, than were true when I entered the field. The general public in larger numbers than formerly recognizes the importance of nutrition to general health and seeks advice from nutrition/dietetics practitioners. The profession is growing in numbers, scientific and social knowledge, respect, and contribution to human health.

My professional style, if I have one, developed as I went along. Some of it came from my family and the community of people in which I grew up; other parts came from students with whom I associated, still others originated with teachers and other professional contacts, and a part I have adopted by trial and error. In some cases I chose to emulate a pattern of behavior that I had observed which I considered to be positively effective, while others were reactions to negative conduct. I grew up in a household that in every way possible encouraged, rewarded, and often demanded socially acceptable behavior. In my home there was no dishwasher, for which I am now glad. There is something very therapeutic about putting one's hands in water (child development specialists call this "water play"). During the time my mother and I daily washed and dried dishes together, she helped me greatly through the conversations we had. I well remember our discussing certain undesirable reactions that I sometimes had in my contacts with a few adults. Mother would explain that some behavior patterns were due to personality traits. When together we analyzed a specific pattern of conduct in this manner, she would always add: "Instead of being so critical of another person, examine yourself and your own personality; the personality of most adults changes very little, it only becomes more exaggerated. You are still young enough to improve yours, to make it more adaptive. Remember, the older you get, the more like yourself you will get; your personality will grow stronger in all its traits. So do something *now* to develop a pleasant, inoffensive manner that indicates concern for others and which you can use for positive communication, both silent and oral." Thus, as I went through school I observed how older students, teachers, and administrators handled themselves and knew which characteristics I would like to emulate and which ones not to use.

Through the long years of my involvement in my profession, I have received recognitions of which I am proud. In certain ways, one might say that I have outlived much of my competition. Some of the recognitions bestowed on me follow: I have been invited to accept membership in eight honorary societies and have been listed in *Who's Who in America*, *Who's Who in American Women*; *American Leaders of Science*; *Who's Who in Higher Education in the United States*; and *Two Thousand Women of Achievement, International*. In addition certain other awards and recognitions are listed chronologically: *1965–68*: named to the Governor's Committee on the Status of Education of Women in Virginia; named to the President's Council (U.S.) of State Committees on the Status of Women; *1968*: named Woman of the Year in Virginia, a *Progressive Farmer* award for ''contributions to the education of girls and women in Virginia;'' named a fellow in the Royal Society of Health, United Kingdom; *1968–71*: named to the U.S.D.A. Committee (Cooperative State Research Service) to review regional research proposals and programs in progress for food, nutrition, fiber, agriculture, and forestry to recommend funding as appropriate to the Secretary of Agriculture; *1975*: Outstanding Alumni Award, College of Human Ecology, Michigan State University; *1976*: received Distinguished Dietitian's Award from the Virginia Dietetic Association; *1977 (May)*: U.S. delegate to the International Dietetics Congress, Sydney, Australia; *1978–79*: member AAUW National Committee for awarding study grants to international applicants; chair, Politics of Food Committee, Virginia Division, AAUW; *1977–80*: appointed to Steering Committee, Governor's Conference on Food and Nutrition in Virginia; *1981*: consultant on curriculum, program, and physical facility development in foods and nutrition, Department of Home Economics, Helwan University, Cairo, Egypt; *1980–86*: FAO/OICD/USAID consultant on nutrition education, curriculum development, and teaching/learning materials for post-secondary agricultural programs in Southeast Asia (Indonesia, Malaysia, Philippines, Thailand) and in Latin American (Chile and Ecuador); *1983 (April*: consultant on a nutrition education project of the World Council of Churches, Dakar, Senegal, West Africa; *1983–86*: president-elect, president, and secretary, American Home Economics Foundation; *1984*: invited speaker, United Nations Women's Day, University of Jyvaskyla, Jyvaskyla, Finland; in commemoration of the American Home Economics Association's 75th anniversary, named one of the Associations 75 leaders; named Lenna Cooper Distinguished Lecturer, The American Dietetic Association: the lecture was presented in Washington, D.C., on October 18, 1984 at the time of the Annual Meeting of the Association (published, JADA, *86*, No. 3, 345–351, 1986 under the title of ''Food, Nutrition and Agriculture: A Liaison for International Development''); named Knight, Class 1, Order of the White Rose of Finland, by Finland's President Koivista, in recognition of the cultural exchange program developed for students and faculty between the University of Helsinki, Finland and the Virginia Polytechnic Institute and State University, Blacksburg; *1986*: received Distinguished Alumni Award, Department of Food Science and Nutrition, Michigan State University; *1987*: at Founder's Day Ceremonies on April 24, received resolution from the Board of Visitors, Virginia Polytechnic Institute and State University, citing long standing dedication and effective service to both the University and the Home Economics Program; *1988*: Invited as visiting professor in nutrition, sponsored by the World Bank to assist with development of graduate programs for nutrition at Institut Pertanian Bogor, Bogor, Indonesia, and at Gadjah Mada University, Yogyakarta, Indonesia.

I believe very strongly that the future of our profession depends on each of its members, both present and future: how well we prepare ourselves for our professional roles; our zeal and effectiveness in keeping ourselves and knowledge in the field of nutrition up-to-date and moving forward through research, education, and experiential study; and the desire and ability to communicate our theoretical and applied knowledge to other professionals in our own field of expertise and in related fields of practice, to clients, to the world-wide political arena, and to the general public here and abroad. Our knowledge base must become more integrative and perfusive. As long as there are gaps in the knowledge that underlies our field, individuals any place in the world who know the facts that support optimum nutrition but do not apply them, people who do not know how to choose foods wisely and well, any who do not have the money or other resources to provide adequate diets for themselves and their families, those who do not see or understand the relationships of what they eat to their physical, social, and mental well-being, or those who have no place to obtain appropriate guidance and assistance in securing, preparing, eating, and storing foods for health and well being, our profession is in jeopardy. To close the gap in knowledge and the desire—or lack of it—of individuals to improve and maintain individual eating patterns that will maintain optimum health and well-being is our responsibility. We cannot be complacent about the future of the profession until the science and art of nutrition are as fully researched as the disciplines that undergird it make possible and people everywhere understand the principles of adequate nutrition and have the ability, both economic and practical, to expedite these principles.

Kathy King Helm

Kathy King Helm, RD is Owner and President,
Kathy King Associates, Inc., Lake Dallas, TX

Entrepreneur extraordinaire would seem to be a fitting description for Kathy King Helm. Boundless energy, unquenchable curiosity and professional vision have shaped her success. This trailblazer managed to receive local television and national radio coverage on her first job at a time when media exposure was not commonplace for dietitians. She became a regular on a childrens' television show, a national spokesperson for Butter Buds and Lean Cuisine, the "NoonDay Nutritionist" for NBC and now has her own nationally syndicated radio show. She began her private practice before it was fashionable and learned early on that marketing was an integral part of business success. Her interest and expertise in sports nutrition led to a consulting position with the Denver Broncos football team before most dietitians had even heard the term "sports nutrition." Kathy King Helm wrote the ADA study kit "Starting a Private Practice" and served as Chairman of the Council on Practice. She co-authored ADA's marketing manual *The Competitive Edge* and is the author of the *Entrepreneurial Nutritionist.*

Kathy King Helm

I never planned on having a career in dietetics. My goal in college was to learn practical information that I might use some day and meet the man of my dreams and marry. My alternative plan was to become a nun and dedicate my life to helping people in a small village in a third world country. Either way, nutrition would come in handy.

My mother actually influenced my decision to choose dietetics. She felt being close to medicine without having to carry bedpans and give shots would be exciting. And besides, preparing beautiful foods and helping ill people recover their health would be so rewarding. I was convinced.

Colorado State University (CSU) was a great place for my undergraduate nutrition education. The nutrition instructors like Dr. Inez Harrill and Dr. Gertrude Blaker were so knowledgeable in their areas of expertise and so dedicated to nutrition as a science I became inspired. Our class of dietetic majors was competitive and highly motivated, so we studied hard.

My clinical nutrition instructor at CSU, Mrs. Gilbert, was especially influential to me for two reasons, first, she showed how nutrition knowledge could be taught in a practical, useful manner, and second, she was the first dietitian I had ever met who had both a family and career. I finally knew it could be done.

The summer before my senior year in college I worked as a Diet Supervisor (Technician) at Methodist Hospital in Houston. It was a very exciting time because Dr. Michael DeBakey and Dr. Denton Cooley at the hospital next door were transplanting organs at a furious pace. I even considered not returning to college in order to work on the transplant team, but my Dad talked me out of it.

Boston was an exciting place for my internship in 1969–70. Never before had I been around so many war protests and locations of historical significance, or so much ethnic diversity and medical power. Beth Israel Hospital (BI) was a Harvard teaching facility which made it rich with excitement in the pursuit of medical knowledge. The BI staff was open to new ideas and allowed dietetic interns to try new food preparation, menu and counseling ideas.

Even with all the positives associated with my internship however, I felt it was a rude awakening into the profession. For the first time I felt the heavy hand of the medical hierarchy molding the practice of nutrition (along with the other allied health professions) and greatly limiting the use of dietitians' expertise. What was worse, everyone appeared to allow it to happen. Patient-centered medical care had not evolved, nor had the concepts of having patients being knowledgeable about their illnesses and taking responsibility for their health.

Through my rotations, I found I most enjoyed the out-patient clinic, metabolic units and Childrens' Hospital. Upon evaluation, what I liked was the greater respect for dietitians' expertise, more visible results when success occurred through nutrition intervention and fewer duties at the diet technician and aide levels.

I know I was both a joy and a headache (along with several others in our class) to Adele Dronsick, Internship Director, and Lorraine Jacoby, Department Head. Upon graduation the staff willed me "an answer to all my questions." I didn't understand why change couldn't happen sooner and why so many people had to be consulted in a hospital setting (two traits that later helped me become an entrepreneur).

Upon graduation, I returned to Denver and became a clinical dietitian at St. Anthony Hospital. I feel fortunate that my boss was Lois Smith, R.D. She was a jewel. The third week I was on staff, she took me aside and said, "You are bored to death. Present me some ideas for programs and we will try them."

We started a journal club and presented a series of therapeutic luncheons for the medical staff. The luncheons received local television coverage on the evening news and mention by Paul Harvey on national radio.

I was chosen after eight months to open St. Anthony's new satellite hospital in a north suburb. I loved the challenge and responsibility. I was the only dietitian and along with two diet aides, we covered seven days per week. The physicians on staff began referring in- and out-patients to me for nutrition instructions. Close relationships developed with the nursing, pharmacy and administration employees, in part due to the size to the hospital, but also because of the type of individuals chosen to start such a venture.

Census was only about 40 beds the first year, and so the decision was made to transfer me back to the main hospital and rotate a dietitian to the small hospital. The anticipation of returning to the large hospital forced me to make the most significant decision of my career.

I was frustrated with the lack of patient teaching in the hospital setting at that time and excited by the future of preventive nutrition. I decided to try private practice for one year, keep my investment and overhead low, work day and night, and then reevaluate. These decisions were not hard to come by since I was single and had nothing of value to borrow against—but I had time and dedication.

I gave two months notice after which I took the next two months off to research my diets and make contacts with physicians. I moved into an inexpensive apartment and paid two months rent. By the time I started work at Dr. Jim Langley's office in September 1972, my only cash was in coins in an old wine bottle. I made $5.00 per hour working two days per week at his office while I cleaned houses and sewed to make ends meet.

After a month in business I started trying to attract other physicians as clients. No one wanted to send their patients to another physician's office, so I worked out of seven different offices that year.

The first year I charged $7 for the initial visit and $2 for revisits—and still had complaints about fees! For every hour I generated income, I usually worked three hours on paperwork, marketing, or projects with no guaranteed income. Now that I am established in my field and wanting to write and break into new areas of practice, I am probably working ten to twenty hours with no income for every hour I get paid . . . but the income is *much* better.

It was difficult getting past office secretaries when I first approached physicians. After several weeks of trying, I finally used Dr. Langley as a referral and got appointments. When I started working out of an office, the secretaries and nurses as well as the physicians acted as patient-referral networks. In the chronic, non-acute care settings of their offices, physicians were supportive of nutrition therapy because the longterm care produced exciting tangible changes.

I found private practice under these circumstances to be very rewarding as far as patient care, but frustrating because of the multiple offices, their routines and patient no-shows due to lack of marketing by anyone, myself included.

Before one year was up, I knew the concept worked. I decided to borrow $1000 from my family (not a sufficient amount even then) and opened an office in a new medical building next to the small hospital where I had last worked.

I loved it. Patients came to me. I marketed to them over the phone when they first called for an appointment and made each one feel special when he or she arrived. Patients seemed more motivated to make change, partly because the effort to show up for an appointment filtered out many of those not ready to make changes. I learned what counseling techniques worked and where I needed more expertise. Patients were giving to me, however, they were also demanding and unforgiving. What a challenge!

When I opened my office I raised my prices to $10 for an initial visit and $3 for revisits. Those prices remained for the first two years. It took a lot of patients to make ends meet. I also made home visits for Home Health Services of Denver.

I learned a good lesson about fees after several years in business. Patients who could not find the cash to pay my paltry fees somehow found $385 cash to pay for the commercial diet programs down the street. What I found out was patients paid according to the "perceived value" they felt they would receive. I did not "sell" my services. I spent my time teaching patients how to calculate diets, while the diet program person sold patients on what that program could do to fill the patients' needs and make them happy. I needed to improve my marketing component.

I carried malpractice insurance from the beginning, but I also wanted to incorporate to better protect my business from lawsuits. My lawyer told me not to worry because I wasn't financially worth suing. I owned nothing of value. I finally incorporated my third year in business.

During my third year I decided to sublease my office two days per week to a speech therapist. That freed me to take consultant positions on the side at the county Head Start and two nursing homes. I also started researching a book on sports nutrition and became a regular guest on a childrens' television show. It gave me a much needed change of pace from constant weight loss and therapeutic counseling.

In 1976 I began approaching all the large employers in the Denver area to offer nutrition counseling at their medical clinics or through their fitness programs. I got jobs at Gates Rubber clinic and at Coors Brewery medical center. For the job at Coors, I was interviewed by Bill Coors, then president of the company and a great believer in good nutrition.

My interest in sports nutrition began to grow as I watched how patients lost weight better with exercise and as I worked (voluntarily) with Marvin Clein Ph.D. and the exercise physiology department at the University of Denver. Dr. Clein called me whenever he had athletes, local or Olympic-hopefuls coming to see him, and I rescheduled my day to talk to them. I also spoke at coaches conferences, at kinesiology and backpacking classes, and to the girls' gymnastics team.

At this time I interviewed with the Denver Bronco Football trainer, Alan Hurst, who asked me to look over their training camp menus and menus for away games. Unfortunately, however, coach John Ralston would not approve me as a consultant, so I worked on an unofficial, unpaid basis until Coach Red Miller came the next year. I consulted with individual players and trainers, and spoke at summer camp.

I was told in the beginning that most professional football players could not relate to "moderation," longterm results, and high complex carbohydrates, especially in the mid-70's and it was true. The job with the Broncos was not my most demanding sports nutrition experience, but because of their popularity it certainly opened a lot of doors for me.

Consultations with other professional and amateur athletes in all sports followed. I served on the medical staff of the Denver Avalanche Soccer Team and continued to speak at coaches conferences and runners' clubs.

In 1976 I invented a natural sports beverage along with the help of a beverage development company in Indianapolis. It contained juice, fructose and natural colors and flavors. It had to be pasteurized because I did not want preservatives. It was far ahead of its time and provided me with a seminar in product invention, food marketing, negotiating skills and power brokering. All of my waking hours for the next few years were spent on trying to develop the product "package," or trying to sell the product to a beverage company, or working jobs to financially support the venture.

The nation's largest convenience store chain contracted to buy the rights to the drink in April 1979. They bought my inventory and continued my contracts with sports teams. However, they then continued to change or renegotiate the contract so many times that their own people finally told me to watch out. I pulled out of negotiations in January 1980 and decided to readjust my priorities. The idea was great, but the timing was off. A stronger lawyer on my side would have helped too.

In the next year I wrote and marketed "Let's Get to Know Vitamin Supplements," produced private practice seminars with Olga Satterwhite, a private practitioner and became a media spokesperson through Gail Becker Associates for "Butter Buds."

My first professional media work came in 1973 as a result of ADA's National Nutrition Month and my position as Colorado Community Nutrition Chairman. While attending a Denver Dietetic Association board meeting several years later, I was suggested as the person to do a "spot" on "Blinky's Fun Club," a childrens' TV show. I did the show, and Blinky and I hit it off (both coming from Oklahoma). I became a bi-weekly guest for four years.

In March 1978, I was asked to do a last minute interview on NBC-TV "NoonDay" show which was number one in its time slot each noon. It worked out well and I was the "NoonDay Nutritionist" each week for the next four years. I met Gail Becker, R.D. on the set of "NoonDay" and she called me several months later to work for "Butter Buds." A year later, I worked as one of the media spokespersons for the introduction of "Lean Cuisine." Working as a media spokesperson was one of the most demanding jobs I have ever performed because of the pressure to please so many people (client, PR firm and each media contact) while promoting a product.

When I married and moved to the Dallas area in 1983, I became a semi-annual guest on the Ed Busch Talk Show, a nationally-syndicated, very popular, radio show. In January 1989 I started my own nationally-syndicated radio talk show produced by Ed Busch Productions. I am on the air live each Sunday morning from 8:00–9:00 AM CST and just love it. The number of affiliate stations increased 40% in the first six months and listener letters are very positive. Finding advertisers to fund the show is the biggest challenge at this time. My skills are improving and I love the challenge.

Over the years I have conducted over 600 media interviews, including ones on "Nightline" and NBC's "1986." Although I like newspaper writing and television, I love the talk show interaction that radio offers.

Writing does not come easy for me. I used to think I had to say everything right the first time, but now I have learned to "just say it" and edit it later. Today, I usually hire a former patient who works as a professional writer to edit my work. Because of her input and informal feedback from family or friends, I may rewrite an article or chapter five or more times before I like it. Years before I would rewrite something even more times and still not like it.

Besides my two consumer booklets on vitamin supplements, I have written an ADA study kit, "Starting a Private Practice," and co-authored much of the didactic information along with Jim Rose, R.D. in "The Competitive Edge" marketing manual. In 1987 Harper & Row published my book *The Entrepreneurial Nutritionist* and John Wiley now carries it. Because I want to break into the public market, I have four book proposals working with a literary agent from the Dallas area. So far no publisher has been interested, but it only takes one.

My involvement in state and national dietetic associations began because I was dissatisfied with our profession and felt I had no right to complain if I did not try to make changes. To my amazement, I found many other dietitians shared the same frustration. My decision to become involved has been one of the pleasures of my life because of the people I have met.

Another reason I attended dietetic meetings when I first started my private practice was because I wanted peer support for my venture, so I knew I needed to get to know people. I took referrals from dietitians for any consultant jobs, non-paid speaking engagements and difficult patients. After about three years, over half of the referrals I received for good jobs and opportunities were from other dietitians.

Opportunities that were crucial to my career besides the ones already mentioned were being chosen by David Nanberg at ADA in 1979 to co-lead the seminar series on starting a private practice with Olga Satterwhite. The series was ADA's longest running seminar and gave me the fantastic opportunity to meet Olga, a dynamic practitioner, as well as other dietitians across the nation who shared my entrepreneurial bent. Being in a solo private practice can be professionally isolating. The seminars gave me a chance to speak, teach, meet people and make money. I really enjoy it when someone who attended a seminar or one of my speeches tells me it made a difference in their careers.

I feel fortunate that I worked three years at The Greenhouse spa in the Dallas area. The spa employees and most guests were dedicated to making that grand "ole" lady function as an exclusive, awe inspiring haven for women. It was like working in a house actress Loretta Young would live in. The experience was great until new owners tried to "fix" the place and I knew it was time to go.

In 1981 The American Dietetic Association was asked to suggest possible dietitians to interview for the Presidential Appointment of USDA Consumer Advisor, and my name was listed. I interviewed in Washington, D.C. with Assistant Secretary Heckler, but decided against making a career change. My good friend and mentor Jean Yancey said, "You wouldn't last two weeks . . . until the first time they wanted you to call ketchup a vegetable serving." I really did enjoy being asked to interview though.

Another opportunity that I have thoroughly enjoyed for seven or more years is my position, through friendship, as the nutritionist for women's wellness and ski and spa retreats in the Colorado mountains. Sometimes I get paid, other times I just get expenses and a vacation out of it. Either way, I do not lose.

The list of special people who have meant the most to my career begins with my parents. My mother has unlimited, but focused energy, high ethics and tenacious loyalty. My father is a cautious deep thinker who is slow to act (which has always frustrated me). But I have to admit he seldom is wrong on his decisions, however, he seldom has to act because the opportunities have died of old age. These two people and I have come to love and accept each other in great part due to the fun and challenges created by my diverse entrepreneurial projects.

One time many years ago when I was at a garage sale at my parents' home, I heard my father ask a couple from Iran who had stopped if they ever watched the show "NoonDay" on channel 4 TV. They said yes. My father then said, "Well, it's just a little bit of Americana, but my daughter over there is the nutritionist on the show." It was the first time I had ever heard him brag about me.

My brother, Nelson, and sister, Coleen, are both talented entrepreneurs today with their own businesses. Nelson is very talented in interior design and graphic art. He designs and builds unique furniture for his showroom in Florida. Coleen is a co-owner of a gift and antique store in Oklahoma, and very gifted in interior design. Both siblings have been my sounding boards, confidants, editors and graphic design artists since I started my business. They developed the servicemark I have registered for my business.

There are literally hundreds of people who have influenced my career and the decisions which lead me in one direction or another. I have been told that I am like a sponge because I like to talk to other people about what they are doing, how they did something, or how I might do something.

Jean Yancey, a small business advisor in Denver has been a mentor, friend and inspiration to me for many years. She is a leader in the business community in Colorado, a popular public speaker and winner of the "SBA Advocate of the Year for Women in Business in 1982." Jean taught me how to prioritize my numerous projects and focus my efforts in order to become more productive, not just busy. She counseled me in negotiations when I first started in order to produce win-win results. She told me to get out of feminine dresses in pastel colors and buy myself a suit. Today, we think alike and I love it.

Olga Satterwhite, R.D. is in a very successful private practice in Houston. We have produced 64 seminars together since 1979. We have learned so much from each others, yet our approach to business is so different. Olga along with a few others taught me not to be afraid to ask for money for the work I do.

Mary Abbott Hess, R.D. and James C. Rose, R.D. are valued critics, sounding boards and friends. They are very hard on themselves professionally and personally, and I always feel that if my projects can pass their scrutiny, I have succeeded. Both are innovative, classy, aggressive, and in demand as experts in their areas of expertise.

My most valued awards or honors were being selected first recipient of the ADA Foundation award for "Excellence in Practice for Consultation and Private Practice," being elected President of the Colorado Dietetic Association and Chair of the Council on Practice.

In my mid-thirties, I made the decision that I wanted to be happily married. I had worked day and night on my career and had achieved some success. I wanted a different set of challenges and priorities. A career is very satisfying and I am not sorry my career came first. But, like I said in the very beginning, I thought nutrition would come in handy some day, and it has. I like consulting, counseling and speaking, but not every day. I am married to a nice Texan named Carter Helm, and we have two young, beautiful daughters. People our age are becoming grandparents and we are getting up for the 2 AM feeding. It is easier to manage a career than it is to manage a family with children.

I feel our strength and survival as a profession will come through the successes of individuals. As highly qualified, exciting, creative dietitians continue to make names for themselves in whatever their practice setting, the image and reputation of the whole profession will improve. ADA can help us through increased national media exposure. We will be most successful when we finally begin to focus our attention on the buying public and its nutrition needs. Public demands for our services and products will produce more revenue and with money comes more power and options.

In a nutshell, my career has been an outgrowth of my love of change and growth. I am more afraid of boredom than I am of risk.

Loyal E. Horton

Loyal E. Horton, MS, RD
is Director of Administrative Services,
Associated Colleges of Illinois, Chicago

If one had to choose a single word to describe Loyal Horton, that word would be committed. Being a male pioneer in a female dominated profession was never easy. Although his early interests in food service and the Association were discouraged by reverse discrimination and female chauvinism, he persevered until he accomplished his goal of becoming a dietitian and active member of The American Dietetic Association. From impacting the length of dietetic internships to the creation of Nutribird, his contributions to the profession have been significant. His activities have taken him from Saigon to a Silver Plate Award. His career included many firsts. He was the first male to be presented a Medallion Award, and the first male Lenna Francis Cooper Memorial Lecturer. His lecture, entitled "The Boys in the Club" chronicled the history of males in the profession of dietetics. An honored administrator and educator, Loyal Horton was aptly named, for he has provided The American Dietetic Association with years of loyal and dedicated service.

Loyal E. Horton

Morris Massey in his theory on "What you are is where you were when" best describes my early start toward a career in dietetics. Dr. Massey expounded the theory that when a person is at the age of about 10 years many characteristics that one carries throughout life are established. The determining factors are the events of that time, worldwide, nationwide, and in the home, family life values, the economy, and the beliefs of your own controlled world. These have a profound influence on one's behavior.

When I was ten years old our country was suffering the debilitating effects of the Great Depression. There were no jobs for the masses. Preparing for earning a living as an adult evidently played a role in my thinking. Those who were 10 years old at that time would be security-oriented and have a strong sense of commitment, according to Massey's theory.

My interest in dietetics, although I could not define the profession, dates back to my early childhood. For as long as I can remember I have had an interest in cooking.

Looking back I realize what an angel my mother must have been. By the time I was ten or eleven years old you could find me in the kitchen asking questions, wanting to help, wanting to cook.

A family friend during the mid-thirties was also a close friend of the Executive Chef at the Detroit News. As I began to indicate an interest in food production, or cooking as it was then known, our family friend would tell me about the world of this executive chef. He was earning $75 per week—fabulous money in those days.

I was thrilled when I had an opportunity to visit this gentleman and observe his operation. I knew then that food service was my calling. I was not yet in my teens but sure of my decision.

My first job was in my junior high school cafeteria where my aunt was cook-manager. My pay was a free lunch, but I would have worked for no pay just to be allowed in the kitchen to try my hand at the tasks.

Throughout my high school years I knew what I wanted but not how to get there. Certainly the guidance counselor, if we had one, didn't know because not once was dietetics suggested. Perhaps this was because dietetics as a profession was not common knowledge at that time. Although The American Dietetic Association was then 20 years old, it is quite possible that many guidance counselors did not know of its existence. My Home Economics teacher could not provide the answer, although she was a friend and gave me much encouragement.

After graduating from high school in Lansing, Michigan, I was propelled into Hotel Administration at Michigan State. This was not what I wanted, but I did not know how or where to go for proper direction. The Hotel Ad faculty attempted to convince me that their curriculum was exactly what I needed. I wasn't convinced.

Uncle Sam interrupted my college days in 1942 and during the next four years I wondered if what I wanted was offered in Home Economics. When I returned home, I immediately went back to campus to seek procedures to follow to transfer into Home Economics.

I called on the Dean of the School of Home Economics and she politely but firmly told me that Home Ec was for girls and that what I wanted was Hotel Administration. I argued but to no avail. Upon her recommendation I went to the next level of administration only to be told that I could not matriculate in Home Economics. It was for girls only. I talked with several people. I could not find this restriction stated in the college catalog.

Finally, in desperation, I went to the President of the college. I had met him as a freshman and remembered his warmth and friendliness. I knew he would talk with me and answer my questions.

Entering the president's office with my now tattered copy of the college catalog I told the president my story and asked him to show me in the catalog where it said that men could not matriculate into the School of Home Economics. I still remember that smile, as he told me every curriculum was open to every student. He reached for his telephone, said a few words, and then instructed me to go back to the Dean's office.

The Dean, a big lady of stern disposition, was not happy to see me. She told me that I would be required to meet all core requirements, including clothing construction, child development and the like. She then gave me instructions on the procedure to follow in transferring to Home Ec with a major in Institution Administration.

I was delighted. In the hallowed hall of the Home Ec building I had noticed many young attractive faculty members. My reaction to the Dean's threat was that I was about the same age as these young faculty members—perhaps I could apple polish those teaching courses and at least get a passing grade.

Woo them I did! In fact I somehow fell into a lot of luck because I managed to woo one into becoming my wife. She just happened to be a dietitian. This kind, generous, understanding lady has been a mentor, a friend, and a professional colleague who has given me continual guidance and assistance throughout my career. It has been this lady who has encouraged me and made many of my accomplishments possible.

My undergraduate work did not meet the academic requirements for membership in The American Dietetic Association. With my wife's encouragement, three years later I entered graduate school, made up my two undergraduate deficiencies and became a member through the Masters Degree program. That was 1952.

I was delighted to be a member of The American Dietetic Association. Having taken a new job I was anxious to become involved professionally. I was working on the campus of Bowling Green State University in Ohio and the nearest district dietetic association was in Toledo.

The Chairman of the Home Economics Department at Bowling Green was an active ADA member and a state leader. She did not want me to participate in the district association and told me that the activities were not for men. She refused to let me know when the group met and discouraged me from expecting to participate. Since I do not give up easily, I called a Toledo hospital and talked with a dietitian. She greeted me warmly and encouraged me to attend the next district meeting.

This initial relationship with a district association gave me an opportunity to learn more about the profession and the Association. When I moved to the Chicago area in 1960 I knew the importance of active participation in my professional association.

I promptly became an active member of the Chicago district association, eventually serving as president. This led to involvement in the state association. I served on several committees and in the mid 60's I was elected President-elect of the Illinois Dietetic Association. In May before I was to take office as President in November, the ADA Headquarters office wrote asking that I submit the name of the Chairman of Delegates before June 1. Thinking to be democratic, I called in the incoming Secretary and asked her to send ballots listing the names of the experienced delegates to the incoming Executive Board. They were to be asked to vote to elect the chairman.

The troops were up in arms! Members of the state hierarchy called my action illegal. I had telephone calls telling me I could not call for a vote before I was officially President. The current Chairman of Delegates called a meeting of the Executive Board to discuss further steps to be taken to stop this action. Ballots came back unmarked—notes attached saying that such action was premature. I insisted that we meet the ADA deadline.

Tempers were roused! I was informed that a secret meeting was called by the current President and Chairman of Delegates. This was to be held in room 1040 of the Sherman House Hotel in Chicago at 4:00 p.m. on a Monday afternoon. I had planned to attend but decided at the last minute that the group should proceed with their plans to set into motion preliminary impeachment proceedings.

I decided that I must meet the ADA deadline. I called my favored candidate and asked her to serve as Chairman of Delegates. She agreed. I was not impeached. This episode was to set the pattern for aggressive and positive leadership.

Involvement at the national level did not come easily. In 1960 at the annual meeting in Cleveland I felt like a minority of one. I am sure that there were other male members present, but they were unknown to me. What I did not expect was the animosity shown to the male member who made himself visible. I was anxious to fully participate. In the small group discussion sessions I did.

These sessions were called "Share and Compare." The concept of the consulting dietitian was just beginning to emerge and at this discussion session we shared views on consulting techniques and report writing. When the subject turned to the fees that dietitians should charge, there was great discussion. The ladies agreed that they could get three dollars an hour, some thought they were worth five dollars an hour. Should this include travel time? Should they charge for expenses? Would anyone hire them if they asked for too much money?

I stood up, addressed the chair and gave a few words of what I considered wisdom. I told the group that they were worth $25 per hour and that if they didn't ask for what they were worth that perhaps they weren't worth very much.

Again, my aggressive leadership pattern was in evidence. A young member arose, addressed the chair and suggested that I be reminded to leave. The color of my badge allowed me to remain.

At the annual meeting in St. Louis in 1961 I was asked to give a paper on the "Shared Dietitian." Since this was akin to my job, I felt well qualified to speak. Little did I realize how frightening it is to stand before an ADA audience and speak. Somehow with the encouragement of my friend and moderator of the session, Fern Gleiser, I managed to deliver the paper. This generated much discussion.

In 1963 I was appointed by ADA President-elect Katherine Hart, one of my former college professors, to serve on the Dietetic Internship Board. This gave me an opportunity to meet many of the leaders in ADA. Serving on the Dietetic Internship Board gave me an insight into the workings of the Association and a feeling of being accepted as a male member.

At the annual meeting in 1963 there were several male members present and I suggested that we meet as a group for breakfast. For several years these breakfasts continued to be a feature of the annual meeting. They were more than social occasions. At each breakfast we discussed our minority status. I believe that in these gatherings we men began to develop an understanding of our role in the Association and how we might offer our talents to the Association. Certainly we identified the need for male members to recruit additional men into the profession.

In the late 60's Mary Zahasky asked me to serve as Chairman of the Dietetic Internship Board. Mrs. Zahasky, a lady with great charm and charisma, recognized that male members could indeed be given responsible ADA assignments. My performance on the DIB indicated that the male member could carry responsibility without constituting a threat to the ladies.

Chairing the Dietetic Internship Board was a demanding and rewarding experience. I took the assignment with a vow that change was needed and I would do my best to make it happen.

My opportunity came at the "Task Force for the 70's meeting. It was to this group that I presented the challenge; did the required 52 week internship, of itself, result in a pre-determined level of learning? Was change in programming of internship programs needed?

Following the Task Force meetings an ad hoc Committee on Education was put to work. As a member of this committee I led the discussion toward recommending more freedom on the part of dietetic educators to plan innovative and effective educational programs.

The report of this committee to the ADA Executive Board recommended that Dietetic Internship Directors be encouraged to shorten their programs from the mandatory and traditional fifty-two weeks. President Frances Fischer, a dynamic leader and a decision maker, accepted this recommendation.

Her instruction to me was to approve at the Dietetic Internship Council the following week any shortened program that would meet the educational and experience requirements. My response was that this could be easily accomplished because the Dietetic Internship Board would be meeting sometime during each day of that week. Miss Fischer exhibited her leadership style by stating that if the Executive Board had wanted DIB as a whole to act, I would have been so directed. Her message was clear— you do the job! By the end of the Council meetings two experimental six-month programs and several nine-month programs had been approved.

At the Dietetic Internship Council meeting, attended by some of the brightest, most able members of our Association, I opened dialogue on the need for this group to provide leadership in implementing shortened internship programs. I offered suggestions as to how this could be accomplished. Many of those in attendance were fearful of playing the leadership role in implementing shortened internship programs. These fears were realistic and understandable. A major change was to be made and this task is not readily accomplished.

My personal conviction gave me the impetus to play the role of leader in this move. The fear of change was stifling creativity. Emotions ran high. Tradition was being challenged and sometimes found wanting. Many of the group felt defensive and my leadership had antagonized some of the more conservative members. I succeeded in arousing enough interest to get some members to think change and take action, a courageous departure from stereotype thinking.

As a result internships were given careful re-evaluation, many were shortened, all were strengthened. Later I was told by Dietetic Internship Directors that this led to improved quality education of the dietitian. For the first time dietetic educators were looking exclusively at learning experiences rather than at time elements for learning experiences.

One person can have an influence on an Association. The concept of shortened internships was a giant step forward in dietetic internship programming.

After leaving the Dietetic Internship Board, President Isabelle Hallahan asked me to chair the Educational Review Committee for Supportive Personnel. As Chairman I was able to encourage this group into eventually developing essentials of education for both the emerging Dietetic Assistant and Dietetic Technician.

In 1971 Mary Zahasky, the grand lady of dietetics, recommended my election to the Board of Directors of the ADA Foundation. This was certainly a highlight of my professional career. I was fortunate to join this group when the time and climate encouraged new directions. The formative years had come to a close, the Foundation was ready for growth and change. It was the beginning of a new era.

Serving as a member of this Board and eventually serving two years as President I saw progress. Fundraising techniques were developed and implemented and Board projects were planned and executed. The most formidable of these was the development of a symbol of good nutrition, the Nutribird concept. I'd like to think that my ability to lead helped to make this possible.

The greatest honor The American Dietetic Association could give me was granted in 1981 when I was the Lenna Frances Cooper memorial lecturer. The thrill of presenting my paper, "The Boys in the Club," an historical review of men in dietetics, to an audience of ADA members can never be forgotten.

Serving the Association has been an integral part of my career. It was with trepidation that I accepted the challenge to serve as Interim Executive Director during a critical transitional period. Although my tenure was short, the experience gave me a new perspective on the working of the Association.

For some years I have served as parliamentarian for the House of Delegates. This is an assignment that sometimes makes me feel like Father Time. I have seen the House of Delegates, where I represented Illinois for two terms, move from a deliberative body to a legislative body, providing leadership and direction for the Association.

Being a male pioneer in a female world has been a professional challenge. I'd like to believe that I played a role in the acceptance of men both as practitioners in the profession and leaders in the Association. In my research for the Cooper lecture several references were found where female members stated that perhaps men would bring strength to the Association. A few years ago, Dr. E. Neige Todhunter, ADA President 1957–58, stated that we need more men in the Association. Dr. Todhunter is a woman of vision, an esteemed ADA member, a distinguished professional leader and a mentor for many.

My professional life has included other professional commitments. I joined the National Association of College and University Food Service in its infancy. Here I have served in many capacities and as the 1966–67 national president.

In recalling the people that have played an important role in my career, I first think of Maybelle Ehlers, my major professor at Michigan State. Here was a grand lady who warmly accepted me into her department and gave me the encouragement to pursue a career in food service. At the time of my graduation when deciding which of two job offers to accept, one in college food service and one in commercial food service, it was Mrs. Ehlers who suggested that I ought to try my hand at college food service.

My first job out of college was a series of frustrations. The university lacked the quality standards and professionalism that I considered imperative. After one year I moved to The Pennsylvania State where I worked for Mildred Baker, a true professional and an ADA member. Miss Baker was a taskmaster, a stickler for accuracy. She had high standards of operation and service and demanded that her staff produce. It was Mildred Baker who polished my academic background into a practical operating background. Here was a tough lady, one who demanded perfection, a lady with little flexibility on the job. She would not allow her standards to be compromised. Off the job that tough and demanding lady was a warm and understanding person with a heart as big as she was. She had compassion for the young family man.

Mildred Baker taught me how to handle professional and personal relationships with my fellow professionals. She was indeed a role model who would affect my professional career.

After graduate school I became Director of Food Service at Bowling Green State University (Ohio). Here two individuals had great influence on my career. The President of the University led with a strong arm. Perform or else seemed to be his motto. To help me meet his expectations I had an immediate superior who led and directed me. This gentleman taught me techniques of administration that proved to be effective. It was the result of his leadership that prepared me for the position of Director of Administrative Services for the Associated Colleges of Illinois.

For 25 years, until retirement, I served in this capacity. In this position it was my responsibility to coordinate all of the inter-institutional activities of the non-academic officers from the twenty-nine member colleges and in addition to serve as an on-going resource person for their food service programs.

My professional involvement and the exposure I enjoyed in my activities with the Associated Colleges of Illinois provided me with many opportunities to accept interesting assignments. In 1963 I was awarded a Ford Foundation grant to study food service operations at six colleges in New York state. Four of these were private colleges and two were state universities. This led to serving as a consultant to more than 100 colleges throughout the country.

My professional association involvement and consulting activities led me into the education of food service management personnel by serving as a workshop leader. For 17 consecutive years I was a member of a distinguished group of educators who presented a week-long supervisory development workshop at Central Michigan University. In addition I have presented workshops in 14 other states. Several of these were sponsored by the U.S. Department of Health, Education and Welfare.

On many occasions I have spoken at professional association meetings. I was invited to give a paper at the International Congress on Dietetics in Washington, D.C. (1969) and Hanover, West Germany (1973). Other presentations include: The American Dietetic Association; the National Association of College and University Food Services; American School Food Service Association; Eastern Association of College and University Business Officers; Association of College Unions, International; Food Service Marketing Association; the National Restaurant Association. Several corporations have invited me to speak at sales seminars.

Being invited to participate in special assignments has broadened my professional perspective. I served as a resource person on the U.S. Office of Education Committee on Vocational Education, serving as a member of the Ad Hoc Committee to study the Role and Responsibilities of the U.S.O.E. Region V office, participated in the American Medical Association USAID project at the Faculty of Medicine (medical school), Saigon, Republic of South Vietnam (1967) and was an Institutions magazine Design Award Judge (1970).

The profession of dietetics has been my total life. This has been enhanced by those leaders in the profession who gave me guidance, encouragement, wise counsel and a shove when I needed it. Isabelle Hallahan, ADA President 1972–73, has been and continues to be a significant influence. The sharing of her on-going interest in the growth and development of the profession serves as a challenge. So many leaders have played a prominent role in my growth and involvement in the Association that it would be impossible to list them all.

Marjorie Donnelly, Col. Katherine Manchester (Ret. USA), Katherine Hart, and others have been most generous in leading me into activities that have kept me challenged. Mary Zahasky was perhaps the most influential in that it was she who gave me the initial push to become involved.

My career in dietetics has been successful because I have always been willing to jump in and do whatever needed to be done. I somehow made time to meet my job responsibilities and also to meet my responsibilities to the profession. There have been times when I have been overwhelmed with the tasks at hand. With perseverance and understanding from my family I have organized the time to meet these responsibilities. I have yet to learn to say "no" when asked to participate.

I truly believe that each of us has a responsibility to serve. My motivation appears to be that I enjoy involvement and sharing my leadership talents. The profession of dietetics has grown from the dietitian with clipboard in hand roaming the hospital corridors to a broad influence in all aspects of nutrition in man's life. This has been made possible because the dietitian has been a contributing influence. We have only seen the "tip of the iceberg."

As I look back on my career I would have liked to have had the daring vision as a young professional that I have today. My career perhaps would have taken a different course if I had anticipated the many facets of dietetics and food service that are available today. Dietetics is no longer gripped in the narrow confines that I experienced as a young man.

What I have accomplished in my career has been a result of not only what I have contributed but what others have made possible through their interest and faith in my abilities. The recognition that I have had from The American Dietetic Association has been more than interesting assignments. I was flattered and proud to be named the 19th Lenna Frances Cooper Memorial Lecturer (1981), the first male member so honored. In addition the Association presented me with the Medallion Award (1984). Other professional associations have been generous in honoring me. The National Association of College and University Food Services recognized my contributions by presenting me the Theodore W. Minah Distinguished Service Award (1974) and the President's Award (1976). In 1974 I received the Silver Plate Award in the College and University category from the International Foodservice Manufacturers Association. The Chicago Food Service Marketing Club presented me a testimonial of service in 1978.

After my struggle to gain admittance to the School of Home Economics at Michigan State University I was particularly honored to be named the 1987 Outstanding Alumni by the College of Human Ecology.

As I look into that "crystal ball" I see the profession of dietetics continuing to grow and be accorded recognition by an even wider public. This will be further enhanced through the National Center for Nutrition and Dietetics. I envision this Center to be the nucleus in providing the public and the total food service industry with extensive resources for all aspects of nutrition and dietetics. I see all of the industry, not just the health care corporations, becoming more aware of the available expertise that the Association and Center can provide.

We have seen a continuous and steady growth in the number of men in dietetics. We can look forward to even greater numbers. The Association has expanded its view of dietetics and recognized the need to involve those serving on the periphery, many of whom are males. There will be no compromise in the educational standards but broader avenues of entrance into the profession.

In these twilight years of my career I can look back with great satisfaction and know that I have given of my time and talents, I have offered leadership. I truly believe that I have left my mark upon both The American Dietetic Association and the profession of dietetics.

Doris Johnson

Doris Johnson, PhD, RD is former Director,
Dietetic Internship Program, Yale-New Haven Hospital
New Haven, CT

Doris Johnson credits her father for guiding her into home economics to offset her tomboy background at a private boys' school where he served as headmaster. Jobs were not as plentiful when she completed her dietetic internship as they are today. After writing over 100 letters and waiting 6 months, she received an offer: room and board; no salary! She is a supporter of quality in education and standards for the profession, once taking on the New York Institute for Dietetics which had been approved by the State of New York to train "dietitians." Dr. Johnson recounts her efforts to establish the dietetic internship at Yale-New Haven Hospital, one of the leading dietetic internship programs in the country which attracts students throughout the world. The recognition and respect she has earned from former students and colleagues evidenced by the numerous times she is named throughout this book attest to her wide range of activities and accomplishments.

Doris Johnson

To be asked to review one's professional life is a sobering experience indeed and also a gratifying one, though one may still feel she should have done more and much better.

I was born and grew up in a boys' private school, The Todd School, in Woodstock, Illinois where my father was the Headmaster. I suspect, that in his wisdom, he guided me into Home Economics at the University of Wisconsin to off-set my tomboy background for I had made known that I did not want to be a teacher since there were already too many in the family.

I was not sure exactly what Home Economics meant but I soon found out that the science aspect, especially chemistry, physics, physiology and eventually nutrition and diet therapy, was the most interesting part of the curriculum. I soon learned that I could not sew a straight seam and had little flair for fashion design. Thus by the process of elimination I ended up as a dietetics major, still not being quite sure to what it lead. In fact I had also had a bacteriology major so that I could qualify as a medical technologist as well. Remember—this was 1932 and jobs were very, very scarce and I hoped to find something to do when I graduated.

After my father, the first person to influence my career was Dr. Abby Marlatt, Dean of the School of Home Economics at the University of Wisconsin who persuaded me to be a dietetic intern at the Johns Hopkins Hospital in Baltimore. I applied. This sealed my professional fate.

The dietetic internship was a memorable experience. We were the first "class" of interns. Up to this time interns came in one at a time and thus left one at a time. We had many interesting classes and assignments and were allowed to audit Dr. Elmer McCollum's course in biochemistry, a real treat. The internship was my first experience in "The South" and my first experience in learning to eat raw oysters, lobsters, soft shelled crabs and other fare of the area. It was also my first experience in learning to work with people in institutional kitchens. I can remember vividly being assigned to the "Doctors' Dining Room" kitchen to get breakfast for the doctors, along side the regular cooks. This was early in the internship and I can remember as I stood there scrambling eggs on a hot July morning saying to myself "Is this what I went to college for?" However, I must admit that this experience did accomplish its purpose of making me realize exactly what went into the art of scrambling eggs in quantity and what it meant to be an employee and to work skillfully.

The Annual Meeting of The American Dietetic Association (ADA) was held in New York city that year and each intern was allowed two days at the meetings. We road the bus at night to New York City and exchanged rooms with the interns who had gone first. We got a little sleep and then on to the sessions. I have missed few annual meetings since, but this first one was most impressive.

There was one experience in my internship which was most influential to my future behavior. Since the interns before us came one at a time we had a party for each one as she left. The party for one intern was planned for the same night as the Maryland Dietetic Association was meeting at the hospital. This was not purposely planned but we did go ahead with our party rather than go to the meeting. We were obviously conspicuous by our absence. Phyllis Rowe, who was the director of the internship "grounded" us indefinitely. We were told in no uncertain terms that professional meetings came first. Miss Rowe later, at a Christmas party, ceremoniously burned the notice of our disgrace and we were again free. I have missed few local or state meetings since. Miss Rowe instilled in us many standards which served us well for the rest of our professional lives. I know that when I directed an internship I felt her influence immensely.

Our class of interns finished in July, 1933 most without any prospect of a job. So the hunt began, but there were few leads since experience was one of the first requirements. One of the things I did, while working on a Works Progress Administration (WPA) project, was to get the copy of the *Journal of the American Medical Association* which listed all the hospitals in the United States and wrote letters—many more than a hundred—until finally after six months I was offered a job at St. Joseph Hospital in Milwaukee by Sister Jovita. She wanted to start a selective menu for the patients which at that time was really revolutionary. This was a new position and all I was offered was room and board—no salary! The room was a patient room on an empty ward. After a few months I was given a room in the nurses' dormitory and a very small salary. I had finally made it!

One of the activities I did while at St. Joseph was to abstract papers from journals as a project of the Diet Therapy Section of The American Dietetic Association. I would go at least weekly to the library of the Milwaukee Medical Society. These abstracts were then mimeographed on 8–1/2 x 11 inch paper and sold at the annual meeting of ADA or on request.

In Milwaukee at the time I was there was a very active group of dietitians. In 1934 the Wisconsin Dietetic Association was founded and became a part of The American Dietetic Association. I was proud to be a charter member and gained much inspiration from the members in Milwaukee as well as those in Madison. I was indeed well indoctrinated with the professionalism which they exhibited.

After a few years at St. Joseph I knew I had much to learn about nutrition, diet therapy, and the administration of Departments of Dietetics and returned to the University of Wisconsin for a Masters Degree with Dr. Helen Parsons as my major professor. I ran the animal laboratory for her and worked with her mainly on the egg white syndrome which eventually lead to the discovery of biotin.

After this sojourn in academia I went out into the working world again for a few years—mainly at the Columbia-Presbyterian Hospital Medical Center in New York City during World War II, first as a clinical dietitian and then as the teaching dietitian. The seven years spent there with Nelda Ross Larsson who was the director of the Nutrition Department were a very broadening experience in many ways. There was the dietetic internship and the various affiliations such as Montefiore Hospital and Lenna Cooper, the U.S. Public Health Service Hospital on Staten Island and Teachers College of Columbia University where I did some teaching under Mary de Garmo Bryan. There was also a very active group of teaching dietitians under the leadership of Hendericka Rynbergen of New York Hospital. We had many interesting sessions especially on writing exam questions for the National League for Nursing.

The members of the Greater New York Dietetic Association and the New York State Dietetic Association were most active professionally and it was a privilege to be associated with so many distinguished members of our profession. One of the great problems which had to be faced at that time was the New York Institute of Dietetics which had been approved by the State of New York and was turning out "dietitians" absolutely untrained to do the work for which they were employed. As a result of this so-called school a great effort was made to establish standards for the profession and even to suggest that licensure might be necessary. Thus this problem has been with us for a long time.

It was while I was at Columbia-Presbyterian Hospital that with the blessing of Miss Ross I became the chairman of the Diet Therapy Section of The American Dietetic Association and began my professional activity at the national level. One of my first assignments was to represent ADA at the annual meeting of the Canadian Dietetic Association in Montreal in 1945.

At the annual meeting of ADA in Cincinnati in 1947 the Diet Therapy Section of which I was still chairman was challenged by Dr. Guest of the American Diabetes Association to do something about standardizing the diet for the patient with diabetes. Of particular concern was the food value figures being used which varied considerably over the country. This became one of the main projects of the Diet Therapy Section for a number of years. Elizabeth Caso was asked to be chairman of the committee to work on this project. The American Diabetes Association, the American Medical Association, and the U.S. Public Health Service participated in the project. After considerable research and much discussion a consensus was reached in 1950 on the term "exchange" and the composition and nutrition value of the various exchange lists. There was also much discussion about whether or not to have preplanned diet plans for several standard diets. It was felt that even though the ideal procedure was always to have an individualized diet to fit each patient's need that realistically there were many doctors who did not have a dietitian to call on and would use diet plans produced commercially. Thus a set of diet plans was developed to be sure that good diet plans would be available, based on the exchange list concept. However, the basic philosophy has always been that a patient should not just be handed a piece of paper with a printed diet but should have an individualized plan with adequate instruction. Dorothea Turner was very adamant about this and a great advocate of this philosophy and never really approved the concept of printed preplanned standard diet plans.

The war years in New York City were an experience in themselves. There were blackouts, drills, rationing, a grave shortage of employees, helped out some by a camp of conscientious objectors assigned to the hospital and teaching Red Cross classes among many other activities. The days were long since we often had to cover all three meals with no time off in between in order to be both dietitian and pantry maid. Nevertheless, we did have the opportunity to go to the Metropolitan Opera, the New York Philharmonic, Broadway plays and to sample New York restaurants, so it was not all work. There was some play or I doubt that we would have made it.

One of the assets of being in New York City was contact with editors and publishers and during this time I made my very modest publishing efforts stimulated by my colleague Corinne Robinson. I helped update the 11th edition of *Nutrition in Health and Disease* by Cooper, Barber and Mitchell published by J.B. Lippincott Co.,; co-authored with Wilfred Dorfman, M.D., *Overweight is Curable* published by the Macmillan Co.; wrote a *Laboratory Manual for Cookery* for the course in food preparation for student nurses published by G.P. Putnam's Sons and redid for them the textbook *Pattee's Dietetics* 23rd edition by Dr. Hazel Munsell, retitled *Modern Dietetics*, with the basic concept that all therapeutic diets are modifications of the normal diet and there does not have to be a separate diet for the treatment of each disease. This is a concept that has many advocates but is not as easily applied as expected. However there has been considerable progress made in getting diets prescribed in specific terms and often as quantitative as possible as a modification of the normal diet, ie., grams of protein, fat, carbohydrate, minerals, etc.

The activity and the stimulation of the profession at this time made me realize again that I did not know as much as I should and returned to the University of Wisconsin to earn my doctorate in nutrition and biochemistry. My major professors were Dr. Helen Parsons and Dr. Conrad Elvehjem. This too, was a stimulating experience in many ways for the University of Wisconsin Biochemistry Department was still making many contributions to the basic knowledge of nutrition in many areas. Again I worked on biotin but my main thrust was on vitamin B12. My first paper at Federated Society meetings was on the absorption of vitamin B12 by male subjects. I had a diet squad of fellow biochemistry students—healthy male subjects—from which to collect my data. To present a paper on one's research at the Federation meetings was indeed an exhilarating experience as well as a requirement.

After completing my doctorate I remained on the faculty of the School of Home Economics for one year as an assistant professor in the Institution Management Department replacing Stella Patton who was retiring. I did not stay longer since my primary interest was in nutrition and clinical dietetics and I knew I must now settle down in my career.

I was fortunate to find the position of Director of Dietetics at the then Grace-New Haven Community Hospital with an appointment of assistant professor in the Yale University School of Epidemiology and Public Health and a promise that I could have a dietetic internship. An interesting note is that I had been promised an appointment in the Department of Medicine at the Yale Medical School but when I came to work it had been decided that they would not accept Ph.D.s, only MD's in the department.

Dr. Albert Snoke was the director of the hospital at that time. He was most appreciative of the profession of dietetics for he had attended a workshop given by the American Hospital Association taught by Margaret Gillam, who had really indoctrinated him! He was always a strong supporter and considered his department heads the experts in their professions and allowed us much leeway in the development of our departments.

Grace-New Haven Community Hospital had just been merged and was in a transitional period at this time, so before I could have an internship I had to develop a Department of Dietetics. A new building was being built, another hospital was being annexed and the institution was doubling in size. Patients were to be in two buildings about a city block apart connected by a tunnel. The kitchen in the new building was to serve both patient units and cafeterias (centralized tray service was to come later) which was quite a logistical feat. The professional staff, as I remember, was all of six so that with the doubling of the size of the patient load, recruiting staff became of primary importance. I visited internships and by the time that the new building was to open I had managed to secure a staff of twenty. A selective menu was instituted for both regular and therapeutic diets. Needless to say this was not accomplished all at once. In fact, it took several years before we were even able to think about developing the internship. Finally we did have a department which met ADA requirements and we could apply.

A Manual of Diets was developed with the approval of the Medical Board. A committee of the Medical Board was appointed as the guiding force in determining the nutritional care of the patients. There were monthly meetings and through these meetings the role and stature of the dietitian was developed and enhanced.

Dr. George Cowgill was at Yale at this time and he lead a monthly seminar in nutrition for the few of us in nutrition. Helen Mitchell would come down from Amherst to attend. I surely felt proud to be in such company.

Dr. Snoke had said that the internship must be cost effective. I was able to justify a class of seven, although my goal had been twelve. So in 1957 our first class began. It was not long before we had classes of twelve or more interns since we did show what an important part dietitians played and the importance of having an internship in a teaching hospital.

During this time the name of the hospital was changed to Yale-New Haven Hospital to make more evident the relationship to the Yale University School of Medicine and eventually to be a part of the Yale Medical Center.

The internship soon was one of the leading internships and had not only students of high academic standing from schools in the United States but from many parts of the world as well. I take great satisfaction in the contributions which the interns and staff have made to the profession and The American Dietetic Association.

Dr. Snoke was a very active person in hospital administration and medical education and a leader in many aspects of health care, and he eventually served as President of the American Hospital Association. Thus he encouraged his staff to be active outside the hospital as well as in, both locally and nationally. We were allowed considerable leeway in our extracurricular professional activities.

When he was president of the Connecticut Hospital Association one of the ideas which Dr. Snoke initiated was a two year project in the hospital association of a position for a dietitian to help the departments of dietetics of member hospitals in the operation of their departments through workshops, individualized consultation, joint purchasing and standardization of procedures particularly in clinical nutrition. This was a very successful project headed by Jane Hartman, but due to a lack of funds it could not be continued. However, the effect of the program was long lasting especially in the areas of joint purchasing and clinical nutrition.

Since Dr. Snoke encouraged his staff to be active in professional affairs I served again as Diet Therapy Section chairman, was then elected to be treasurer and eventually President of The American Dietetic Association in 1959, which became a two year term when the President-elect, Cora Kusner resigned for personal reasons. These were eventful years to say the least!

Probably one of the most eventful things to happen during this time was the changing of the tax status of the association from non-taxable to taxable. For years great care had been taken to have the association be an educational and professional association and not do lobbying, licensure and other such activities which would jeopardize the tax status. With this change both national and the state associations were now able to carry on programs which up to then had been prohibited. One of the outcomes of this tax change status was the formation of the ADA Foundation to protect the Association's funds. I was the first treasurer of the Foundation but the office required little work at first since the funds were few.

Another outcome of the changing of the tax status was the possibility of some type of registration or licensure. I was chairman of an ad hoc committee to work on this problem. After legal advice and much discussion the committee recommended to the House of Delegates that registration should be the procedure of choice at this time, thus setting off a whole new era for ADA.

Another outcome of the change in tax status was the recommendation that a legislative representative should be employed for the purpose of lobbying in Washington. Here, too, an entirely new activity for ADA was begun. Isabelle Hallahan was our first representative.

In 1960 another organization, the Hospital, Institution and Educational Food Service Society (HEIFSS), was begun. There was an ever growing need to have a forum for the food service supervisor who had been trained during the previous years as an assistant to dietitians to relieve them of many routine chores. This organization grew rapidly and has been an important factor in our profession. The training of food service supervisors had gone on for a number of years and correspondence courses were developed at several universities. The W.K. Kellogg Foundation gave ADA a grant to develop a correspondence course for food service supervisors. This project was ably carried out first by Myrtle van Horn and then Sallie Mooring.

In 1961 Lenna Frances Cooper passed away. There was an Executive Board and Coordinating Cabinet meeting in Chicago at the time. In her memory we established the Lenna Frances Cooper Memorial Lecture to be given at the annual meeting each year. I have always been proud to have been instrumental in bringing about this memorial to Miss Cooper whom I considered a real friend and mentor.

In an attempt to have better communication with the membership it was decided in 1961 to send the "Courier" to all members as a part of membership. Up to this time it had been by subscription only.

Continuing education was also one of our concerns. There had been requests that ADA be the source of workshops and other avenues for membership to keep updated in the various aspects of the profession. First Bessie Brooks West and then Dr. Bruce Kirk were employed to carry out this program, which lead eventually to the now extensive continuing education activities of the association.

Recruitment was also a priority for us but funds were a problem. Lucille Refshauge, when she was president and I was treasurer, was able to get a commitment from the H.J. Heinz Co. for a film on the profession. Under the guidance of Thelma Pollen, "A View from the Mountain" was produced. This film, a first for ADA, received wide circulation and lead to many other recruitment activities.

It was my privilege to represent ADA at the Third International Congress of Dietetics held in London, England in 1961 and to invite the Congress to hold its next meeting in the United States. There was much pomp and circumstance to the entire meeting and a most memorable experience, and I have been most grateful for the privilege.

The opening session of the annual meeting of ADA was always a very formal occasion. Gloves and hats were to be worn. In fact the gloves, according to the parliamentarian, were not to be taken off until after the invocation and the singing of the national anthem. One annual meeting at which I was presiding provided a bit disastrous. Since I am not known for my ability to carry a tune as it came time to render the Star Spangled Banner I stepped away from the microphone so as not to throw people off key. As it turned out the organist did not know the music. A more dismal rendition of the national anthem has never been heard before or since. Needless to say one of my recommendations was that hereafter there be a competent leader to sing the national anthem.

The Executive Director of an association is a most valuable asset to the president. I am ever indebted to Ruth Yakel for all she did for me as president. Her knowledge of the association, its role in the health care field, her insight into problem solving, her high standards and thoroughness and her dedication to the profession and the association were outstanding and a tremendous help to me. I could not have done it without her.

One of the results of being President of The American Dietetic Association is serving on committees or as a representative to allied organizations. Over the years it has been my honor and privilege to have been an ADA representative to the American Hospital Association, the American Heart Association, the American Medical Association, the Veterans Administration, and the National Health Council.

While on the American Hospital Association liaison committee one of the projects accomplished was the preparation of a "Menu and Diet Guide" for the use of departments of dietetics of small hospitals especially.

As a cooperative activity in 1961 the American Medical Association and ADA formed a committee to bring about some common understanding and standardization of the diet therapy as related to gastrointestinal function. This was a most difficult assignment but we were able to debunk many practices and to make some important recommendations. We did get rid of the Sippy Diet, etc. A joint paper was published.

One of the obligations of a member of ADA is to serve on committees and boards of the association. I have served as Diet Therapy Section chairman several times, on the *Journal* Board, the Dietetic Internship Board, the Legislative Committee, and a number of other ad hoc committees.

One special committee funded by the W.K. Kellogg Foundation was the Study Commission on Dietetics under the chairmanship of Dr. John Millis, which, after two years of deliberation, resulted in the publication of *Dietetics as a Profession* in 1972. This was an unique experience for it was indeed enlightening to have a very objective look at the profession by essentially outsiders and "to see ourselves as others see us," and to view what should be done in the future for the growth of the profession. One of the more lengthy discussions held was whether or not the dietitian should be a generalist or specialist. Space does not permit the pros and cons of the discussion, but I do hope that we do not become so specialized that we are no longer dietitians in the full meaning of the profession.

At the annual meeting of ADA in 1971 the Michigan Dietetic Association made a resolution in the House of Delegates that ADA prepare a manual of diets which would be well documented and would be used as a basis for standardizing diet therapy procedures. I can still remember sitting there in the House of Delegates as an observer and thinking that is an interesting resolution and that it would be quite an undertaking if it were to be done properly. We already had *The Handbook of Diet Therapy* but it did need to be updated. After a few months of not giving a thought to the Michigan resolution a letter came from ADA asking me to be chairman of a committee to carry out the mandate of the resolution. We were allowed a budget large enough to employ a dietitian to do the research and the basic writing of the text. As a result *The Handbook of Clinical Dietetics* was published in 1981 by the Yale Press. There was one delay of more than a year waiting for the latest revision of the Recommended Dietary Allowances. Thus revision of the entire manuscript was necessary adding to the delay in publication. *The Handbook* was well received and was soon in second printing.

I was a member of the Nutrition Committee of the American Heart Association for a number of years. During this time we developed both the restricted sodium diet booklets and the controlled fat diet booklets as well as patient education materials. We used the basic concept of "exchange lists" as had been done with the diet for the patient with diabetes. Much research and discussion were held before a consensus on terms and content of the lists of foods was reached. These booklets and the other patient education materials made a valuable contribution to the education of patients with heart diseases of various types.

One of the more interesting experiences I have had was to serve for three years on the Scientific Advisory Board of the Campbell Soup Company. A suggestion I made at one of the meetings that there was a place in the market for single portions of soup, especially for the elderly and other single people, led to the development of the single serving can now popular in the grocery store.

Retirement from Yale-New Haven Hospital lead to other activities, mainly teaching part time at the University of New Haven courses in nutrition and food science for the Hotel and Restaurant majors though the courses were also open to the entire school. During this time we developed a program for Dietetic majors to meet ADA requirements. It has also been my privilege to serve on an advisory committee to this program as well as to the dietetic technician program at the South Central Community College and the dietetic internship program at Yale-New Haven Hospital. I have served on the Board of the Regional Visiting Nurse Association (along with Dr. Snoke) and have continued to espouse the role of the dietitian in this agency. I guess once a professional, always a professional.

Since my retirement gives one so-called more leisure time I am an active volunteer for FISH, an emergency food agency; a "stalwart" in my church and a member of Quota International, a very active service club with especial interest in the hearing impaired. In my spare time I do a variety of craft activities and am a Red Sox fan.

One of the great rewards that has come to me professionally is the host of friends I have made over the years. My profession has been very good to me. I recommend it heartily!

Edna P. Langholz

Edna P. Langholz, MS, RD is President,
Langholz Consultants, Inc., Tulsa, OK

Edna Langholz was earmarked for leadership from an early age. As a youngster, she received her grade school's annual leadership award! This 58th President of ADA personifies the qualities needed for a pacesetter—a sense of mission, enthusiasm, willingness to take risks and challenge the status quo, optimism, and common sense. During her Presidency, there was an internal reorganization of the ADA headquarters operation to make it more responsive to members and the external environment. Project Image was initiated which resulted in the ADA Ambassador Program. Continuing education activities were broadened, including the launching of monthly education articles as a regular part of the ADA Journal. Both Edna Langholz and her husband have been instrumental in laying the ground work for the campaign to establish the National Center for Nutrition and Dietetics. She credits her supportive family for nurturing her career in the days when the "working wife and mom" was more the exception than the rule. Edna Langholz was the recipient of an 1987 ADA Medallion Award, honored for her futuristic thinking and unique contributions to the profession.

Edna P. Langholz

I have often said, "Life is like a cafeteria. I want to sample everything; then I'll know what to go back to for seconds." I have had many wonderful experiences in my life, and I am still sampling new ones. A few I continue to go back to for seconds. One of them is the profession of dietetics.

I spent the first few years of my life in a small town in Georgia where my father, and his father before him, were pharmacists. When I was six years old we moved to Jacksonville, Florida which was home until I married. My father owned a small drug store, and I have fond memories of the old-fashioned marble tables with wrought iron chairs where people would come to sip ice cream sodas or indulge in banana splits. It was always fund to sit on one of the stools at the long marble counter and watch the creation of wonderful things at the soda fountain. Even producing a Coca Cola was an art in those days because one had to know just how much syrup to mix with the carbonated water in the fountain. At the back of the drug store was a series of booths where hot lunches were served to the business people in the neighborhood. These booths made wonderful desks for my brother and me as we did our homework in the afternoons, while our parents both tended the store. As I reflect on my life I believe these early exposures planted a seed of interest in both food service and medicine.

I was always a serious student, but I also wanted to be involved in whatever was going on around me. My friends were always very important to me. When I graduated from grade school I received the annual award for leadership . . . and I liked the feeling of this kind of accomplishment.

In high school I studied music (piano and clarinet), played in the high school band, served as president of my high school sorority, and involved myself in many other school and church activities. Typical of most teenage girls, I loved parties and clothes and decided that I was destined for the fashion world!

When I arrived at Florida State University I immediately declared a major in fashion merchandising. I was assigned to the School of Home Economics where I was told that I must complete a core curriculum which included courses in other areas of Home Economics. One of the required courses was a basic nutrition course, which I enrolled in at the beginning of my sophomore year along with a clothing construction course. Everyone in the clothing course knew how to sew beautifully . . . except me. I made an A in my nutrition course and a C in the clothing course . . . the first C I had ever made in my life. I decided a career in the fashion world was probably not for me! I made an appointment with the Career Counseling Department, took a series of aptitude tests and was told that I should pursue a career in science. I considered a career as a physician, but medicine was not a very viable option for women in those days. I found subjects like chemistry too "non-people" oriented, and math was never my greatest strength. I decided that dietetics could offer me a challenging and interesting career with many options and opportunities. I was on my way . . . and I've never looked back or regretted my decision.

My college years were exciting and busy. To help finance my education, I worked as an assistant to the Dean of the School of Journalism during the school years and in the dining room of a large resort on a lake in Canada during the summers. These work experiences provided good background for the career path I was later to follow.

I chose the University of Iowa Hospitals for my dietetic internship because I wanted to pursue graduate work under Dr. Kate Daum, a former president of The American Dietetic Association (ADA) who was widely recognized for her outstanding research in nutrition. I spent two and a half years in Iowa City during which I completed an internship, a Master's degree in nutrition, and worked as a clinical dietitian at the Veteran's Administration Hospital.

I enjoyed every minute of those years even though studying under Dr. Daum was not for the student without a strong constitution. She demanded the very best from her students and we all learned to "walk the extra mile" just to keep up with what she expected of us. Our days began at 6:00 in the morning and ended at midnight. It seemed as though we were always working in a classroom or research laboratory. Dr. Daum taught us discipline, professional ethics and mental toughness. She taught us to question and to never accept the status quo. We learned to persevere when there seemed to be no answers or solutions to our questions and problems. Under her direction and tutelage I developed character strengths which would serve me well throughout my professional career.

While at the University of Iowa I met Robert Langholz, a law student who, in addition to a full class schedule, was working as a research assistant in the College of Law during the day, in the dietary department of the university hospital at mealtimes, and at the hospital for handicapped children in the evenings. I'm not sure when either of us found time to get to know each other but we did, and we were married at the beginning of his senior year in law school. After graduation in 1956, he accepted a position with an oil company and we moved to Tulsa, Oklahoma for what both of us thought would be only a few months—and we've been there ever since.

My professional activities led me to Tulsa's Hillcrest Medical Center where I worked in numerous capacities ranging from clinical dietitian to chief dietitian to coordinator of nutrition education with the School of Nursing. Between 1966 and 1972 I became a visiting instructor in nutrition at three nearby colleges and universities—Tulsa Junior College, the University of Tulsa, and the University of Oklahoma. This was before the days of public interest in and awareness of the importance of nutrition . . . and it was a challenge to keep students interested. It soon became a subject which most young people wanted to know more about. Although the 70's brought about the popularity of many bizarre and faddish ideas about food, I believe it was the beginning of the explosion of interest in health and nutrition which we have witnessed in the 1980's.

In 1968 I was asked by Mary Zahasky, another former ADA president, if I would like to work for the Oklahoma Regional Medical Program. The Regional Medical Programs, signed into law in October 1965, were intended to implement innovative programs and to foster cooperation among the various elements of the health care system. Under Mary Zahasky's direction we established the first nutrition segment of a Regional Medical Program in the United States and under her leadership led the way for dietetic involvement in these programs in other parts of the country. The next four years were indeed exciting! We planned continuing education events which included not only dietitians but registered nurses, physicians, physical therapists, and other health care personnel. Continuing education was not an important issue in those days . . . and certainly not on an interdisciplinary scale. I shall never forget how difficult it was for many of these health professionals to think beyond their own role and to learn to share their continuing education experiences with those outside their own discipline. Soon they came to appreciate the value of this approach. As I reflect on those years I realize that we were ahead of our times as we participated in many "new" approaches to health care. We worked with educational programs for dietetic assistants and encouraged the leadership of The American Dietetic Association to follow a new movement which was emerging in several disciplines . . . the development of associate degree programs for support personnel. We were convinced that the day would come that in order to be cost effective the dietitian would have to delegate many of her routine duties.

Very little attention had been given to feeding programs for the elderly prior to 1968. From 1968 to 1970 I served as a nutrition consultant for a pilot project being conducted in Tulsa by the University of Oklahoma Extension Division, Office of Urban and Community Development. This study was entitled "Nutrition and Social Interaction Among the Aged," and it focused on the nutritional as well as the social needs of senior citizens. This program provided community dinners for the elderly long before the feeding programs as we know them today existed.

Mary Zahasky's influence during these years in instilling in me an interest in becoming involved in activities of The American Dietetic Association was significant. I do not know that anyone has ever been really successful without having had some role model or mentor. We have all been helped. For some the help comes with more warmth than for others, and with some it is done with more forethought, but most persons who succeed in a profession fondly remember individuals who influenced and helped them in their early years. I shall always be grateful for the encouragement I received from Mary.

I had always been an active participant in dietetic association activities and had served as president of both my district and state associations. In 1969 I was asked to serve on my first American Dietetic Association committee, the Diet Therapy Section Advisory Committee. A year later I was elected to the ADA House of Delegates where I served for seven years in many capacities including that of area coordinator.

During these years I also became involved in the educational programs of the profession as a member of the accreditation board from 1971 to 1975, serving as its chairman for two years. I was a site evaluator to internships and coordinated undergraduate programs from 1972 to 1978 and was on committees which worked with traineeships and educational programs for support personnel. These were exciting times in our profession because we were seeing the development of the movement of the coordinated undergraduate programs. There were only six in existence when I first became involved. I had many opportunities to visit and consult with emerging new programs, and I was challenged by this pioneer involvement. At the same time we saw the emergence of the technician movement with initial efforts in the development of associate degree programs in dietetics. I served on the advisory committee for the first dietetic technician program approved by The American Dietetic Association. Not only were changes occurring in the education of our students, but continuing education for members was determined to be essential for the future of the profession. In 1977 I was asked to chair a committee to develop a master plan for continuing education efforts of The American Dietetic Association.

In 1972 I formed my own company, Langholz Consultants, Inc. and began a limited practice with small hospitals. I pursued a number of activities over the years including corporate consultations, public speaking, and development of publications. A large part of my time, however, continued to be spent as a volunteer with The American Dietetic Association.

In 1978 the ADA Board of Directors was expanded to include members at large, and I served in this capacity for two years. I was elected President of The American Dietetic Association, and when I took office in October 1981 we had a very ambitious Plan of Action. I could not help but wonder how we would accomplish everything we had set out to do. Enthusiasm was high, and I soon discovered that those with whom I was to work that year did not believe gradual change was an effective way of moving toward a different future. I found myself on a fast-paced track, surrounded by people who were innovative, dedicated, and productive, and who initiated programs which have had a lasting impact. They had strong wills and invincible determination. They put into action qualities needed for leadership . . . a sense of mission, enthusiasm, willingness to take risks, creativeness, optimism, and common sense. They were willing to challenge the status quo and try something new. We began with an internal reorganization of the headquarters operation to make it more responsive to the members, the volunteer leadership, and the external environment. With this in place we set about implementing and improving the continuing education activities for members through satellite telecasts, sponsorship of workshops in many areas of the country, production and promotion of audio and video cassettes, development of study kits and launching continuing education articles in regular issues of the Journal of The American Dietetic Association. A major undertaking was the initiation of Project Image, a joint activity of ADA and Ross Laboratories to develop nutrition spokespersons who could project through the media the ideal image of the dietitian. We selected and trained 16 registered dietitians to become spokespersons, and this was the beginning of the now widely recognized Ambassador Program of The American Dietetic Association. This program would prove to be a major step in improving the ability of the public to make informed nutrition decisions. During the year many volunteer committees made great strides in working on bylaw revisions, ethics, improved dietetic practice and education, and role delineation studies.

A new volunteer group, the Council on Research was established and began to fulfill its charge of advising the Board of Directors and the headquarters staff on research needs and activities of the Association. A high priority was placed on the study of the role and function of dietetic practice groups which had been formed but not properly integrated into the Association. We worked very hard to establish the relationship of these practice groups within the structure of The American Dietetic Association in terms of fiscal management, incorporation, participation in legislative and public policy activities, headquarters support to be made available, and the implementation of a communication network among the practice groups. Issues which were identified as legislative priorities were third-party reimbursement, home health initiatives, maternal and child health, nutrition labeling, and nutrition education for the public. Major strides were made in strengthening our legislative process and in communications with members, government agencies, allied organizations, and policy makers.

During my year as President of ADA I also represented the Association on the Board of Directors of the ADA Foundation. It was an exciting year. For the first time, the goal of awarding 200 scholarships was reached, including 25 Silver Anniversary Mead Johnson Nutritional Division Scholarships which commemorated that corporation's 25 years of support of dietetic education. The Foundation Board also awarded the first (1982) and the second (1983) Frances E. Fischer Memorial Nutrition Lectures to The American Dietetic Association. The premiere gala of the Foundation, "The Friends of the Foundation Dinner," was held at the Annual Meeting and was so successful that it became an annual fund-raising event. Of great significance was the awarding of a grant to the Foundation from the W.K. Kellogg Foundation to again take a look at the profession and what it had done since the first study in 1972 and to project future needs and directions for dietetics.

In December of 1981 something happened which was to greatly influence the direction that the next five years of my life would take. My husband, who had over the years become not only an attorney but an entrepreneur and businessman, began discussion with the ADA Foundation's president, Audrey Wright, about the possibility of the Foundation acquiring a building which could be leased to The American Dietetic Association, thus enabling the Foundation to earn money otherwise paid by the Association as rent to third parties. This could provide a permanent source of income to the Foundation and enable it to have predictable funds to carry out its mission. This idea was expanded by the Foundation Board of Directors to encompass the concept of a National Center for Nutrition and Dietetics with a primary thrust to support activities in nutrition education and research for both professionals and the public. We began planning and laying the groundwork for the Let's Build Our Future Campaign which was to make possible the subsequent investment in a permanent building and the establishment of the National Center for Nutrition and Dietetics. Because my husband had made the initial "kickoff" gift in my name, I was committed to a successful campaign. I remained on the Foundation's Board of Directors until 1986 working on the many aspects of the campaign and serving as the Foundation president for two years. Beginning in June of

1986 I became the interim Executive Director of The American Dietetic Association and the Director of the National Center for Nutrition and Dietetics for what I thought would be a few months. I functioned in this capacity, on a volunteer basis, for a little over a year, living in Chicago during the week and on weekends going home to Tulsa to see my husband or some other location to see my three sons, who were in undergraduate or graduate schools at the time.

Balancing a career and family is not easy. When I was a young professional, few married women worked outside the home. I shall never forget the day that a well-intentioned friend sat me down and told me that as the wife of an aspiring young attorney, it seemed inappropriate for me to work. However, it was from an exceptional husband that I received the encouragement to continue. In an interview during my year as ADA president, he summarized so well what many young working couples must experience today when he said: "What is it like to live with Edna? Simple question, easy answer—Yes? Well, maybe not. We have been married for more than 26 years. Anyone with a scintilla of experience knows two people encounter some periods of strain over such a period, even without the normal joys and concerns resulting from the birth and rearing of three sons—Bob, Larry, and Kris. Edna, in addition to being a mother and wife, has worked or had other outside activities during our entire married life—and always on what one would consider a full-time basis. The problems arising from all this were numerous, as they must be for every working woman. How often I used to hear her express her inner conflict of mother versus working woman. How many times did tempers flare because one or both of us seemed to reach that point where the unaccomplished tasks seemed too great for the time available. How many times we used to envy others, who seemed to have a much easier time and were not so involved with other activities. Time and again we would ask each other—are we doing the right thing for our children?

In addition to her self-imposed demands on her time, I also created certain demands. Every aspiring young professional or businessman does. There are always the normal social functions, but during the early years my business took me away from home for extended periods of time and often outside the United States. This meant Edna was not only a full-time working mother with three small children but also often could not depend upon me for even the simplest of father-type duties.

Through all of this Edna persevered—and grew. The old adage is true—there is no better teacher than necessity. She developed a tremendous ability to organize. She had to. All meals and activities were planned at least a week in advance and committed to writing. Heaven help the person who fouled up the schedule! She also continued to fuel her unquenchable thirst for knowledge, progress, and success. I must admit that here we are both alike. Edna has always had great curiosity and a continual desire to learn. Once she acquires certain knowledge and skills, she sort of "chafes at the bit" to use them. That, coupled with her competitiveness, brings about a desire to contribute and succeed—sort of making it all worth while.

What is her greatest single attribute? I would have to say her love and compassion, along with her ability to place everything in proper perspective, considering the circumstances at the time.

Have there been sad times? Certainly. Have there been difficult times when it seemed touch and go? Yes. Have there been moments of utter frustration? Absolutely. But we always worked them out and then (and most importantly) continued growing. It's difficult to remember the times. In fact, I don't think of them as hard at all—just the building blocks we each needed to put in place to enable us to gain the necessary experience to grow and climb up to the next block. We have had many marvelous experiences together.

Edna has always been very supportive of me and our boys when such was earned or sometimes just needed. We tend to support each other—not always toward a common goal but often toward one of our separate, individual goals. I believe we have learned that although we live together as a family, it is a family of individuals. This is why we are so supportive of each other and our individual goals. I have the right to pursue my goals within certain constraints we place on ourselves. Edna also has that right. Our belief is that the price each of us pays is the obligation to support the other in the pursuit of his or her goals. She has been largely responsible for my happiness—I only hope I have made some contribution to hers.

What is it like to live with Edna? Great. Couldn't be better!"*

I never saw these remarks until they were printed in November of 1981, but I have treasured them since, as they serve to remind me of a wonderful family without whose support I could never have served my profession. I include them here not only to share a part of my private life, but to inspire young working mothers to appreciate the opportunity to remain professionally involved.

I am humbled by the recognition I have received from my professional colleagues. In 1983 I received the Distinguished Alumna Award from the School of Home Economics at Florida State University. The year 1987 brought two awards: the Distinguished Service Award from The American Dietetic Association Foundation and the Medallion Award from The American Dietetic Association. In 1988 I was honored by the Oklahoma Dietetic Association with the Distinguished Dietitian of the Year Award. Whatever I have accomplished has never been done alone but was the collective effort of many dedicated professionals. I owe a huge debt to persons far too numerous to mention for the wisdom, patience, help and support they so readily and generously lent me during my years of volunteer service to the profession. These years brought me large measures of challenge and excitement, but most importantly they served to remind me that The American Dietetic Association's greatest strength is in its members who have given of their time and shared their talents.

*Watson, DR: Edna Page Langholz, RD, President, 1981–82, The American Dietetic Association. Copyright The American Dietetic Association. Reprinted by permission from JOURNAL OF THE AMERICAN DIETETIC ASSOCIATION, Vol. 79:575, 1981.

I believe it is the members of a profession who make or break it, who make it respected or ridiculed, and who ultimately build its image. We must not be afraid to venture out and try the untried, and we must have the courage to take risks. If we think we always have to be right, always have to win, must be liked by everyone, and criticized by no one, then we are doomed to mediocrity. People who try to do something and fail are infinitely better than those who do nothing and succeed. My personal philosophy is that high failure towers over low success and that it is better to fail endeavoring to accomplish something great than to succeed at doing something of little consequence or value. A favorite saying of mine by Theodore Roosevelt expresses this philosophy well: "It is not the critic who counts; not the man who points out how the strong man stumbled, or where the doer of deeds could have done better. The credit belongs to the man who is actually in the arena; whose face is marred by dust and sweat and blood; who strives valiantly; who errs and comes short again and again; who knows the great enthusiasms, the great devotions, and spends himself in a worthy cause; who at the best knows in the end the triumph of high achievement; and who at the worst, if he fails, at least fails while daring greatly; so that his place shall never be with those cold and timid souls who know neither victory nor defeat."

Dietetics is a profession with strong roots in the past and unprecedented current strength. We have a treasured heritage from the past, but we must ask ourselves how we can meet the challenges of tomorrow, how we can prepare for tomorrow, and what factors will determine the direction of tomorrow's road? To the young dietitian who will travel down that road and who will create and mold our profession's future, I share the following message. Your expectations must be great. Frustrations there will be, but it takes great expectations to make great careers, and it is that measure of greatness you must seek as you work with your dietetic colleagues toward common goals. You can possess all the knowledge and know-how and have all the resources to work with, but, when all is said and done, it is who you are, what you are, what you believe in and what you are willing to stand up for that really determines how effective you will be as a profession. Unless you strive for the very best in your profession, you will never know how good you could have been! To influence the future of The American Dietetic Association or your professional may not take much . . . a single person or a single thought. *You* may be that person or have that thought.

Miriam E. Lowenberg

*Miriam E. Lowenberg, PhD is former Head
of the Department of Food and Nutrition,
Pennsylvania State University*

Dr. Miriam Lowenberg began her illustrious career teaching high school home economics for several years before pursuing graduate work in nutrition and child psychology. She earned her doctorate in child welfare and pediatrics. Her career has included college teaching, researching the relationship of food to history and culture, and working in various consulting positions. Except for two references to forced retirement because of age, it is difficult to imagine that this woman is 90+ years old. Forced retirement from Penn State opened another door—consulting on the dietary requirements of mentally retarded children. A second forced retirement left her with more time to conduct nutrition workshops on campuses around the country, travel, and write. Two of her most notable works include *Food and People*, and *Feeding Your Baby and Child*, which she co-authored with Dr. Benjamin Spock.

Miriam E. Lowenberg

Two years ago, after several friends had urged me to do it, I wrote down a number of stories about events which have occurred to me in my life. A pediatrician with whom I had worked, and who has remained a close friend, asked me to record why I had chosen to pioneer a new field in child nutrition.

Dr. McLean had come many times to the lectures in which I discussed this for the pediatrics students as they came into our program at the University of Washington. I asked him why he kept coming and he said, "I always learn something new each time. Something I think a practicing pediatrician should know."

My particular interest, from early in my career was children's food likes and dislikes and how these affect their food behavior. This is, to me, important if we are to be able to improve their food habits so that they eat happily the foods needed for healthy growth and well-being.

Now I will happily describe here the developments of my career for a professional audience. I had written two years ago, about this in "Letters to a Friend" style, just for my friends.

I must admit what to my friends say, that I believe that I have always been goal oriented. True, my goals have changed as I matured and worked with many professional co-workers during my life. Part of this drive toward a goal, undoubtedly, came from my inheritance and early training.

Even before the time that many girls left a small midwest farming community to go to a large city university I did go to the University of Chicago. I know that my father expected that all his children would finish college; my brother took his bachelor's degree; my two sisters took bachelor's and master's degrees and I took my Ph.D.

Two of my favorite high school teachers were very influential on how I approached my college years. Florence A. Gates, my sophomore botany teacher epitomized to me the great teacher; I fully intended then to teach botany as she did. Later a cousin, the only college graduate in my immediate family, urged me to consider the then called domestic science, which he thought more appropriate for a woman. L. B. Mull, my senior year Physics teacher, in whose class I did well, encouraged me by saying that he believed I would be a success in college and in life. I exchanged Christmas letters with Miss Gates for 44 years and I still have her letter written 35 years ago in which she complimented me, whom she called her "little sophomore," when she saw a review of the book *Feeding Your Baby and Child*, written with Dr. B. J. Spock, which appeared in Time magazine.

There was little choice as to where I would go to college; I must live with my Chicago aunt and uncle because I could not afford room and board. This aunt was the only survivor then of my mother's immediate family and she and her husband welcomed me to live with them. So, on October 1 of 1914, I entered the University of Chicago as a freshman, then a great university, as it has been since then. My entire sum of $1500*, which I had inherited from my mother's estate, must finance four years of tuition, books, supplies, lunches, street car fare, clothing and at least a little recreation. In addition, I must pay railroad fare to and from my Iowa home so I could spend my summers at home. My mother had died when I was two and one half years old. I wish she could have known how well I used what her adopted parents had left to me.

During those four years my aunt sometimes gave me her ticket to the opera and the woman with whom she went also gave her niece her ticket. At 17 to 18 years of age we braved the "big bad" city to come home late at night on the street car after hearing such famous singers as Madame Melba, Caruso, Galli Curci, Lily Pons, and many others. It was worth our fright.

Many of my friends were on as tight a budget as I was. I remember that I early settled on having for lunch a dish of mashed potatoes and a glass of milk for 13 cents.

I can also remember being grateful that I was at a great university studying to be a teacher; I wasted no regrets that I was on a very limited budget. My breakfasts and dinners with my aunt were very generous and delicious, so I certainly did not suffer. My uncle made then a princely sum, from the commission firm he owned in the U. S. stockyards. They had catholic tastes and I soon learned to appreciate the delicious, though new to me, foods such as the unusual cheeses which the Chicago market afforded. We had excellent meat which my uncle was allowed to buy at wholesale in the lockers of the great packing companies. My food selection became, fortunately enlarged. I say this because later I was discouraged when college students in food preparation classes refused to try new foods. Perhaps learning to eat new foods then formed the basis of my belief that children's food habits can be changed. The weight gain I needed then, but I did start my lifetime struggle with gaining weight.

At barely 17 years of age I enrolled in what was then called the Department of Household Art. After I took my first nutrition course under Dr. Lydia J. Roberts, I had no question at all as to what my field of study would be; I would become a child nutritionist, as she was. She certainly imbued my best friend and me that we must have this as our major. She had taught in elementary schools in Montana where she saw malnourished children who ate inadequate carried lunches and cold warmed over suppers, mostly of fried foods. These did not furnish them with the foods needed for healthy growth. She could see the effects of this poor food on young minds. When good

---

* Charles Montandan, Houston, Texas, the husband of a former student of mine, graciously computed for me how much the $1500 ($375 approximately per year) would be in 1988 dollars.

year	1974 dollars	Worth of $1 in 1988 dollars	Approximate cash in 1988
1914–15	$375	0.089925 (.09)	$ 4125
1915–16	375	0.095902 (.10)	3750
1916–17	375	0.112467 (.11)	3375
1917–18	375	0.131648 (.13)	2875
		Total	$14,125

How much the accrued interest on this would be I have no way of knowing.

school lunches were put in those schools Dr. Roberts said that she saw the effect of these good foods on young minds and bodies.

She came to study nutrition at the University of Chicago so she could become more effective in instituting programs to improve children's food habits. When her biography was written, after her 1965 death, I found that when I took my first nutrition course she was working at the time on her bachelor's degree. She took her Ph.B., that is bachelor of philosophy degree, the year before I took mine. She constantly inspired me to do the same thing to which she was dedicated and later I never wavered from the goal I set for myself then; I have never been sorry for this choice.

After my best friend, Ethel Maloney and I were graduated from the university, Dr. Roberts hired us to grade the 40,000 Gary, Indiana children's diets she had collected on a study financed by a grant from the Children's Bureau. As I read that study now I am amazed at how well-planned and executed it was, even before modern statistical methods and computers. Later I taught four years in high schools and three years in two small religious colleges. In 1927, I accepted a teaching graduate assistantship at the Iowa State University, then Iowa State College (ISC), in preference to an offer of an internship in dietetics at a large Chicago hospital. At this time I made a real career choice.

In 1929 I received my Master's degree from ISC in Child Nutrition and Child Psychology, which gave me a greater understanding of children's food behavior. In one of the courses, students, among other things, prepared and served the children's food, observing how they ate. Later Mrs. Lancaster, then head of the department there, asked me to supervise this food preparation, serving on a volunteer basis; at the time I was teaching one half time in the foods and nutrition department.

The next year, when Mrs. Lancaster was able to put the position of a nutritionist in her budget she asked me to take the position. I happily accepted and now I was really entering the career I had envisioned. I very much wanted the children to like our food. I believed that I could find out what foods children liked and that I could change the preparation to suit their tastes. I had a background of the science of how foods react with heat and cold and physical manipulation from wonderful courses which I had taken under the great Belle Lowe, my mentor and friend. I had also helped cook our family meals at home from the age of nine years. I really tried to prepare the food so that the children would like and accept it gladly. For instance, it was easy to cook the disliked strong-flavored vegetables in an excess of water, discarding some of the strong flavor. It did not matter if thus we threw away some of the minerals and vitamins if we helped a child to learn to eat that vegetable. We served meat, largely either ground or in small tender pieces so young teeth could chew it easily.

During my second year of my teaching assistantship and work on my Master's I placed in the upper 2 percent of good teachers on a college-wide survey. I had tried very hard to do the best teaching I could and I truly liked my students and felt they liked me. This student rating had caused then President Hughes to recommend to my dean that she hire me on the permanent staff, which she did. Now I had my golden opportunity. I would have a real group of young children to feed on a long-term basis. Of course I did other teaching besides that.

For twelve years I had observed closely children's food behavior at the nursery school lunch and worked with parents to monitor their children's food intake at home. Then, as now, I saw the noon meal as a part of the whole day's intake. We measured the food onto the plates in the kitchen in exact tablespoonfuls and cupfuls. This was all carefully recorded, as were second servings and food not eaten. Thus I could study from these written records what foods children liked and what they rejected. I also solicited the teachers' comments on how and what the children ate. One year I asked each teacher and student who was eating with the children to record their opinions of the menu combinations and the way children accepted them. From these records I revised the menus the next year when I again asked for their written opinions. From these, for instance, I found that a menu that had one crisp food, one soft food and only one chewy in the main course was most popular. These twelve years of careful and close observation led me to see some general principles in children's food behavior.

This work became known outside by observers such as Gladys Denny Shultz, then Child Development editor of the Homes & Garden magazine in nearby Des Moines, when she visited us she asked me to write an article for her magazine. I was also writing articles and having them published in other woman's magazines about what I had learned.

Our local college radio station had a five-day-a-week woman's program. I liked to talk on this to spread more widely what I was learning, and I was often asked to speak on this program. I gradually became known as the "Liver Loaf Lady" from the recipe which I gave out often. These were 12 wonderful years, but I began to see that I would not advance without a doctorate, so in 1941 I resigned after I had spent the summer of 1940 trying out the University of Iowa as a place to study nutrition and child psychology. There I had such teachers as Dr. P. C. Jeans, Dr. Amy Daniels, Dr. Ruth Updegraf and Dr. Howard Meredith, Dr. George Stoddard, and Dr. Robert Sears. Encountering these brilliant minds was indeed stimulating and in June 1943 I received a Ph.D. degree.

When I had resigned at Iowa State University one nutrition staff member asked me whether I was afraid I would never get another job because I was then 44 years old. To encourage brave young souls now, let me say I hadn't thought about it because I was forging ahead, learning more and more. After I received this doctorate I never sought another job, they always sought me.

In 1934 I had published with the Iowa State College Press a book, *Food for the Young Child*. In the late 1930s Whittelsly House, then a part of McGraw Hill & Co. (doing their popular books) asked me to redo this locally-published book. They brought out *Your Child's Food* in 1939, so now the work which I had done at Iowa State was in a nationally published book. I found this all worthwhile because later several of the positions I accepted came to me because people had read and liked what I had written. That is, they liked the philosophy of making the needed foods acceptable to the young child. Somehow, I always had faith that I had something to say which parents needed to know.

In a recent Seattle newspaper article about me a good friend is quoted as saying that self-confidence and persistence are some of my most outstanding characteristics. I say this not to boast, but to say that a goal pursued with hard work and then public appearance can build self-confidence. I can hardly imagine how I came to have it from the days when as a college student I was too shy to answer in class, even when I knew the answer.

This same friend said that once I had an idea I follow through. I realized that I had always thought that to be important, and I still do. Now it may be to promote something which she, as a Seattle City Councilwoman is doing. I say all of this not to say, "Look how good I am," but to honestly analyze why I did what I did.

My Ph.D. work included courses in pediatric nutrition in medical school, as well as child development and child psychology courses; my major was in the relation of diet to physical growth of children. All of this deepened my understanding of children in relation to the needed foods.

After the awarding of my degree I taught a course on how to feed children in wartime day care centers at the Vassar Summer Session in 1943. Dr. Mary Fisher, head of this section, said she liked what I had written on feeding children.

After the Vassar session, Dr. Lois H. Stolz asked me to come to the Portland, Oregon Kaiser Shipyard Child Service Centers to feed 2,375 preschool children on a 24-hour basis. Actually, we never had, fortunately, more than 1,000 children in our two Child Service Centers and there were never many children on the so-called "graveyard shift." I accepted because the position sounded challenging and I had not been given the final word on another position I had been offered as director of the Women and Children's Program in the U.S. Civilian Food Requirement Branch in Washington, D.C.

I arrived in Portland in early October 1943 and the first center was to open November 7. No one scarcely believes me that on Friday afternoon the Center's kitchen floor was not laid and hence, no large equipment was in place, but my Kaiser bosses told me to get ready to serve breakfast the next Monday morning. The so-called "expeditors" could work wonders. Serve that breakfast we did! I often wish now that I had such powerful creatures to call on when something needs doing.

The Center served the children of the workers, mostly ages eighteen months to six years; few "after school" six to twelve year olds were enrolled. We required in these two centers, 100 nursery school teachers. There were 26 on the kitchen staffs in the two centers to handle all the food preparation and serving. Each kitchen had a well-trained supervisor and an assistant to cover the 14-hour days. It takes a lot of doing to cut up fruit for dessert in bite-size pieces for so many eighteen month to two or three year old children. The older children could cut up their own.

Why did I get this offer to take charge of this feeding program? Dr. Elda Robb, who had been Dr. Stolz's nutritionist at the Child Development Institute at Columbia

University, told her that I knew more about feeding young children than anyone in the country. I probably did, because no one else had done the years of careful study of children's food likes and dislikes and patterns, which I had. It was a case of being ready for a job when it was offered.

I was especially gratified that what I had learned from the 12 years of meticulous study and observation at Iowa State College worked for the 1,000 children who were in the Kaiser Centers.

Our centers had the largest population of preschool children in the United States, and they attracted even international attention. One day when Edgar Kaiser, the one in charge of the 110,000 men in those three Kaiser shipyards came to the Swan Island Center. I was called from my shipyard office because he had important guests with him. I expected that it was an entourage with Eleanor Roosevelt, who had been the most influential person in Washington, D.C. in getting the money to establish those centers under the Maritime Commission. The principle visitor in that group turned out to be the woman in charge of U.S. wartime housing. The third Kaiser shipyard, in Vancouver, Washington had Lanham Act schools established before we were.

We also started Home Service food, where parents could order food to take home for their next meal and pay only the cost of food. We began preparing an entree and dessert, but due to later demand, salads were added in what proved to be a very popular service. By including suggestions for food to serve with our foods, I could hope, thus, to influence what the children ate at home.

In the summer of 1945 orders for ships, now not needed after the Japanese armistice, were cancelled and our Centers were no longer needed. One of my most poignant memories of this entire experience was tearful parents coming to the Centers even after they were closed to their children.

I was capping my 14 years of studying children's food likes and dislikes, when on any day I could observe many different children to see how well they ate our food. Now, when I read research articles on children's food behavior done by a person who has never really fed children, I, who had at the end of the Kaiser experience supervised the feeding of over a million meals to young children, have little faith in their conclusions. For instance, I could only laugh at one woman who fed children spinach every day for seven days and concluded, when the children did not eat it better on the seventh day, than on the first, that familiarity did not cause acceptance, as I had said it did.

Several months before I left Portland, Oregon, Dr. C. Anderson Aldrich from Rochester, Minnesota contacted me, and paid my way from Portland to try to entice me to join his staff as Nutritional Supervisor for his Rochester Child Health Institute, financed largely by the Mayo Clinic. This project was set up to study how a small city, as Rochester, could improve its facilities and services to better serve children. After I visited them I was very excited over the possibilities and joined the staff gladly.

Dr. Russell Wilder, who had offered me the position in the Civilian Foods Requirement Branch in Washington, D.C. then had returned to be head of Metabolism Nutrition in the Mayo Clinic. I was glad to work under him, also.

This six years that I was in the Rochester project were happy and fulfilling years, though the last two years after Dr. Aldrich's untimely death in 1949 were less satisfying because he had truly been a great leader. It was here that I knew Ben Spock so well while he was our psychiatrist. Our small staff had eaten brown bag lunches together and had many good discussions.

My first efforts were directed toward doing a survey of what pregnant women in Rochester were eating. Dr. Aldrich asked me to study this because he said that in his Winnetka, Illinois pediatric practice he had seen unhealthy babies born to women who had eaten inadequate diets, living mostly on coffee and sweet rolls during their pregnancy. This research was planned by a committee I chose, consisting of an obstetrician, nurses and nutritionists, with whom I would be working. We selected one half of the women from the Obstetrics Department in the Mayo Clinic and one-half from the Public Health Maternity Clinic. The results showed many less than adequate diets in both groups.

The public health nurses could hardly wait until the survey was done so I could get started with dietary counseling for their patients. With a device called "Score Your Diet" which we had designed, I helped these women to evaluate their own diets and to determine how they could bring them to adequacy. Finally women began complaining that at the Mayo Clinic, where they paid for their care, they did not receive the services of a nutritionist, while the women at the free clinic did. When Dr. Hunt, who was in charge of obstetrics at the Mayo Clinic asked me why, I said, "Just ask me to work in your department and I will."

I also did nutrition counseling in all the Rochester well child clinics as well as serving as a consultant to the skillful but untrained supervisor of the school lunch program. In addition, I was welcomed when I offered to teach nutrition in the elementary schools. There I mostly answered the children's questions on nutrition at rewarding sessions. One student coming to his own conclusion when he used "Score Your Diet," said, "Look, when I drink cola all I get is calories."

In 1949 I was able to have a demonstration kitchen in the new public health building. I asked the General Mills Company of Minneapolis for $4,000 to buy the food supplies for several years for that kitchen. When some of the executives of that company came down to see how their money was being spent, they were much interested in my demonstration, "Food As Children See It." At this time they decided that they should do a film on it so more people than the women in Rochester could profit from my advice. This film later received wide acceptance and use and even some prizes as an educational film.

In 1952, I left the Rochester Child Health Institute, which was truly "Camelot," as Dr. Aldrich's oldest son, Dr. Robert Aldrich, later of Seattle, has called it.

In early 1952 I became the head of the Department of Food and Nutrition of the Pennsylvania State University. This was an excellent department with very good courses and staff, whose main interest was in the biochemical and physiological aspects of nutrition. I thought, however, that a course about the people who eat the food was needed and this I wrote and taught to receptive student groups. One Ph.D. student well-trained in the biochemical aspects, said that this course opened her eyes to the "other side of nutrition."

In the late 1950s Dean Grace Henderson and the faculty voted to institute six general courses in as many departments to form what was called the "core curriculum." She asked me to plan and teach the first of these courses. This might be, for majors in other areas, the only course in nutrition which they would take, so I planned a course which attempted to show the worldwide importance of nutrition. To prepare for teaching this course, I requested and received a sabbatical leave so I could travel around the world to see firsthand what I would be talking about in class. I needed to see malnutrition, especially in children, and to see what national and international agencies were doing about it. This course also dealt with the determinants of food patterns and the history of these.

After I had taught this course for two years a number of other colleges and universities had put in similar courses. A textbook was evidently needed, so I with several other prominent nutrition friends who wrote chapters, produced this. In 1968 the first edition of *Food and Man* was published by John Wiley & Company. Heavy revision in which I now had written 60 percent of the text brought out a 1973 edition. In 1979 the so-called sexist word "man" was changed and the book called "Food and People" was published as a third edition.

On my 1959 world trip I had scheduled conferences with 115 world leaders, some of whom I still correspond with at Christmastime, keeping up with what is happening.

In 1963 age forced my retirement from Penn State and I joined the staff of the Child Development and Mental Retardation Center at the University of Washington in Seattle as Chief Nutritionist. This was the first and the largest of the ten Kennedy University Affiliated Training Centers, the purpose of which was to train professional people to work with the mentally retarded.

In 1967 we expanded under a grant to the Nutrition Department and began training nutritionists. Dr. Deisher, the director, asked that I be allowed to remain two years after the then required retirement age of 70 so I could get this program well on its way. As my friends point out, I didn't really retire in 1969; after that I wrote most of the two later editions of *Food and Man* and taught 13 workshops in as many states on the idea of *Food and Man* most of these were two weeks in length. Many of my friends remind me that I was 80 when I really retired to enjoy my house and garden, with only a part-time interest in writing, travel and a bit of lecturing.

I would like here to say that I had seen Dr. Roberts at many American Dietetic Association annual meetings when I sat with her and talked to her about her work. In March of 1965 I visited Puerto Rico and was able to spend much time with her. Dr. Roberts had worked there for some 20 years. She took me to see her favorite project at Donna Elena. After she had, at 75 years of age, walked ten miles over the mountains to get to the Donna Elena district, she enticed then Governor Munoz to appropriate money for community improvement. She told me that good roads, better housing, a good water supply were first priorities, even before she could mention better food. There I saw a reformed, colorful, beautiful community of happy people, some of whom kissed the hem of her dress when they saw her. How fortunate I was to have her pass on to me then so much of her wisdom. I didn't know, until I heard of her sudden death two months later.

I have chosen to discuss my activities in The American Dietetic Association separately. Soon after I joined the association, when I was at the Kaiser Child Service Center I moved to Rochester, Minnesota, where I was elected as a state Delegate, serving three terms. Later in Pennsylvania, I served two terms as a Delegate and one term as state president. After this I was elected a Delegate at Large and in 1963 I served as Speaker of the House of Delegates. The next year when I was asked to be president, I had to decline because I was retiring from Penn State and going to a new job. During all these years I have served on numerous committees.

I was greatly honored in 1970 to receive the Marjorie Hulsizer Copher Award and in 1973 to be asked to give the Lenna F. Cooper Lecture.

Now, in my 92nd year, when arthritis and knee surgery plague me and without a car, I am somewhat grounded. I do, as a friend says, bring the world to me; I enjoy serving simple tea parties and having friends and what meetings I can in my home and garden. With lots of good and faithful help I can keep "in charge." Perhaps I am, as one friend said, still "the administrator." I have a parade of flowers in my garden, some of which I can have for bouquets inside almost year-round and to give to friends.

During my 90th birthday party, given for 63 guests by six especially close friends, my good friend, Margaret Till called from Auckland, New Zealand to greet me. What a thrill that was!

I am very glad that I chose the career I did. No one could have had a better mentor than Dr. Lydia J. Roberts.

Without the help of kind, caring and giving friends, both professional and personal, I could not have accomplished as much of my goals as I have. I am fortunate to have had and to have now a wide circle of friends. To them and to my family, I am forever grateful. I truly believe that no bird flies high on its own power alone, nor can a human go far alone. The pure job of friendship has always spurred me on.

So I developed a career which I have found interesting and very rewarding!

Roy S. Maize II

Roy S. Maize II, PhD, RD
is an Associate Professor in the Department
of Human Nutrition and Hospitality Management,
The University of Alabama.

Dr. Roy Maize has the distinction of being the first male ever to be elected to the ADA Board of Directors. His career began with a 20 year stint in the Army where he attained the rank of Lieutenant Colonel and moved his family 12 times in 19 years! Among his many Army positions were those of Dietetic Internship Director at Brook Army Medical Center and Chief of Food Production at Walter Reed. He also worked on the development of the Army's Combat Field Feeding System. Dr. Maize combined his love of management and education in his doctoral research at Ohio State, focusing on the relationship of job orientation/training and job turnover. He has received numerous honors including the Legion of Merit Award, the highest service award given during peace time. Upon retiring from the Army in 1985, Dr. Maize became General Manager of Personnel for Valley Food Service and then went on to his current position as an Associate Professor in restaurant and hospitality management at The University of Alabama. He offers his reflections on the challenges ahead for dietitians and the need for more dietitians in management positions.

Roy S. Maize II

College Years

After graduating in 1962 from a small high school in Brownsville, Pennsylvania, a coal mining community with a population of about 5000, I entered The Pennsylvania State University. Attending Penn State was a family tradition since my father, sister, two uncles, and an aunt had previously graduated from this institution.

My goal entering college was to become a hospital administrator. This decision was influenced by the community hospital administrator who attended our home church. I had talked with him and had visited the community hospital and felt that this was a career I would enjoy. After my first semester in Business Administration, I discovered a major called "Institution Management" and went to visit the Dean of the College to pursue my ultimate goal. I transferred from the College of Business to the College of Home Economics and began my major in Food Service and Housing Administration. I enjoyed my classes very much and found the faculty particularly helpful, especial Ruth Eshelman, Jim Kaiser, Ruth Eccleston, Helen Guthrie, and Ruth Pike. Little did I know that Ruth Pike and Helen Guthrie would become nationally known experts in the field of nutrition. In addition, Ruth Eshelman and I have remained friends for life. It was Ruth Eshelman that helped me understand the advanced nutrition principles and concepts that Dr. Ruth Pike was conveying in her class. I will forever be indebted to Ruth Eshelman for her time, interest, and support during these years.

Early in my junior year I visited The University of Pittsburgh Hospital Administration program to determine entrance requirements. I was told that I needed to be at least 29 years of age, and have several years of work experience in health care before being considered. At this time Hospital Administration was offered in only twelve universities in the country and only at the Master's level. With this new knowledge, and somewhat frustrated, I began to explore options which ultimately would allow me to achieve my goal. I explored hotel management since I had worked during the summers at a resort hotel, the Mount Summit Inn, in Uniontown, PA, about 15 miles from my home. This had a great appeal since it would allow me to work with people, making decisions, develop management skills, etc. However, during the second semester of my junior year, a representative from the Army Medical Specialist Corps came to campus recruiting students for their student dietitian program. After hearing MAJ Janet Hammill, an Army dietitian, discuss program requirements and benefits, I applied. I felt that this would give me experience in health care and would also pay for some of my education. Also, on a personal note, being selected would allow me to get married to a young lady I had been dating since a sophomore in high school. Student dietitians received pay as a Private First Class, were entitled to commissary and health care privileges and best of all, were guaranteed a dietetic internship. As fate would have it, I was selected for this program and enlisted in March, 1965 as a PFC. I was in the student dietitian program until graduation in March, 1966. My career was set, at least for the next four years.

Dietetics Career

In March 1966, I graduated from Penn State and was commissioned a Second Lieutenant in the Army Medical Specialist Corps. I reported to Brooke Army Medical Center, Fort Sam Houston, Texas to begin my twelve month dietetic internship. I knew very little about dietetics, and even less about the Army. Most new officers received a six week orientation before internship, however, because of my late graduation from college, I was unable to experience this orientation—how to wear a uniform, how to salute, proper protocol, etc. In fact, by the time I got to San Antonio, the internship was already in its second week. I was excited but also apprehensive; a new city far from home, a very large hospital, new people and a new career. My salvation was that I was not alone, for my wife had accompanied me, a friendly face in this strange new land.

From March 1966 to April 1967, I received the best training that any dietetic student could possibly receive. The internship provided hands on clinical care to patients, community experiences, management experiences, educational opportunities, etc., enabling me to develop a broad base of knowledge, skills and abilities necessary for dietetic practice. During my internship COL Nannie R. Evans was Chief, Hospital Food Service. She proved to be a mentor, friend, and disciplinarian. COL Evans' standards were exceptionally high, sometimes they appeared unattainable. While not always appreciating her values at the time, I have since come to appreciate her ability to set, maintain and achieve high standards and goals. The internship was intense, working many long days, nights and weekends. The lessons, values, and standards learned during this twelve month experience formed the basis of my professional practice today, and I am grateful to those individuals that guided me in my early years. I might add that it was during this time that I became semi-involved in the local dietetics association. COL Evans required that all interns attend every district meeting, and we did. While many of my peers dreaded the experience, I found it enjoyable. This experience set the stage for my continued involvement in local and national dietetics.

After completing my internship in March 1967, I completed a six-week basic training course at the Medical Field Service School, San Antonio, TX. This was the orientation to the Army that I should have received prior to internship. Even though I had learned quite a bit from the internship program, I still learned much about Army organization, protocol, etc. Because I was more senior than most of my classmates, I was made a platoon leader during the six week program. This meant that I was responsible for the other officers' behavior during the orientation and during marching drills. From dietitian to drill sergeant in less than one year. What more could I ask for.

In August 1967, after graduation from basic training, I was assigned to Walson Army Hospital, Fort Dix, NJ as a clinical dietitian. My primary duties for the first two months involved patient care, outpatient counseling, ward rounds, general supervision of dietetic technicians and other patient care functions. While interesting, my real love was food production and other management activities. After three months an opportunity arose to move to the kitchen and be the Assistant Chief, Production and Service Branch. I immediately requested the change. It was really exciting. Here I was in a 300 bed hospital with no recipes, no production worksheets and a group of employees who were old enough to be my parents, if not my grandparents. I was shocked. During the next three months I established a recipe file, production worksheets, nourishment schedules, solved day to day people and operational problems and had a wonderful experience. The employees and I learned to respect each other, even though they were unionized and this did present some challenges.

After six months at Walson I was asked to move to Fort McPherson, GA to a 90 bed hospital to become Chief, Hospital Food Service. Never having lived in the South I was not sure whether I should move or not, but I accepted the challenge and my career in dietetics too a new direction.

As Chief, Hospital Food Service in a 90 bed general hospital, I was responsible for all aspects of dietetic services: food ordering, inventory, financial accounting, employee hiring, training, food preparation, patient counseling, writing of modified diets, out-patient counseling, tray line activity, etc. During this assignment of two years I grew both personally and professionally. My first task was to reorganize the diet kitchen. Approximately 60 to 70 trays were served to patients per meal. Employees would place all patient trays on tables around the room and then go from tray to tray placing food items on them. After installing a tray line system, the workload became much easier for all employees and patient trays became more accurate. I knew from this experience that I wanted to focus my career toward the management aspects of dietetics. Many exciting experiences happened to me while here, but perhaps the most exciting professionally was my involvement with the Atlanta Dietetic Association.

The dietitians in Atlanta were wonderful. I met wonderful individuals who are still my friends today, such as Mary Bauer, a dietitian who was married to the Third Army Surgeon at Fort McPherson. Mary and I became friends and went to meetings together and to this day stay in touch. Pat Hodges, another dietitian I met in Atlanta, is now on faculty with me at The University of Alabama. While in Atlanta, I was elected Treasurer of the Atlanta Dietetic Association, my first elected position. This early involvement and the caring of other professionals encouraged me to continue my involvement in local dietetic association activities. I was awarded the Army Commendation Medical for exemplary performance upon leaving Fort McPherson.

In 1969 I was selected by the Army to attend graduate school and moved to Columbus, Ohio, home of The Ohio State University. I chose Ohio State since it was close to home for my wife and me. While majoring in Food Administration I became very close friends with my advisor, Rachael Hubbard. Rachael, an administrative dietitian for many years, gave me much insight into the profession. I gained much respect and admiration for Rachael because she made time for me and encouraged me in all my endeavors. While at OSU I also met Joan Sharp who was very active in The American Dietetic Association. This association would influence me more than I realized. After completing my master's degree in August 1970, I was stationed at Darnall Army Hospital, Fort Hood, TX as Chief, Hospital Food Service Division.

Darnall Army Hospital, a 300 bed hospital, was located at Fort Hood, TX and about 60 miles north of Austin, TX. I was fortunate to have two other Army dietitians working for me, one recently finishing her dietetic internship at Brooke Army Medical Center in San Antonio. One dietitian was responsible for the Clinical Dietetics Branch (patient care activities) and the other for the Production and Service Branch (food procurement, production and service activities). My first experience at managing other professionals proved exciting and rewarding. We established a monthly Journal Club to review professional journal articles, attended local dietetic meetings, developed new a la carte menus and held a county western buffet luncheon which proved to be a great success. At this time, September 1970, the Viet Nam War was at its peak. In March, 1971 I received a call indicating that I would soon leave my position to go to Viet Nam. About two weeks later, I received a second call telling me that I had been selected to be the Dietetic Internship Director at Brooke Army Medical Center in San Antonio. I didn't argue the point, since San Antonio looked a whole lot better than Viet Nam and the far East. Thus, in July, 1971, after completing a short ten months as Chief, Hospital Food Service at Darnall Army Hospital, I was assigned to Brooke Army Medical Center as Dietetic Internship Director and Director of Education and Training.

At 27 years of age, and with five years of operational experience I found myself developing, planning and coordinating learning experiences for 8–12 dietetic interns each year for the next four years. The Chief, Hospital Food Service was none other than COL Nannie R. Evans, my mentor from internship days. While I thought I knew what needed to be done and how to do it, COL Evans' years of experience and innovative ideas proved to be most beneficial. During this experience I went to a national dietetic educators meeting in Chicago where I was asked to serve on the Program of Work Committee for the Section on Education Preparation. Thus, my initial involvement with The American Dietetic Association. I was also elected Secretary-Treasurer of the San Antonio Dietetic Association and served on the nominating committee. The association with other professional colleagues helped strengthen my values, and helped me realize the administrative dietetics and training were the aspects of the profession I enjoyed most.

In 1975, while internship director, I was nominated and selected to receive the Recognized Young Dietitian of the Year Award from the state of Texas. This is an honor I cherish and one which encouraged me to continue my involvement with The American Dietetic Association.

Working with dietetic interns was perhaps one of the most rewarding experiences of my career. It was during this time that I realized that I wanted to work toward a doctorate degree and began attending night and weekend classes at Southwest Texas State College in San Marcos, TX. I attended classes on Tuesday and Thursday nights and all day Saturday with the intent of leaving the service to work full time on the doctorate degree.

In 1975, the Army Medical Specialist Corps selected me for long term schooling. I was elated that my goal of obtaining a doctorate degree was now within reach. I went back to Ohio State to work with my friend, colleague and mentor, Rachael Hubbard. Since I had been going to school part-time, I would be able to complete the Ph.D. in two, instead of three years. Since I had determined that training was an area of interest, I chose to do my dissertation on the relationship between job orientation and training and turnover rates among hospital dietary employees. In collecting data for the study, I visited over 30 hospitals in Ohio and was able to observe different operating systems, training programs, and styles of management. This was a most beautiful experience.

During my last year of graduate school, Joan Sharp, Director of Dietetic Services at The Ohio State University Hospital, was President of The American Dietetic Association. Joan asked me if I would be interested in serving as Chair, Division of Management Practices, Council on Practice. This position had recently been created as a result of a bylaws change which created a new organizational structure for The American Dietetic Association. I accepted and served in this capacity from 1977 to 1979. During my tenure, the Council on Practice defined its role, worked to establish numerous dietetic practice groups, and developed policies and procedures. This experience helped me learn how to work with people of differing opinions and arrive at a consensus. I might add that the experience was challenging, usually fun, but sometimes very frustrating.

After graduating from The Ohio State University in 1977 with my doctorate degree in Food Administration, I was stationed at The Academy of Health Sciences, US Army, Fort Sam Houston, TX. As Chief, Hospital Food Service Branch, Health Care Administration Division my primary duties involved developing continuing education programs for Army dietitians, developing self-paced learning modules for hospital food service specialists and teaching a number of courses to enlisted and officer personnel. It was during this assignment that I was elected Secretary-Treasurer of The American Dietetic Association, a job that I thoroughly enjoyed and one in which I grew professionally. As Secretary-Treasurer, I was on the Board of Directors, the first male member to be elected to the Board. In this position I became extremely familiar with the magnitude of The American Dietetic Association, its budget, its membership and most importantly its organizational structure.

In June 1981, I was assigned to the U.S. Army Command and General Staff College, Fort Leavenworth, KS for nine months of schooling. During this program of instruction I learned how the Army really works, from air defense artillery to military intelligence. Information presented was totally foreign to me and it was a *difficult* year.

After graduating from the Army's Command and General Staff College in June 1982, I was assigned to the U.S. Army Natick Research and Development Laboratories, Natick, MA where I was Military Assistant to the Director, Food Engineering Laboratory. I worked with researchers in the development of the Army's Combat Field Feeding System, and was program manager for the Tray Pack Ration, a new concept for feeding one hot meal a day to troops on the battlefield. Again, I found myself using the skills gained in college and internship—planning, coordinating, evaluating, staffing, organizing, and writing. While in this assignment, I was nominated for Director at Large,

The American Dietetic Association and was fortunate to be elected for a three year term, from 1983 to 1986. While serving in this position it was apparent that the profession of dietetics was changing rapidly. Younger members were wanting to be more proactive in nutrition issues and be more visible to the public. It was during this time that much effort was placed on marketing of the profession and making the dietitian more visible as a recognized nutrition expert.

While at Natick I was awarded the "A" professional designator for continued demonstration of exceptional professional ability in Hospital Dietetics by the Department of the Army. In addition, the Meritorious Service Medal was also awarded for my performance as Military Assistant. While awards in and of themselves mean very little, it does help provide a sense of satisfaction that hard work is valued and recognized.

After one year at Natick Labs, I was assigned to the Nutrition Care Directorate, Walter Reed Army Medical Center, Washington, D.C. as Quality Assurance Officer. Quality Assurance was gaining much attention in the health care community and I was excited about developing a quality assurance program. From 1983 to 1984 I developed policies and procedures related to QA, developed monitors, trend line information, and implemented a comprehensive QA program. This was an exciting time. I was able to use the talents I had developed over the past 18 years to develop mechanisms to enhance patient care activities. As Director at Large for ADA, I was asked to assist in the selection of a new executive director for The American Dietetic Association. After numerous trips to Chicago to select a search firm, and to interview prospective candidates, the Board selected Dr. Julian Haynes, Provost at MGH Institute of Health Professions, Boston, Massachusetts. This too was a new experience and one I found most educational.

In June 1984, my best friend at Walter Reed, MAJ Jerry Shaffer, received orders for Panama. I was asked to assume his duties as Chief, Production and Service Division. Thus, I became responsible for the procurement, preparation, distribution and service of food to all hospitalized patients (about 400–500 per meal) and to all customers and guests in the cafeteria (about 1200 daily). I directly supervised five dietitians and indirectly supervised over 120 civil service food service employees. Walter Reed's food preparation system was a combination of cook chill, cook freeze and conventional. New menus for patients and cafeteria were developed and plans for a major renovation of the kitchen and cafeteria were reviewed and implemented.

In July 1985, I made the decision to retire from the service after serving 20 years and moving 12 times in 19 years. By this time I held the military rank of Lieutenant Colonel in the Army Medical Specialist Corps. At this point my oldest son was in the eleventh grade, my youngest son in the fifth grade and my wife and I wanted more stability in our lives. I was awarded the Legion of Merit, the highest award given during peace time, upon retirement. Thus, after 20 exciting, challenging years I left the service to become General Manager of Personnel, Valley Food Service, Jackson, MS.

In my new role, I would recruit food service managers and dietitians, develop and implement training programs for managers, develop management salary schedules and incentive compensation plans, develop performance evaluations systems and develop and implement a company wide quality assurance program. My involvement in ADA continued as a Director at Large through October 1986. As Director at Large, I was Board liaison to the Marketing and Public Relations committee and the Publications committee. A marketing plan for dietetics was developed and implemented during this period of time.

In August 1987 I left Valley Food Service to join The University of Alabama as an Associate Professor in the Department of Human Nutrition and Hospitality Management. My primary focus is the development of a strong, visible Restaurant and Hospitality Management Program. After two years at the University, enrollment has increased from 30 to 100 students. Funding support from industry has started to develop and there is a great deal of enthusiasm from students majoring in this field. I teach management courses to dietetic, restaurant and hospitality majors in their junior and senior years. From the experience gained in the Army and industry, I am able to relate "real life" situations to students, making the learning experience more realistic. Working with Betsy Barrett, R.D., a dietitian who worked with Morrison Corporation prior to joining the university, we developed instructional strategies for the Quantity Food Production and Service course that are unique. Operating a full scale cafeteria, J.J. Doster Cafe, we offer a full range of entrees, starch, vegetables, salads, desserts and beverages. The cafeteria is open three days a week during the Spring semester and serves an average of 170 customers per day with average sales of $456.00 per day. Thirty-seven students operate the cafe working one day per week, rotating through twelve positions from manager to dishwasher. This course integrates theories of menu planning, personnel management and financial management and allows students to apply the theories in a non-threatening, real-life environment. I also serve on the Council on Research, the Quality Assurance Committee, the Educational Standards Committee of the Council on Education , and the 1989 Nominating Committee of The American Dietetic Association.

Reflections on My Career

Over the past 23 years, I have experienced a number of different jobs with a variety of duties and responsibilities. I have worked for, and with, numerous professionals from administrators, educators, comptrollers, company presidents, physicians, nurses, Army officers, and dietitians. In each endeavor I have felt fortunate that my educational background at the undergraduate and graduate levels provided me with a set of knowledge, skills and abilities required to function effectively in any assignment.

Certainly a main factor for choosing a career in dietetics was that the Army offered experience, a guaranteed dietetic internship, pay while in college and numerous benefits. I hadn't planned on a twenty-year career in the Army, but because of my quest for more information through education, I chose to stay. I doubt that I would have obtained a Ph.D. had it not been for the Army Medical Specialist Corps. For this opportunity I am most appreciative.

I believe a primary factor in any career is that of continued learning. Through new knowledge comes new opportunities and new challenges. I was fortunate to be at the right place at the right time in many instances. However, I also believe that when presented with an opportunity, one must seize the moment for the opportunity may never be available again. I like new challenges and new experiences and my career in dietetics has afforded me this opportunity.

Dietetics has provided me an opportunity to learn, experience the wholesomeness of life and provided me a comfortable living. Had I desired to become wealthy, I probably would not have stayed in dietetics, for it is not a career where financial reward is the norm. However, because I like working with people, enjoy planning and implementing new ideas and enjoying the results, dietetics has and continues to be a good career choice for me.

My career is now at mid-point. I am searching for new directions and new challenges. I am certain that whatever direction I take, the foundation gained in dietetics will continue to be beneficial in the future as it has in the past.

Perspectives on the Profession

I entered the profession of dietetics in 1966 not really knowing what it was or where it would lead me. My personal perspective is that the profession has changed greatly in the last 23 years. The greatest change has come within the last ten years. Today, professionals entering dietetics want to become more involved in professional activities and move the profession forward. Young professionals want to be heard, they want to have a voice in policy making which can positively influence the nutritional knowledge and practices of the public.

Today, dietetics offers over 23 areas of practice from food systems management to pediatric practice. Dietitians can begin in one area of practice and move into other areas of practice rather rapidly. In addition, dietitians are in relatively high demand throughout the country so relocation is an asset to career advancement.

My greatest concerns, however, are that young dietitians need to understand the necessity to continually learn new information, be willing to work the number of hours it takes to complete the job and be willing to take risks. While in the position of General Manager of Personnel, I became concerned that young professionals were seeking a 40 hour workweek while expecting relative high entry level salaries. The two are not compatible. High salaries are paid to professionals willing to take risks, make unpopular decisions, work 50 to 60 hours per week, supervise others and consider their work a career, not just a job.

Dietetics, like many other professions, requires some degree of flexibility and mobility. Professionals not willing to move to other locations for more responsibility and growth should not expect employers to continually increase levels of compensation unless they can demonstrate increased profits, cost savings or improved services to their employers.

Another concern is the lack of dietitians who desire management positions. It seems there are fewer and fewer practitioners wanting management positions in health care institutions, in industry and in education. To move up the corporate ladder in any organization, practitioners must be willing to take risks, seize opportunities and sacrifice short term rewards for long term gains. The future of the profession will be determined in large part by the competence of today's practitioners. If we choose to relinquish management positions our competition will be happy to fill the void.

I believe the 1990's will bring more change to the profession of dietetics. Dietitians are becoming more entrepreneurial. More will enter business and industry, consulting and other innovative practice areas. There will continue to be a demand for dietitians in traditional health care settings, but a greater need will be for practitioners in new and different roles with food equipment manufacturers, restaurant chains, and in areas involving fitness and health. This new role will require individuals who are willing to take risks, who think about new ways of doing old things and who continually want to learn new strategies to improve organizational efficiency and effectiveness.

I am personally ready for the challenge.

Beula B. Marble

*Beula B. Marble, BS, 16th ADA President
and Recipient of the 1964 Marjorie Hulsizer Copher Award*

Imagine these as choices for your first position: teaching at the University of Washington, a therapeutic dietitian at the American Hospital of Beirut, or research in the Metabolic Research Unit at the Massachusetts General Hospital! Beula Marble chose the latter and thus began her professional career on Ward IV. She describes experiences such as preparing constant metabolic diets, experimenting with rats and ketogenic diets, planning food supplies for Admiral Byrd's first trip to the South Pole, and marrying one of the medical residents. She successfully combined marriage, family, career, and commitment to dietetics, serving as 16th President of ADA. Life has come full circle for Beula Marble; her career began on Ward IV and decades later she returned as a volunteer subject in a study on osteoporosis.

Beula B. Marble

This poem written in 1964 contains a synopsis of Mrs. Marble's first six decades. It was her response when she received the Copher Award, the highest honor bestowed by The American Dietetic Association.

It might be you—so singled out
    and pondering what to say.
The joy, the thrill which came at first
    to soberer thoughts give way,
To moments of reflection long
    to try to understand
What does this mean, this honor rare,
    and why it comes to hand.

It could be parents, now away,
    who gave me "vigah" (credit J.F.K.),
And made me think that work is fun,
    that almost anything can be done—
    if one tries.

The guiding hand of wise Kate Daum,
    of Quin and Mary P.*
were A.D.A. insurance
    in the fledgling days of B.**
The callowness of youth, perhaps,
    when all this started out,
Gave courage blind to take some steps
    which later rise with doubt.

A husband, great, who sets the pace
    in paths professional,
Who tact and patience has
    with foibles quite unmentionable.

There was a day, I well recall,
    when marriage and past-presidency
were double strikes against a gal
    and to the shelf the tendency.
    A shelf at thirty-four!

* Quindara Dodge
  Mary Huddleson
** Beula Marble

But afterwards our notions changed
    and there was more to do;
So back we came occasionally
    to do a job or two.
And now this hour. But why for me
    to be a spokesman? Possibly
To cite again our heritage
    of service to humanity.
Because we share ideals and goals,
    this honor is not mine alone,
But ours, —as inspiration for
    a future yet unknown.
QUAM PLURIMUS PRODESSE[1]

Soon after I started my first job in Boston in 1928, I met Frances Stern, an idol in Dietetics. Talking with her was a challenge—partly because I was awe-struck but chiefly because her sentences were often incomplete as her thoughts raced ahead of her tongue. My sentences may be incomplete too, albeit for a less worthy reason. My pen is headed for a chatty, informal style with many asides and digressions.

As I watch my grandson choosing college and career, I'm grateful that my choices came in the 20's when there were fewer options. Where to go to college was an easy choice after I won our county scholarship for the University of Illinois. [What good fortune for the oldest of six children during the Depression!] It covered all classes, even electives; lab expenses were covered, but I did have to pay for piano and organ practice rooms—not for lessons. [Required subject, gym, with minimum competency in swimming—passed with flying colors.]

Music was not my major—just icing on a Liberal Arts curriculum of English, history, math and science. Chemistry became my primary interest, particularly biochemistry. A dilemma was looming. This was a man's field. To compete, a woman had to be half-again as good as a man.

The Science of Nutrition was beginning to flourish. The leaders were Chittenden, Osborn and Mendel, McCollum, Francis G. Benedict. *THE* textbooks were written by Henry C. Sherman and Mary Swartz Rose.

Dr. Benedict was the only one of the ''greats'' that we knew. His Carnegie Nutrition Lab with its room-size and other basal metabolism apparatus was in Boston. Once a year he invited the Joslin Diabetes Clinic staff and wives to a party—a magic show. Dr. B. was a full-fledged member of the National Society of Magicians (I don't remember its correct terminology). After he retired from the laboratory, he was invited by university psychology departments to lecture about scientific observations as influenced by perceptions and preconceived ideas. Dr. Benedict had three ''long suits''—science,

1. Beula Becker Marble receives 1964 Marjorie Hulsizer Copher Award. Copyright The American Dietetic Association. Reprinted by permission from JOURNAL OF THE AMERICAN DIETETIC ASSOCIATION, Vol. 45:351, 1964.

magic, and circus. You may remember his monograph on the Physiology of the Elephant. We learned a lot from Dr. B. about the people involved in the Ringling Brothers Circus as well as how to make tests on an elephant.

Before the "famous people" interlude, I was about to say that a nutrition major in the Home Economics Department solved the gender dilemma for me. At this juncture, I was a junior with time for only a part of the Home Economics curriculum. It took later adult education courses to catch up with tailoring, arts and crafts, etc. To my regret, I am still delinquent in interior decorating.

I wanted to do graduate work and to have an internship. The University of Iowa was the only place where one could do both at the same time. But, I was advised not to apply. Why? The Department of Nutrition in the University Hospital had an outstanding reputation. It was organized and directed for several years by Dr. Ruth Wheeler, a physiologist. In 1925–26 she decided that the department should have a director with a long suit in administration. A well-qualified successor from the East survived in Iowa City for one year. She thought the doctors should have baked beans every Saturday night. There was a crisis with baked beans on the dining-room ceiling and a resignation.

In the summer of 1927, Dr. Kate Daum, new Director of the Nutrition Department, welcomed her first small class of interns—I was one of three. Dr. Daum had been doing nutrition research in the hospital and knew it well, so the transition was achieved without incident. She proved to be a good manager with uncanny ability to spot a potential problem and to head off trouble.

The word "internship" was peculiar to Iowa as was the name of its department. The usual terminology was "student dietitian" in a "Department of Dietetics." We made rounds with doctors and spent time with our patients on therapeutic diets. In this era, freedom to work on the wards one-to-one with patients was an extraordinary asset—not achieved in Boston for several more years. Our post-graduate courses were chiefly in the College of L.A. and the Medical School. My thesis work in mineral metabolism of infants honed my laboratory techniques, tested my ability to work 16-hour days, and gave me a taste of stage-fright—the oral exam. The Children's Building was an entity with its own kitchen. One of my last assignments was vacation relief for the administration dietitian. I planned an out-of-the-rut Sunday Supper, borrowed waffle irons, and blew the fuses in the dining room. In spite of this debacle, I was allowed to graduate from an internship with an M.S.

A choice of jobs was next. A Ph.D. candidate in our department invited me to teach with her at the University of Washington. The American Hospital of Beirut wanted a therapeutic dietitian. The Massachusetts General Hospital in Boston had an opening in its special research ward. Dr. Daum invited me to stay on in Iowa City. I wanted to try my wings away from the Middle West.

After 15 busy, happy months in Iowa City came 2 1/2 exciting years in Boston. I arrived, as scheduled, on September 1. For some reason, I don't remember what, Ward 4—the Metabolic Research Unit—would not open until a week later. I borrowed money and hopped the train to Ann Arbor for my first American Dietetic Association (ADA) convention. [This happened in 1928. ADA was founded in 1917.] Here were the dietetic pioneers in person. What an experience to be in their company!

On Ward 4, patients accepted CONSTANT diets, weighed on old platform balances, —with encouragement and cajoling— for several weeks of study (and monotony). Part of the routine for low-calcium diets was to bake our own bread and to make fudge for calories. An extra loaf of hot bread, followed by many residents and nurses, sometimes made its way into my "office" with its big hand-me-down roll-top desk. This "office" was a big room used for storage and occasionally for an extra patient or two. Caring for eight patients was a comfortable workload for one dietitian and her student. Twelve patients created a big challenge. Even with a second student dietitian, we were working from 6 A.M. to 10 P.M. This was when I started a life-long custom—reading in bed to unwind.

Most of our patients were studied for mineral metabolism. I was not a complete novice on the team because of my thesis lab experience and summer jobs during college in a cement mill laboratory, analyzing limestone and cement—quantitative chemistry— and in the mill pond, trying to learn to dive. [My chest was black and blue all summer.]

There were some children on Ward 4 who were on ketogenic diets for epilepsy. I was so concerned about their bone growth on low mineral intakes that I started a group of rats on ketogenic diets. One of the Residents helped me in the Animal Farm. Results:

1. The rats did not become ketogenic.
2. I married the Resident.

Teaching Harvard medical students was a new venture for a dietitian at M.G.H. We used the nurses' food lab, preparing and eating the diets they prescribed and wrote for patients.

Another side-line venture during my Ward 4 years was planning food supplies for Admiral Byrd's first trip to the South Pole. How much of the plan was used, I don't know. I shudder mentally as I remember this experience. [How could I stick my neck out so far? I hadn't even had camping experience!] The courage of youth is now tempered by the caution of age.

Harvard Medical School awarded a Moseley Traveling Fellowship to Dr. Marble. Boston was blustery in January, 1931 as we set sail across the North Atlantic to warm and sunny Madeira, the Mediterranean, Monaco and Italy.

A few of many memories: children alongside the ship diving for coins, a gambling casino, art, architecture, the Coliseum, hillsides of orange trees—oranges in profusion! As a child, the only orange I saw was in the toe of my Christmas stocking.

After a few days in Naples, Rome, Florence and Venice, we took a train trip over the Alps to Vienna and saw moonlight skiers on the mountains. Getting our first meal in Vienna gave us our first German lesson. Restaurants and our landlady were our language teachers. Memories: feather beds, tiled Kackelofen, giant bathtub (baths by appointment and fee) —palaces, bent-over beggars (sequelae of WW I)—overrated Sacher Torte, opera (standing at the rear of the fourth balcony)—Lippinzaner horses in the

Spanish Riding School, the Boys' Choir in St. Stephens—Schubert, Beethoven, Strauss. A bus holiday in the Tyrol was a scenic delight with one shocking night. Our neighbors had a prolonged vociferous argument—my first and only exposure to a marital fight.

After three months it was time for study in Wurzburg. The professor's wife came to call. Looking askance, she advised us to move. The room we had found was in the red-light district. The next room was on Roentgenstrasse. (Dr. Roentgen discovered X-ray in Wurzburg.) Our landlady's son was a "brown-shirt," training undercover in Hitler's Youth Movement. We heard Hitler speak at a semi-clandestine meeting. Nine months later we saw and heard him rabble-rousing in the open in Berlin.

German classes at the University combined with private lessons enabled us to read fairly, not very, well. We boarded a crowded train in a half-empty coach and were summarily ejected. It was for Kriegsvershadicte (war wounded). A summer day of boating on the Main River with German friends resulted in fatigued gray cells [conversing was still difficult], aching muscles [our rented craft was a rowboat, not the intended Faltboat], and a scalding sunburn.

Dr. S. and Professor G. invited us to their homes for a taste of German family life. The friendships formed there lasted over many years with happy reunions at later international meetings. The best and best-remembered parts of other trips to Europe, South America and Japan are the hours spent with people in their homes.

Margery Abrahams was our "god-mother" for six months in London. She was an Oxford graduate intrigued by the new profession of Dietetics which was further advanced in the U.S. than in England. She did graduate work at Columbia with Dr. Sherman and Mary Swartz Rose and visited dietetics departments in the U.S. She had heard about Ward 4 and came to learn about diets in metabolic research. Margery then opened and directed a Dietetics Department in St. Bartholomew's Hospital. She welcomed me as a volunteer member of her staff.

Tinned tomatoes, all canned foods, were unacceptable in Britain. Mutton, well aged on the hoof, and over-cooked Brussel sprouts were frequent fare atoned for by delicious steamed puddings, especially the upside-down ones with treacle or strawberry jam. We loved having tea with good goodies at four and dinner at eight, huddled close to our shilling-fed fireplace, toasting on the front side and freezing on the back side. Central heating in England was still anathema.

Margery entertained us many times in her flat and at her country estate in Amersham—[She even took us to the resort hotel in Brighton, where she chose to go to recover from a bad case of adult measles.]—tea served in bed to start the day, strawberries in February from her greenhouse. Stimulating conversation at her dinner parties was accompanied by smoking—no ill effects suspected at that time. I tried it but didn't have my own holder for serious smoking until my early 30's.

The pound took a tumble during our six months in London. This stretched our dollars enough to pay for six weeks in Berlin at the University's Institute for Auslander with students from 39 countries. All of us were struggling with the language. Morning classes used a magazine—similar to *People* with lots of pictures—newspapers, and elementary school textbooks. One showed maps of Europe with the areas lost by Germany in World War I colored bright red. German children were learning that the red areas should again be part of Germany—seeds of World War II. Afternoons were spent in the theater, museums, and sightseeing with our teachers. Chinese and American students were worst of all in speaking German—we swallowed our L's. Finally I was able to get by in beauty parlor conversation without being recognized as a foreigner.

It was spring. Students could fly "stand-by" at 3rd class rates. On a beautiful sunny day we saw acres of flowering tulips in Holland on our way to Rotterdam and our ship to the States.

In 1932 Dr. Marble started his 60-year tenure at the Joslin Diabetes Center in Boston. I found a job in a mini-Ward 4 with Dr. Joseph C. Aub, who had started the research ward at the M.G.H. In his move up the academic ladder at Harvard Medical School, he succeeded Dr. George R. Minot [Nobel Prize—pernicious anemia—raw liver cocktail] as director of a small cancer research hospital. There I spent part time working with patients and part time in the laboratory where my course in histology at Iowa City helped me learn to prepare slides and count mitotic figures in regenerating rat liver. Tissue culture was an entirely new skill for me to learn. Aluminum poisoning from cooking utensils was a popular concern (early thirties). Rats again! I fed them bread made with different levels of aluminum. No cancer. (1989—Aluminum concern again).

In 1939 I was President-elect of The American Dietetic Association—and pregnant! I was happy to give up lab work for several months. We were giving 20–40 hours a week to ADA work. Except for time abroad, I had been involved in professional activities: Program Committee, Diet Therapy Section Chairman, and President of the Massachusetts Dietetic Association; Membership Committee, Secretary, Diet Therapy Section Chairman, Vice-president, President-elect, and President of ADA (Dull reading but fun doing.)

Past Presidents were expected to pack up and disappear from professional activity. I did for a while. Later I was invited to work in the House of Delegates, Journal and Internship Boards, Nominating and History Committees and on a Code of Ethics Committee.

Ethics and professionalism are of abiding interest to me. The latter, to a classicist, is now history. Today anybody with a special skill calls himself professional. Service to others was primary to the original professions—theology, medicine and law. Dietitians cherished the concept of service for many years. We used to have a participatory class with about 50 Boston interns. It was called "Professional Perspectives." Annie Galbraith wrote this encouraging comment: "Interns are richer for this all-too-brief session—discussion does not end with dismissal of class."

Students in many guises have been a source of inspiration and rarely of headaches. Who wouldn't admire women in a two-hour dinnertime class at the end of a hard day's work or a medical student who became a Nobel Prize winner? Headaches: a dishonest student and another who borrowed a rare book and kept it.

155

Combining family and career responsibilities was not the norm when I did it. It was a bit queer, but logical with a husband who worked 12–15 hours a day. I expected to play second fiddle to patients and was happy and out of mischief when I was busy too.

Soon after our daughter joined the family, World War II was in the offing. Her father went on active duty before Pearl Harbor as Chief of Medicine in an Army hospital on Cape Cod. When he was transferred, we went with him to Texas and later to Chicago. Moving meant leaving friends (a bit traumatic for a child) and making new ones (easy). Otherwise we have pleasant memories of Army life.

As the war was winding down, Betsy and I came home to start first grade and part-time teaching of nutrition to junior and senior college classes. Part-time help was available for teaching mornings. Betsy had care and company in case she couldn't go to school. I could do most of my work at home. When reading of papers palled, the garden called.

Gardening in New England is a challenge. We came home from a New Hampshire week-end with small birch and pine trees, expecting to plant them the same evening. We couldn't even dig holes—rock, rock, rock.

We acquired a pick ax and laboriously dug some holes only to find very little soil and that was poor. So, off to buy loam (called loom here) and fertilizer. Over the years we learned enough about gardening to have an all white hillside rock garden as backdrop for our daughter's wedding reception. Nowadays I am content with lighted shelves and a condominium balcony for container gardening.

Eight decades is enough time for lots of hobbies—singing [E. Power Biggs was our organist and choir director], piano, organ, painting, embroidery, three-dimensional decoupage, crosswords, bridge, and enameling.

It's strange how things dovetail. My best enameling was inspired by a guest lecturer in an advanced nutrition course. I taught at Simmons College. Dr. L. showed us some of the marvelous and beautiful secrets hidden in a cell as revealed by the new electron microscope. On my tile top table: fat globule with mitochondria, DNA double helix, RNA amino acid formation, insulin granules and mitochondria, etc. . . . .

Church work has run the gamut of "women's jobs" followed by a few "men's jobs." Civic involvement included the National Nutrition Advisory Committee during World War II, a few years as Consumer Consultant to the Food and Drug Administration, Fred Stare's committee to enact legislation requiring enrichment of bread and flour in Massachusetts. Local involvement—Advisory Committee on Adult Education, Health Council, Health Fair, and the League of Women Voters. [League work is like Church work—both have a propensity to become full time.] It was League experience in town affairs that occasioned my appointment to a Selectmen's Committee to study Appointment vs Election of Assessors in Brookline. There was a young lawyer on this committee who ran for President of the United States in 1988—Michael Dukakis.

The editors asked about honors. I thought it was an honor to be invited to appear in a "Who's Who." I don't remember which one. Our daughter has copies of "Women of the World'' and ''Who's Who in the East'' which lists both of her parents. At first we dutifully bought the books as they appeared. The number of Who's Whos proliferated, each with frequent revisions and high prices. I felt suckered. My feeling of honor succumbed to admission of vanity.

Here are examples of pride—the Seal of The American Dietetic Association and an idea for a Refresher Course in the Nutrition in the 30's. As far as we know it was a ''first,'' a forerunner of Continuing Education.

Valued honors include Phi Beta Kappa in my junior year, Omicron Nu, Iota Sigma Pi, the Copher Award, and Honorary President of the Massachusetts Dietetic Association.

In 1975, I fell victim to a vicious attack of shingles in my left shoulder. Despite excellent medical care, I still have constant pain—post-herpetic neuralgia. Anything touching or moving on the shoulder exacerbates the pain, so clothes are anathema. Bare is best, but I do not want to hibernate. A combination of elasticized tops, cashmere sweaters, gritting my teeth and distraction allow me to go about my business.

My life has come full circle. My first job was on the research ward at the Massachusetts General Hospital. Sixty years later I am a patient on the same ward, a volunteer subject in an osteoporosis study.

Here's to the future! Yours and ours, especially yours.

Marion Mason

*Marion Mason, PhD, RD is the Ruby Winslow Linn
Professor of Nutrition, Simmons College, Boston*

Goal setting, mentorship, networking and team playing are all important considerations in the establishment of a successful career according to Dr. Marion Mason. Well known as the senior author of the textbook *The Dynamics of Clinical Dietetics*, she is a renowned educator and professional. Through her early work with the Visiting Nurse Association, Dr. Mason was responsible for the grant which funded the first meals-on-wheels program in the city of Chicago. She has served on the editorial board of the Journal of The American Dietetic Association and is herself an avid writer. Her dedicated work as Chairman of the Ambulatory Nutrition Care Research Study Committee shed invaluable light on how cost benefit and cost effectiveness techniques could be applied in clinical settings. This resulted in the publication of ''The Cost and Benefits of Nutritional Care: Phase 1,'' which raised the consciousness of ADA members in the areas of fiscal accountability and reimbursement for services. Dr. Mason was director of the graduate program in medical dietetics at Ohio State and now holds the Ruby Winslow Linn Endowed Chair in Nutrition at Simmons College in Boston.

Marion Mason

A good friend of mine, Dr. Margaret Hennig, is the senior author of *The Managerial Woman*. Over the years, I have learned a lot about career planning from her. Goal-setting, for example, is of primary concern to women starting out in their careers; establishing a five year plan to lend direction to a career is another concern. Finding and cultivating a mentor, establishing a network and learning to work on a team are other important considerations in the establishment of a successful career. I know that I have broken a few cardinal rules (i.e., goal setting and five year plans), but I've managed, through very little concerted effort on my part, to find mentors, network and to work on teams. My career has developed and flourished over the years through a series of happy accidents, encounters and circumstances. The net result has been that I have had a wonderful time and feel richly rewarded about my great good luck in my career over the past 35 years.

As far as my family is concerned, I have two claims to fame. One is that my cousin Tommie was Walt Disney's private secretary. The other is that my great aunt, Mary England Cranwell, was an assistant (today's dietetic technician) to Lenna Frances Cooper at the Battle Creek Sanitarium during the period of time when Miss Cooper was busy in Cleveland writing the constitution of the upstart group, The American Dietetic Association. My Aunt Mary was a 'presence' in my life until her death soon after I finished my master's degree, so I had ample opportunity to learn from her.

I entered Miami University in Oxford, Ohio, in 1951. It was the school of choice because my family knew a successful graduate, it was reasonably inexpensive ($50/semester for in-state tuition) and the Admissions Office was willing to take me. As was the fashion of the day (the decade following the end of World War II), young women who were college bound most often elected majors that were "traditionally female" and this is exactly what I did. I enrolled in the program in Vocational Home Economics Education and discovered in a relatively short time that I hated it. Before much time had passed, however, I was presented with an opportunity that seemed at the time to be a major defeat, but turned out to be a turning point for me. At the end of my freshman year, my father died and harder times came to my family. In the fall, I went to work for my room and board; my job was to dry the glasses and silverware at the end of the meal for two dining rooms, each serving about 100 people (I guess I *am* from the dark ages—this was the days before Miami installed large dish machines in its food service facilities.). I worked three meals a day, six days a week. The biggest liabilities to this job were that I was unable to have meals with my friends and the work was boring. The latter liability turned out to be the greatest asset, however, since as I stood there, bored to tears, I began to watch all the workers in the kitchen. Over time, I became fascinated with what they were doing, watching and making mental notes. In a matter of months, I was launched in my career in Dietetics and I have never looked back.

My next encounter with the world of Dietetics turned out to be one of the major milestones of my career. I was lucky—I was only 19 years old, but I applied for and got my first job in the profession as a summer student, working as a food service supervisor at the University of Michigan Hospitals (my family had moved back to Ann Arbor during the previous academic year). It was during that summer that I met a number of people who have been important to me both personally and professionally over the past 35 years. On the staff at the time were both Dr. Virginia Vivian, now retired from the faculty at The Ohio State University, and Dr. Margaret Wilson, the first Director of Education at ADA and now with the federal government in Washington; the dietetic interns included Darlene Erlander, once of the faculty of the School of Nursing at Cornell-New York Hospital and now deceased, and Joan L. Sharp, to become president of the professional society a quarter of a century later and now retired as Director of Dietetics at The Ohio State University Hospitals. Each of these people helped me, in one way or another with my career over the years. In addition, Dar Erlander taught me an important lesson in living and that is how to cope with the death of a friend.

I had a number of interesting experiences at the U of M, not the least of which was watching the birth of a baby. A physician whom I had fed at odd hours at the Women's Hospital made arrangements for me to sit in the spectators' gallery in one of the delivery rooms. This was pretty heady stuff in those days, too! I was so encouraged by all of my experiences that I applied for a summer intern's position for the next year at the Ann Arbor Veterans' Administration Hospital. Lucky me again, I got the appointment and met up with one of the more memorable people in my life, Grace Stumpf, Director of Dietetics. I began to learn about dedication to the profession from Grace; I also learned something about horses and dogs, the latter one of the major passions of her life (and mine, too, I guess).

Eventually I graduated from Miami, having survived student teaching in the University school where I had a class of eighth grade boys and girls for an entire semester (the longest 18 weeks of my life). Since I was a small town girl (so to speak), from a small town college (Oxford, Ohio isn't much even with the 5000 undergraduates who were underfoot when I was there), I decided to head for the big city. With great good luck, I landed in Boston at the Massachusetts General Hospital and had the most wonderful year of my life, bar none. What was even luckier, I knew it was a great year while I was living it! Wow! I got to live in a brownstone mansion on the corner of Commonwealth and Berkeley; I shared a room on the front with two other dietetic interns, one of whom is still in my life on a regular basis. I got to work in one of the most historic hospitals in the world; I went to lectures in the Ether Dome; I made trips to Quincy Market at 7:00 in the morning to buy fruits and vegetables for the entire hospital; I went to MDA meetings in a hat and gloves (yes, a hat and gloves, even to the fish market at 6 in the morning!); I went to the theatre and to Orchestra Hall for the Boston Symphony and to the Esplanade for the Boston Pops and to THE OCEAN! And, of course, I had the opportunity to work with Louise Hatch, Director of Dietetics and Copher Award Winner in 1976, and other professionals on the staff. All in all, it was a great year and I was sorry to see it come to an end. Seventeen years later I returned to Boston, partly because of my positive feelings about the city and the MGH. I left the General with a commitment to the profession, and to the professional society, but with a rather narrow view of the world (the same narrow view that almost every other 22 year old in the world has). I didn't realize that my education had hardly begun.

My first job, started in the fall of 1956, was in the School of Nursing at the University of Rochester in upstate New York. I was an assistant instructor (a rank so low that I think its been abolished in more humane institutions today), hired to teach nursing students something about nutrition and dietetics and paid the handsome sum of $280/month plus two meals/day (not such a bad deal when you think about it). My home base in the hospital was the diet kitchen, where I was in charge of teaching the students how to prepare simple, nourishing meals and snacks for the patients when there was no one else around to handle the chores. Shades of my Aunt Mary! The nursing students weren't too happy about this phase of their training, but I tried to ignore their opinions on the subject. I also treated myself to an education in the medical center. I went to grand rounds; I found the observation booth for one of the operating rooms and watched countless surgical procedures; I spent hours in the medical library. I finally decided that I couldn't spend my life working in the diet kitchen, so I went off to graduate school at The Ohio State University after two years on the job. Again, a smart move that turned out to be more significant that I would have ever dreamed.

When I arrived in Columbus on the first of July 1958, I discovered there friends from my Michigan days. Jo Sharp was in the same Residency and Master's program, and Marge Wilson was a doctoral student, housed in Preventive Medicine with Jo and me. Jo and Betsy Biggar Holli and I were "the" nutrition students for the year; other students were in the occupational medicine and aviation medicine programs in Preventive Medicine. The chairman of the department was Dr. William Ashe, one of the finest physicians with whom I have every worked; the guiding light of the nutrition program was Martha Nelson Lewis, without a doubt the most important mentor I ever had. This department became the initial home of the Ohio State Medical Dietetics program, the first coordinated undergraduate program in the country. Medical Dietetics eventually became the backbone of the School of Allied Medical Professions at OSU; I was lucky, again, to be around during the incubation time. With me in Columbus at that time was Burness Wenberg, now of the faculty of Michigan State University, and to be my co-author twenty years later. Grace Stumpf was Director of Dietetics at OSU Hospitals.

I learned three important lessons in Columbus. The first was that the profession of Dietetics and the professional society are, in the scheme of things, very small worlds. I had not anticipated that people I knew in Ann Arbor would turn up in Columbus; this was my first lesson in networking. I continue to network to this day, a practice which I consider paramount for getting things done in the world and, not incidentally, for getting ahead in my own career.

The next lesson resulted in a healthy respect for research. The degree required a thesis, so we were all up to our eyebrows in one or another of Mrs. Lewis' pet projects.

It seems to me now that the topic of the day involved the gastrointestinal tract and that we were all feeding each other or innocent patients something or another, followed by data collection in some form. Nothing we ever did made a difference in any lives, except our own. I was expected to write an article for publication, which I did. It was published, too, as a filler in the JOURNAL. I was thrilled! The darned thing hangs on my office wall to this day. It was this experience which led me to the realization that the value of a master's thesis is that it serves as a practice for the doctoral dissertation.

The third lesson I learned was that Mrs. Lewis was henceforth in charge of my professional life. The same is true for all of Mrs. Lewis' "girls," as any one of them would be quick to acknowledge. Mrs. Lewis, Copher Award Winner in 1968, was a past master in the art of arranging a life before the occupant knew what had hit. The "arrangements" were always for "the best"—an additional course, more subjects, another paragraph, more consultation, more responsibilities, a new job, a new town. It's safe to say, that on the whole, Mrs. Lewis' students, current and former, were in agreement with her and just about did what Martha Nelson thought best. For me, it meant three new jobs and another degree. Further, I believe there is not any one of Mrs. Lewis' students who would not have given her the moon if she had asked. Oh, to be so regarded by one's students!

A year later, when Mrs. Lewis let me venture out into the world again, I took the most important job of my life. Since I considered myself an authority on working with nurses, and an educated(!) nutritionist as well, I went off to Chicago to serve as the first nutrition consultant with the Visiting Nurse Association (VNA) of Chicago. The VNA is a private public health nursing agency which, in 1959, had a staff of 125 nurses and perhaps two or three physical therapists, ten sub-stations (neighborhood offices) and a headquarters office in the Loop. The ten offices were spread all over the city of Chicago; it was my job to visit each of them on a regular basis. I worked with all of the staff nurses in group in-service education programs and then consulted with many on an individual basis to discuss particular clients and appropriate ways to handle nutrition related problems. I also had my own case load of clients, whom I saw on a regular basis for one reason or another. Most of them had been discharged from area hospitals with inadequate preparation for dealing with the significant changes in food intakes which were dictated by their health (or lack thereof, as the case may be).

Since my "territory" was the entire city of Chicago (which can be a pretty big place when traveling via subway, bus and foot as I did for the first 18 months on the job), I went into the homes of people in all socioeconomic brackets. I visited very nice apartment units on the near north side (the "Gold Coast") and I visited the worst tenements the city had to offer. I was not usually afraid, however, as the blue VNA uniform was known and respected throughout the city. I never knew such poverty existed and I was never the same again. I no longer cared about total compliance—I was thrilled with one small change for the better. The staff nurses, in my opinion, performed heroics on a daily basis. I no longer cared if they knew much about sodium restricted diets—I was thrilled if they had a chance to talk about salt or baking soda with their patients and, in the most dire of circumstances, referred them to me. At last I became a human being.

I was housed in an office near 47th and Halstead, in a neighborhood known as the "Back of the Yards," just down the street from Mayor Daley's home. On a warm August day, when the wind was blowing just right, the smell from stockyards was overpowering. My office companions, physical therapists and nurses responsible for other aspects of staff education, and I would escape from the smell and the heat as often as possible. Mostly, though, we were "out in the field" supporting the staff nurses in their daily activities.

These were heady days for me and I partook of what life had to offer. Since the agency offered tuition benefits to the staff, I enrolled in a foodservice course with Fern Gleiser, an ADA past president, at the near north campus of the University of Chicago. The only thing I remember from the classroom was that one should always choose china that is a food color (i.e., never select black plates)! After class, which met once a week, we adjourned to a local watering hole for the most important part of the course.

We were also expected to write a term paper on a subject of interest that had some remote relationship to foodservice management. Since I had lived in Rochester, NY, where Elizabeth Henry had started one of the first meals-on-wheels programs in the country (at the Rochester VNA), I decided to take on a feasibility study of meals-on-wheels in Chicago for my paper. The 125 staff nurses, at my behest, set out to count how many clients would agree to benefit from such a program. I took their data and turned it into my term paper for Fern Gleiser. From there I took it to a committee of the Welfare Council of Metropolitan Chicago. Since this group was chaired by a member of the Board of Directors of the VNA, I had a hearing. Eventually the data served as the basis for a successful grant application which brought to Chicago almost $400,000 to fund the city's first meals-on-wheels program, a lot of money in those days. I remain proud of this achievement.

Not long after I joined the VNA staff, I was invited to a meeting of the Chicago Nutrition Council. This was a small group of nutritionists who were united originally, I believe, because of their affiliation with the University of Chicago. The members included Ethel Austin Martin, author and nutrition educator with the National Dairy Council for years; Lydia Roberts, author, member of the first Committee of Dietary Allowances of the Food and Nutrition Board, educator and mentor of some of the leading nutrition professionals of the day; and Anna Boller Beach, nutritionist in the ambulatory unit of St. Luke's-Presbyterian Hospital, first executive secretary, Cooper lecturer and past president of ADA. Mrs. Beach's living room was the first headquarters office of ADA; Mrs. Beach, then Anna Boller, and her mother were the staff. Well, since I had grown up with a person associated with the founding of ADA (my Aunt Mary), I was aware that I was in the presence of "history" and I had a wonderful time with these women, the super achievers of their day. Even today I stand in awe of the fact that *I* knew a member of the first RDA committee. Wow!

The Chicago Nutrition Council met on the first Monday of every month at Wieboldt's department store in the Loop. Since they had a cafeteria and gave us a private dining room for free, it was a great deal. We had a secretary, who, on occasion, gave us an update on the financial health of the organization and then asked us for a quarter to pay for mailing (no, I am not kidding). The speaker, whenever there was one, was a person in town for other purposes (there was no way we could finance a speaker on 25 cents per month). It was a time for information sharing and story swapping and networking. I thought it was the grandest time of all.

As an aside, I might add that Wieboldt's did not have a bar. Mrs. Beach and I, therefore, met at 5 pm at a nearby restaurant. It was during these occasions that I heard the stories about the early days of ADA. Mrs. Beach and I remained pals all the days until her death some years later.

One winter's day in 1963 I was invited, again, to join the faculty of the University of Rochester (U of R), this time as an assistant professor (up the academic ladder at last). Since I was never really happy living in such a large city, Rochester looked good to me and I was pleased to be invited back to an academic environment in a quality medical center. In addition, I missed being around young learners. I was sorry to leave Chicago, but I looked forward to Rochester.

I hadn't been back in academia very long when it came to me, that in order to stay in teaching, I needed to go back to school for the doctoral degree. So I applied to a number of graduate schools and finally settled on Cornell University, primarily because of the presence of Charlotte Young on the faculty of the Graduate School of Nutrition. I then spent the better part of three years taking tuition-free courses on a parttime basis at the U of R (a great faculty benefit because a course then cost the magnificent sum of $400). Among other things, I took quantitative analysis one semester; it met two nights a week for 2 hours each and every Saturday from noon to 6 pm. I decided that if I could pass quant, I could do a doctoral degree and, eventually, I did.

I arrived at Cornell in the fall of 1966 and immediately plunged into the life of a new graduate student. Since I was a novice, and hence, did not know the system, I let my temporary advisor sign me up for the worst possible course load. I shared an office on the fourth floor of Martha Van with a number of veterans who finally took pity on me and told me how to manage the work load; I immediately dropped a course. Biochemistry met four mornings a week at 8 am, including Saturdays. The lab met all day on Thursdays, except for an hour out to go to Statistics (big deal). Sometimes we finished up in lab at 5 or 6 pm and sometimes at 9 or 10 at night. It was an exhausting experience but I learned a valuable lesson and that was that I did not want to spend my life as a laboratory researcher. (I might add that the laboratories of the world breathed a sigh of relief!)

In the spring it was "suggested" that I put together a doctoral committee and I chose for the chairman Dr. Jerry Rivers, researcher and scholar in the area of ascorbic acid metabolism. Since I was in Food and Nutrition, a unit then separate from the Graduate School of Nutrition, Dr. Young could not chair my committee and, as it all turned out later, it was just as well. The third person on my committee was a nationally known authority on intergroup relations, Dr. Robin Williams, Jr. I happily took a minor in sociology under Dr. Williams; I learned a lot about the discipline and found the research techniques fascinating. Jerry Rivers turned out to be a great chairman as she allowed me to develop my thesis problem with minimal interference on her part. She also helped me finish the degree in a humane period of time.

I was lucky more than once during my time at Cornell. Not only was I a graduate student in one of the best departments in the country, able to study with famous and accomplished people, I competed for and won graduate awards from the professional society, from the US Public Health Service and from Cornell. In 1967, I won, along with Eileen Matthews of the University of Wisconsin, the Mead Johnson Award for graduate studies in Dietetics. The next year I won the Hazel Hauck Fellowship for graduate education. I was really thrilled at the honor of the ADA awards and, needless to say, happy to have the money (I recall one time that I had 12 cents in my checking account).

In the fall of 1967, Mr. Mead Johnson wrote to me, extending congratulations and offering his support in the future. Seizing the opportunity, I wrote back and asked for 4200 ascorbic acid-free prenatal vitamin supplements, packaged in bottles of 30. Since the supplements were crucial to my research, I was pretty happy when they arrived, air express, in time for me to start my work in the prenatal clinic at the University of Rochester in the summer of 1968. My exchanges with Mr. Johnson only served to reinforce my view that its often useful to start at the top.

In the spring of 1969, Mrs. Lewis and faculty of the Medical Dietetics Division of the School of Allied Medical Professions at Ohio State invited me back, this time to join the faculty and I accepted. I arrived in the fall of 1969, shiny new degree in hand, to start work as an associate professor (once more up the academic ladder). My job was to serve primarily as the leader of the group looking after the graduate program but I worked with the undergraduate students as well. Mrs. Lewis had retired in the summer, but Jo Sharp was in place in the service unit in the hospital and Burness Wenberg was doing the bulk of the administrative work to keep the undergraduate program going. We were still housed, at that time, in the old hospital building, where my non-air conditioned office faced west, affording me the benefits of the hot afternoon sun and giving me a great view of the morgue entrance. (We did move, a year or so later, into a building which was funded by federal monies awarded on the basis of a grant authored primarily by Burness.) Linnea Anderson, of Anderson, Dibble, Mitchell and Rynbergen fame, was the pediatric nutritionist in Medical Dietetics. Sally Seubert and Gail Harrison, friends from Cornell, were also on the faculty.

A small parade of graduate students marched through during my days at Ohio State. We worked on a number of research problems and published a few papers, none of them earth shattering, but nonetheless we did useful work and tried to share it with others. I enjoyed the graduate students as they brought interesting life experiences with them and they were usually serious about being in school. They caused me to become curious about problems that I never before considered. I worked hard to create environments in which they could learn and equally as hard not to be a hindrance to their learning.

After I had been at Ohio State for while, I volunteered for the Board of Editors of the Journal of The American Dietetic Association. This was my way of making some effort to repay the professional society for the support given to me as a graduate student. And talk of happy encounters! Members of the board during those days (1971–74) included Myrtle Brown (of Pike and Brown fame), Grace Ostenso (now a ''staffer'' on the House of Representatives' Committee on Science and Technology) and my Mead Johnson award pal, Eileen Matthews. I felt privileged to work with these women, and with Dorothea Turner and Harriet Sankey. I gained a lot from the Board meetings and from the actual reviewing of the articles sent me; it was a great opportunity to learn about what other people were thinking. I would guess that my interest in writing dates from my first term on the Board (I served a second term in the mid-80's).

In the winter of 1972, the provost of Simmons College wrote to me out of the blue, asking if I would consider coming to Boston to join the faculty. No, I replied, I would not. A very little time passed when I heard from him again, this time offering me the endowed chair in nutrition; on this occasion I paid more attention. An endowed chair, after all, was nothing to be scoffed at. More time passed while I thought about returning to Boston and undergraduate education, and leaving the graduate students and the medical center and my Ohio State friends. Eventually the lure of undergraduate teaching and the reward of the endowed chair won out and I returned to Boston in January, 1973, to start the major phase of my career (once more up the academic ladder). Simmons started a new phase, too, since the Department of Nutrition came into being with my arrival. Some time later the endowed chair was named for its donor, Ruby Winslow Linn, Simmons College class of 1932, distinguished for her long career in the military and Copher Award winner in recent years.

One of the first new courses added to the curriculum soon after my arrival was a beginning clinical practice course, based a great deal, of course, on my Ohio State experiences. Our practice site was the old Boston Lying-In Hospital, located just up the street, on the same block as the College. Our purpose in offering the course was to give the undergraduates some sense of what it would be like to practice dietetics in a clinical setting, focusing primarily on client counseling. Although we have shifted the practice site to an acute care facility one block away, the course remains just about the same in purpose. And, of course, in 1973, there was no text; I discovered that my colleague, Burness Wenberg, by then on the faculty of Michigan State, was thinking the same great thoughts as me—Write the book!

Write the book? Surely you jest, we said to each other. And soon we were sketching the outline, drafting a proposal for publishers' considerations and adding a third author, P. Kay Welsch, then a graduate student in education at Michigan State and working for Burness, and now an ordained minister with her own church in rural Wisconsin. I asked for and received a year's leave from Simmons (a year which eventually became two). On the day after Labor Day in 1975, I started in; I delivered the finished manuscript to our editor on St. Patrick's Day in 1977. *The Dynamics of Clinical Dietetics* was a labor of love, not a labor for financial return. It has had extraordinary success, I believe, for a text written for such a limited audience. The biggest thrill for me is to be recognized, by a young practitioner, as the senior author of a familiar book.

The second edition, published in 1982 following my sabbatical leave, is probably the last edition as well. There are two reasons for this development: One is that I grew weary of spending my leave time in solitude (successful writing of first drafts is done alone). The second is that there are now available a small number of equally good books, covering much of the same material. One, in fact, is authored by Betsy Biggar Holli, my classmate at Ohio State 30 years ago. I like to think, though, that Mason, Wenberg, and Welsch set the pace and the standard; I believe that few would argue with me. Writing about philosophy and practice in clinical dietetics has probably been the most rewarding experience of my career; I think this is so because we have helped to guide the practice of a whole generation of dietitians.

As an aside, I would just like to mention how scary Day 1 was! There I was, all set up in my finished attic loft, big dining room table to write on, file cabinets full of old reprints and class materials, a very large dictionary, a rebuilt standard typewriter (these were prehistoric times), years worth of JOURNALS, a box full of sharpened pencils and 1500 sheets of clean paper. Wow! It took until Christmas to write the first chapter. Once I got going, a good day was a whole new page—and revisions of the previous day's work. Not every day was full of writing, however, as I was teaching parttime, once again at the University of Rochester, this time as a Visiting Professor (a far cry from Assistant Instructor).

I returned to Simmons in the fall of 1977, just after the Department had moved into new quarters in the Park Science Center. The chairman at the time was Dr. Pat Kreutler, now working in the food industry; on the faculty was Rena Mendelson, a Cornell graduate and doctoral student at Harvard, and Nancie Harvey Herbold, doctoral student at Boston University. Eventually Rena returned to her home in Toronto and Carole Dichter, also a Harvard doctoral student, arrived to replace her. As a department, we have spent years on the new baby-graduate student routines, but it was rewarding and we had a good time. At the time of this writing, the faculty all hold the terminal degree and the youngest offspring is approaching 11 years. I have been richly rewarded from my associations with the Simmons faculty, both within the department and throughout the college. It has been particular joy for me to work with Nancie Herbold, my professional alter ego.

The next decade at Simmons brought a number of challenges for me, including a four year stint on the Committee on Tenure and Appointment (two as chairman), a semester at the National Institutes of Health in Washington, major curriculum revisions and a protracted defense of nutrition as a science on the floor of the all-college faculty meetings. In 1984, I was invited to be part of a two person program for the annual Mary Swartz Rose lecture of the Greater New York Dietetic Association. Anita Owen, since then an ADA President, was charged with looking at the future; I, because of my white hair, I guess, was charged with an examination of the past. Since I couldn't narrow the topic and still do justice to the professional society, I used Simmons as a microcosm of the profession's history. Imagine my delight when I discovered three ADA presidents had once been members of the Simmons faculty (Beulah Becker Marble, Quindara Dodge and Margaret Ross). Marjorie Hulsizer Copher, she of the Copher award, graduated from the college in time to serve in Europe with the Red Cross during World War I. Ellen Swallow Richards, founder of the American Home Economics Association, taught at Simmons in its early days, just after the turn of the century. The college archives are named for Miriam Perry Goll, class of 1930, first dietitian in the US Air Force. The tradition goes on today, as witnessed by examination of current candidates for office in professional associations, both on the local and national levels, a review of the authors of papers in scholarly journals, and textbooks, and the roster of individuals in top positions in a variety of educational, health care and food industry organizations. To say that I am proud of Simmons alumnae and their accomplishments is a vast understatement!

At the same time that I returned to Simmons from my writing stint, I was asked by Jo Sharp, then ADA President-elect, to chair a national committee charged with the task of studying the application of cost benefit and cost effectiveness methodologies to dietetics. Since I didn't have the slightest idea of what she was talking about, I immediately enrolled in a course in health care economics at Simmons. The instructor was Dr. Harriet Tolpin, then on the faculty in Economics and now chairman of that department and a member of Nutrition's advisory committee. We struck a great deal—she served as a consultant to the committee and I helped her launch her career outside of Simmons.

The committee came to be known as ANCRS, the Ambulatory Nutrition Care Research Study committee (pronounced ''answers'' by the ADA staff, or so I was told). The membership of the committee changed now and again during its four year life span, but Dr. Patricia Mutch, of Andrews University in Michigan, Isabelle Hallahan, past ADA President and Copher award winner, and I hung in for the entire duration. We worked very hard to understand how cost benefit and cost effectiveness techniques could be applied in the clinical setting, resulting ultimately, we hoped, in third party reimbursement for dietetic services. Our first efforts resulted in the publication of a monograph, THE COSTS AND BENEFITS OF NUTRITIONAL CARE: PHASE 1. (We called it, among other things, ''The Purple Passion.'') We generated some data out of limited clinical studies, but nothing of significance. We were handicapped from the start by lack of funding for research and by the fact that we, as volunteers, were expected to take on a work load more appropriate for a staffer. The latter problem we caused for ourselves as the committee became more knowledgeable in defining its task. Since that time, the Council on Research has been established to give direction to ADA's efforts in investigational work.

The committee was disbanded in 1981, both to my sorrow and to my joy. I had spent enormous amount of time over the four years working on behalf of the committee, speaking and writing and traveling (I began to know O'Hare as well as Logan). I was tired, but I was so committed to the work that I could not bring myself to resign from the committee. Thus, the joy was an end over which I had no control. The sorrow I felt stemmed from the same end, an ending caused by a lack of understanding and appreciation of the yet undefined tasks that lay ahead. The committee drew a lot of attention over its lifespan; I would venture to guess that we were instrumental in raising the consciousness of the membership in the areas of accountability and reimbursement for services. Times change, however, and the advent of the DRGs in the management of acute care facilities has made cost benefit a moot point. That there is still a future for cost benefit studies in ambulatory settings remains to be seen. The one big point that has never been understood by the membership in general and the leadership in particular is that cost benefit and cost effectiveness studies are extremely difficult to do and, regardless of what we say to one another on the subject, that point remains irrefutable.

As I begin to think about winding up my career, and particularly as I have had my memory jogged by the writing of these passages, there are a number of observations which I may make. One is that the professional society has made enormous strides toward its recognition by the public as an authentic source of health information. Only this morning I saw an ad for a food product which proclaimed that "the American Dietetic Association recommends that. . . ." A second note is that the members of the society *look* better—we look and act the part of achievers (the "dress for success" generation is alive and well in ADA). And as we come to believe more in ourselves, we are seen by outsiders as a force to be reckoned with. Our journal's stature has been greatly enhanced by the quality of papers now submitted for publication and the criteria which are used to select those that are published. Our "public" face has improved vastly over the past couple of decades.

The average practitioner of the late 80s is much better educated than was her counterpart a generation ago. Undergraduate education is much more demanding in 1989 than it was in 1959. That news is both good and bad. Its good because practitioners are better equipped to handle the complex problems presented to them; its bad because many young women who are capable of handling the sciences represented in the discipline of Nutrition are capable of doing the science associated with more financially and socially rewarding careers in medicine and dentistry. Hence, we are loosing good people.

As a result of all the public recognition and because of the introduction of credentialling 20 years ago, the professional society has grown enormously. Such growth is generally viewed as a step forward in many circles and I tend to agree in most instances. Certainly size is an important factor when exerting influence in political arenas. Size is a liability, however, when the professional society cannot effectively communicate with smaller segments of the membership. The Council on Education has grown so large and, with such a dramatic increase in size, has assumed a posture of authority which is unresponsive to the particular needs of one group as they differ from the entire population of educators. The Council no longer recognizes its members, the college and university faculty, as scholars. College and university faculty, on the whole, are not in the business of preparing entry-level practitioners; they are in the business of educating undergraduate and graduate students who chose to do many things with their lives, one of which is further education in the field of Dietetics. College and university faculty are responsible to their academic units first and foremost; they tend to be unresponsive to systems which are seen as punitive. Norms and standards affecting college and university faculty, put in place by others, inhibit the role of faculty as scholar. Educational programs, developed by college and university faculty, designed to be implemented in colleges and universities, deserve assessment by other college and university faculty, not by other kinds of educators or even ''interested'' practitioners. In my opinion, the system has gone haywire. While the Council on Education purports to ''protect'' the interests of students, it has abandoned the educators that it is in business to serve. Scholarship has a low priority on W. Jackson Blvd. these days, resulting in educators like me who feel like Don Quixote fighting deaf and blind windmills.

This is a glimpse of what I've done over the past three decades and how I now look at the world. My career has been rewarding in a number of ways—I've met some wonderful people and made a few good friends over the years. I've traveled some, written a lot, listened even more, and talked and talked. I've been proud to be a member of a profession which serves so many people for such great benefit to them. I've been thrilled to be a teacher, scientist, counselor, author, trail blazer. Most of all, I hope to be remembered as a person who cared so much about her profession that she was willing to accept the stigma of being the lonely voice of the opposition.

Kristen McNutt

Kristen McNutt, PhD, JD is President of Consumer Choices Unlimited, Inc., and Editor, the Consumer Magazine Digest

Kristen McNutt chose to develop her biographical sketch with a different yet refreshing style which serves to reflect her own personality and appreciation for others. As she writes not so much on what she has accomplished but on what she has learned from others, she invites each of us to reflect on memories and to appreciate how those around us have helped to shape our lives. Family, friends, and colleagues whom Kristen McNutt honors through her own reflections and whom she credits for shaping her life have most assuredly done an admirable job. Consumer Magazines Digest which is published by Consumer Choices Unlimited, Inc., is written by Kristen McNutt. Her experience includes service as Associate Director of the Good Housekeeping Institute and Vice President for Consumer Affairs of Kraft, Inc. She authors a bimonthly editorial column for Food Engineering as well as another for Nutrition Today.

Kristen McNutt

The assigned purpose of this autobiographical sketch, "to be both informative and inspirational to colleagues and future leaders of the profession," is quite a challenge. I am accepting the invitation to contributors to use our own style and adapt the bio to our personal priorities. Since my curriculum vitae chronicles my training and work experience, I have chosen to reflect not so much on what I have done but on my learnings from others. A few of their lessons I have mastered; many I am still trying to incorporate into my life. Perhaps their wisdom can provide the inspiration requested by your editors, more than can mine *de novo*, along with a few chuckles.

A serendipitous benefit of my recollections may be that readers will dust off the memories of their own learnings from others and, as had happened to me through this writing, renew their appreciation of the people who have shaped their lived. The risk of taking this approach is leaving out many people who have helped along the way. With apologies to them, let's start down Kristen's memory lane.

Lessons from Home

Mom taught me to cherish education. She is responsible for my never considering not having a career. Our relationship changed for the better during grad school days when she let me know in no uncertain terms that family members deserve the same consideration and kindness we more consciously give to friends. Dad's expectations were softer and his aspirations for me more personal than professional. He showed me how to use hardware before computers redefined the word and to delight in the grain of natural wood. When we stopped filling the silence with words as we took walks together, I learned to appreciate the value of a precious type of communication.

My brother and I taught each other respect for choices different from our own. Our lives are worlds apart but we tenaciously defend against outsiders' criticisms each others' values and lifestyles. Aunt Dorothy who has been Executive Secretary of the National Democratic Committee since I was a baby taught me that voting is a precious responsibility, even if I flip the lever for a Republican. Uncle Peter was the richest and most generous person I knew as a kid; he paid me a nickel for every day lily stalk I removed from the garden but took back a quarter for each one I missed. M'dear, my mother's mother, was my closest link to my roots. Born in Mississippi before this century began, her ability to adjust to change is a model of progressiveness which helps me look with excitement into the next. Southern Baptist Training Union and Mormon Testimony Meeting on fast Sunday probably explain my growing up with the assumption that standing up and speaking out about "right and wrong" is not a big deal, that's just what you do.

High school/college summers working at Grand Canyon and in Maine planted the seed, or nourished what had been planted earlier, of my wander lust. My Mormon friends in Utah taught me to be more sensitive to others when they, rather than I, are in a minority; this time it was a religious one. My Duke roommate interested me enough in history that I audited a Saturday morning class she took for credit. As a student in Vienna, Nancy now-Eustis convinced me that "No friendship deserves to be called that unless it can withstand a difference on ideas" and we've had more than a few over the years.

What Wasn't in the Books at School

Diane Climo who lived down the hall at International House when we were grad students at Columbia and her family opened to me the rich world of Jewish traditions. My friends in Cairo who took me to their villages showed me the personal heartache caused by their version of nutrition problems which is quite different from our U.S. perspective. When we were with Project HOPE, a Brazilian medical student countered my lecture on infant diarrhea as a cause of malnutrition with a far stronger argument that the problem is due more often to washed-out roads and grain-eating rats; he envied our processed foods.

George Briggs' translation of food production numbers into train cars spanning miles sensitized me to the importance of putting our messages into a realistic perspective. Bill Darby would spank me if I left out his instilling in me an appreciation (for him, it's a love) for the history of nutrition. But I remember equally well his lessons on how to save time by getting to the airport no more than thirty seconds before they closed the plane door. Dick Stalvey proved to me that the way you learned to write is to write and rewrite and rewrite and rewrite . . .

Senate Ag and the Consortium

Dale Stansbury was my political process tutor at the Senate Agriculture Committee but it was from Marshall Matz that I learned to agree and disagree with the same person on different issues. I often recall Herman Talmadge's reminder, as the Committee debated U.S. Department of Agriculture (USDA) and Department of Health and Human Services (DHHS) authorities, that we are supposedly talking about one government.

The Nutrition Consortium Fellows gave me far more than I instilled in them. Many of them continue to stretch my mind. Carol Fletcher challenges me to be true to myself, every moment of every day. Donna Porter is a model for what I probably need most to learn—how to have an outside-the-office life as rich and exciting as what one does on the job. From environmental sensitivity to journalistic excellence, Patty Long is a special inspiration. Michael Goldblatt whetted my appetite for law school but it was Mahlon Burnette who helped me make the final decision. He simply asked if I would forgo being a lawyer for the next thirty years because I wasn't willing to study for four.

Consortium Board members have become some of my closest friends. Marge Devine taught me always to include "other" as a multiple choice response on questionnaires. Bob Olson taught me that some people's bark is bigger than their bite; hang in there and you'll discover a person well worth knowing. Gil Leveille and Dave Hurt have doubly enriched my life because their wives, Carol and Judy, are people I would seek out as friends even if their husbands were not professional colleagues.

From the Windy City to the Big Apple and Return

Chicago corrected my misconception about there being no life beyond the Washington beltway and made me realize the dangers of Potomac Fever. There Merryjo Ware, a School of Public Health student, taught me to think twice before I try to help others less fortunate because I might do more harm than good. Elliot Abramson, my contracts professor, flipped my mind back and forth about interpretation of the law. Should it bend to do justice or be strictly applied for fairness?

Good Housekeeping provided a feast for learning. Liz Sloan-Bubrick is the most creative person I know. She taught me to let the wildest and best ideas flow before reality testing. Willie Mae Rogers made me even prouder of my Southern heritage and asked questions that led to better answers. John Mack Carter is a model for capturing what you do well and constructively recognizing mistakes so you don't repeat them. When Lynne Leone leaned over my typewriter, looked me in the eye and waved, I vowed never again to get so wrapped up in a project that I missed the person. Laurie Cybul in the Beauty Clinic taught me what other co-eds learned at Duke while I was in chemistry labs, how to put on eye makeup.

Don Davis at Kraft helped me learn how to drive in the Chicago snow. Steve Kapur taught me that FSI's are those pages that fall out of the Sunday newspaper. My friendship with Susan Pearsall is close enough that she tells me what I'm *not* good at, routine, repetitive tasks and others things I don't confess so willingly. When my position was eliminated, Dennis Gallitano who had been in my law school study group and is now corporate counsel for Consumer Choices explained the first three phases—denial, anger, and humiliation—which most people experience under such circumstances. His advice and friendship helped me reach the fourth phase, highly motivated objectivity.

Positive from Negatives

I've had lots of opportunities to learn from things I've done wrong. But Marilyn Kruse insists I start with what went well before trying to understand what did not. Karen Scott, another small business owner with whom I regularly lunch, has the most positive attitude of anyone I know about mistakes. A market researcher through and through, she pries every possible learning from things that did not work. When we've already paid for a project with money that otherwise would have gone for the mortgage or groceries, we better figure out how not to throw dollars away again.

Eleanor Beckley-Crouse watched me flippantly say something dumb that hurt a third party. Her advice was to wallow in my embarrassment and pain, rather than trying to forget it. Only by hurting hard would I be sure never to do that, or anything close to it, again.

Ridge Associates, a management education firm, analyzed my Myers Briggs responses and taught me things about myself that I only wish I had learned twenty years earlier. Recognizing not only my own personality type but also that of others can help me build a strong, complementary team which balances each other rather than allowing natural differences to create frictions and frustrations.

Association Acquaintances

Professional association activities, not only The American Dietetic Association (ADA) but also Society for Nutrition Education (SNE), Institute of Food Technologists, American Institute of Nutrition, and now Chicago Nutrition Association, have been mini-universities for me because they brought me friends who continue to help me grow. I frequently recall Kathy Kolasa's SNE presidency speech about the need to pat ourselves on the back. I'd been speaking frequently for a couple of years before Ferg Clydesdale explained that almost everybody who is on the circuit has only three speeches; they just change the intro and ending for various audiences and add-one/drop-one when a new topic becomes a focus of greater interest.

Helen Guthrie who comes from a science-educator perspective and Bee Marks who excels in public relations have led my thinking for almost two decades on the benefits and risks of public-private sector cooperation. Johanna Dwyer is my model for being willing to take risks in this arena while fastidiously observing safeguards to avoid conflict of interest.

Elizabeth Alston, editor of Woman's Day, laid the groundwork for my believing that nutrition knowledge doesn't do much good if people don't know how to cook. With little luck, Mildred Ying of the Good Housekeeping kitchens patiently tried to improve my culinary skills but her cookbook has gotten me through many a dinner party. Sue Huffman of CPC, Karen Morgan of Nabisco, and Pat Quarles of ConAgra taught me the things that no one would put in writing about Consumer Affairs. Lutheran General's Parkside Medical Services, for which I serve as a voluntary Board member, has proven to me that a major corporation can use its fiscal resources effectively while respecting the whole person, its employees as well as its patients, and seeking the guidance of a Higher Power.

Old Ideas

Some of the most useful words of wisdom have come from friends who admit now being over the four decade mark. Colonel Barber who went to Columbia after retiring from the Army and loves to refer to me as a classmate, warned me never to be possessed by my possessions. Keith Garrison who is exactly twice my age shares his theories of how seniors can continue to live now that science can extend their lives. At the Oxford seminar honoring her ninetieth birthday, Cicely Williams who described kwashiorkor in the medical literature half a century ago was still hammering away about how physicians and nutritionists should see the whole person within the family and community environment before deciding what therapy or services will really help.

Job Tips

Debbie Nordstrom who worked with me at the Consortium and Kristin Donnan, the magna cum laude who was more a partner than a secretary at Good Housekeeping, proved the wisdom of taking a job beneath your skills when you know you are good enough to make the job grow into a challenge. On the other hand, Neige Todhunter cautioned years ago not to take any job, if I already knew how to do everything it demanded.

Anita Lauterstein retired twice before forming the graphics design company which does the layout for Choices' Consumer Magazines Digest. She stretched my vision of that publication and showed me how presentation can enhance an editorial message.

A high school buddy of my husband's who is now a top executive for a Fortune 500 company gave me the rule of first getting in the trenches to learn every detail of a task. Then pass that responsibility on to someone else even if I seem to be giving away my job. Only then will I stretch myself to learn another skill that makes me an even more valuable employee.

Houses and Hobbies

Restoring Victorian homes, first in Washington and now in Evanston, has been one of the joys and challenges of my life. As I strip off coats of paint, imagining what life was like for the people who ate and slept, birthed babies and mourned the death of loved ones there a century ago, gives perspectives to my life. I've learned from carpenters and electricians, plasterers and landscapers. Jay Zeebooker in DC taught me all I know about plumbing. Hot on the left, cold on the right and sewage doesn't run uphill.

Bob Crownover, the lifeguard at Cumberland Mountain State Park, taught me to swim when I was four. The Egyptian Olympic team tried to improve my diving when they practiced where the Americans swam. Mark Hausler at Arizona did more for my pool game than my techniques for separating vitamin D metabolites by column chromatography. I love tomatoes from my garden but they don't get much help fighting weeds from me.

Nobody has been able to teach me to carry a tune, something I do with vigor while playing the piano which I do equally badly. I'm pretty good at foreign languages but Karchy Turcsanyi whose English is better than my Polish made me appreciate how difficult our language is for foreigners when he questioned anybody's being able to translate "Do you still steal steel?"

Laugh and Learn

The lessons that have been easiest to learn have been laced with laughter. My sister-in-law cross-stitched for me "This ain't stress. This is life" and the coffee mug from her at Christmas reads "Pushing fifty is exercise enough." A birthday card from Star Campbell-Hottenstein which I framed is itself now yellow with age. It shows a pig in a ballet dress, trying to get her chubby leg over a fence; the message, "to someone of remarkable ambition," helps me laugh at myself at least once a week.

My best teacher is the one who married me almost twenty years ago. Many couples have "their song;" we have our disease because our first discussion was his lecturing me about lupus over coffee in the Vanderbilt cafeteria. His attempts to teach me to differentiate folate from B-12 deficiency failed because all I could see in the binocular microscope was my eyelashes. He wouldn't marry me until I'd finished my research because he didn't want a half-baked Ph.D. hanging around his neck for a lifetime. The same lesson, finish what you start, was re-applied when it came time to take the New York bar which I would never have attempted without his believing me and insisting I take it. When I periodically search for meaning in life and want to see that I've accomplished something, he smiles and sends me to the kitchen to scrub the sink!

It's Your Turn

The list could go on and on. I've enjoyed refreshing my memories. Perhaps you are beginning to do the same with yours. I hope my friends have provided a few ideas which help others along life's way. I thank your editors for their invitation which is yet another example of how richly my life has been blessed.

Jean B. Minskoff

Jean B. Minskoff, MA, RD is Consultant,
The Minskoff Organization, New York City

To those who remember the early days of licensure efforts in the late seventies, the name Jean Minskoff comes immediately to mind. Her pioneering work in the state of New York became a model for other states to follow. She authored "In Pursuit of Licensure" and became the first Chairman of ADA's Licensure Advisory Committee. Her professional involvement in ADA has also included many years in the House of Delegates. She has been a consultant for the Italian Trade Commission and has worked with famed artist Milton Glaser (who created "I Love New York" theme) on the re-designing of Grand Union Supermarkets. Her greatest professional commitment is to see that the National Center for Nutrition and Dietetics becomes a reality. She blended her expertise in real estate and nutrition by helping with negotiations for the new ADA headquarters at 216 West Jackson Boulevard which will house the Center. She credits her success to being proactive and never being afraid to take a risk!

Jean B. Minskoff

In 1976 I completed my undergraduate work at New University, I knew I was going to be a Dietitian/Nutritionist. I wanted to work hard, I believed I would do well. I was not 21 years old, I was the thirty-three year old mother of twin boys age 14 and a daughter of 12.

My children and I lived in Greenwich Village and my children were in school there for the years it took me to complete a Bachelor of Science with honors attending college at first part-time and then full time. Initially, I was accepted into Washington Square College of Arts and Sciences (WSC) at New York University (NYU). I had no clue of what I wanted to be or what I wanted to do. After graduating from Harrison High School, I went to Cornell University. I was in the Home Economics program which evolved into the College of Human Ecology. I attended Cornell for one year, during which I married my first husband and became pregnant with my twins. I was too young, but as with others of the rebellious 1960's, I suffered from the teenage malady described as being ''seldom right, but never in doubt.''

During my first consultation with my newly appointed advisor, at NYU I learned that WSC, did not permit part-time attendance, but I could attend classes on a part-time basis in the School of Education. That is how I found myself in the Department of Home Economics (now Home Economics and Nutrition). After several semesters of focusing on the core courses; History, English, Art History, and Expository Writing, given by WSC, my advisor suggested it was time I took something within the department.

I will never as long as I live forget my first day in Nutrition. I was with the famed Dr. Henrietta Fleck, with whom I still correspond. Everything I knew about nutrition came from my mother an enormously intelligent and well read woman. Unfortunately, she like so many others during the late forties and fifties, relied upon self-help books like those by Adele Davis and Gaylord Hauser. Much of what they said was good information, but they were not then nor are they now recognized authorities in the field of nutrition and dietetics.

Dr. Fleck asked for the names of people who were considered ''experts'' in the field of dietetics and nutrition. I shot my hand up and announced ''Adele Davis.'' Dr. Fleck then treated me to my first, but no my last stunning humiliation. For what seemed like an hour, she discussed who was and who was not a professional, credentials, the scientific method, refereed journals and the description of an authority. Adele Davis clearly did not qualify as an expert in her eyes. My own mother had failed me. Today I can laugh about it. On day one of my first nutrition class I was stunned and unhappy.

From those less than auspicious nutrition beginnings, I came to love the science and the art of nutrition and dietetics. I was tremendously fortunate. In addition to Dr. Fleck, my teachers included Dr. Margaret D. Simko, Dr. Ruth Linke, Dr. Judith M. Gilbride, Dr. Dorothy King, and Dr. Jenene G. Garey, Dr. Mildred M. Cody, and

Dr. Mabel Chan. These women while all different in their style and teaching methods, set high standards for performance and gave tremendously of their personal time and energy. I worked hard, did well and was rewarded with admission to two Honor Societies, Omicron Nu and Pi Lambda Theta, later with an assistantship, and good jobs. Over the years I was invited to submit articles for publication. When Margaret Simko, Judith Gilbride, and Catherine Cowell were assembling what was the first definitive book on Nutrition Assessment, I was privileged to be asked to submit a chapter on the role of the dietitian on the health care team.

One of my first favorite stories involves my writing of that piece. My younger brother Alan, a magazine editor, edited the chapter for me, he did a most professional job with one minor exception he corrected the word "parenteral" to read "parental" assuming a typographical error. This makes the case for editing the editor.

I was a student at the same time as Julie O'Sullivan-Maillet, now Dr. Maillet. We have been close friends ever since, having shared major life experiences both personal and professional, I respect her today and I did then—when everyone who knew her was confident that she would emerge a leader in the field, she has certainly proven us right.

In 1977 I began a Dietetic Internship at the then College of Medicine and Dentistry (currently, the University of Medicine and Dentistry) in Newark, New Jersey. At that time I believed that it was the most challenging work experience of my life, at this time I know that is true.

We were the fifth class of interns under Dorothy Brooks the Director. Three of us were married, two of us had children, all were women. The most rigorous experience in the internship was the three week clinical pediatric rotation with Claudette Austin. That is where I began to learn the field of dietetics first hand, to discover what it meant to be a clinical dietitian, to start my career. I was not having any easy time in that experience. My sense was that Ms. Austin took her responsibility very seriously, she intended that this experience was going to prepare me for the rest of the internship. I worked very, very hard, but it was not easy to tell if she was pleased. During the first one-to-one counseling session with a young mother I had to excuse myself during the interview. I was in extreme discomfort and had been trying to convince myself it was psychosomatic. It was not in my head, I had a ruptured ectopic pregnancy. During my post-operative recuperation I worked on my projects for Ms. Austin and though I had to make up the time I was out, I graduated with my class.

The internship year was demanding, painful, seemingly endless, extraordinary, enlightening and exciting. With each year of distance I put between me and the internship; I found myself saying that as hard as it was it was well worth it. Phyllis Kaskel and I were the two interns with children. This year I was delighted to have a chance to work with her on the New York State Dietetic Association (NYSDA) Annual Meeting Committee. She is now the outstanding Assistant Director, of Food Services at New York University Medical Center. We had a chance to reminisce about our year in internship. It is a special thing to share a pivotal life experience with someone and equally special to be able to relive some of the times together.

I promised myself a reward for surviving that nine months and so when my children were released from school, we piled into the family station wagon; four children, one dog, me and Gail Wilson, a friend from the internship. We headed west to Idaho and stopped at wonderful places along the way.

My three children and John, my son's Richard and Michael's friend, were only bearable for this journey with the CB radio to occupy them. We chatted across this country with truckers and travelers. We learned the lingo and became quite proficient in our communiques. Our "handle" was "big dipper."

I had only two trip rules, the first was that the car came to a complete halt, if the kids did not behave, and the second was that we never drove more than 500 miles per day. It was a great trip, Mount Rushmore, Craters of the Moon, the Badlands, Yellowstone and Jackson Hole. Amos, the Shetland Sheepdog won the prize for the best behaved under 15 years old.

Fall of 1977 brought me right back to reality, job hunting. There were two jobs I was applying for. One at the Bronx V.A. Medical Center and second at the New York Infirmary Hospital, now The New York Infirmary-Beekman Downtown Hospital where I had been a student and a volunteer.

The New York Infirmary, was a great place. The staff was bright and accomplished. They worked very hard and made a difference. Louise Cariotti, the Director of the department was a visionary. She was always willing to listen and try new ideas, and support you 100%. I was anxious to work there. Funnily, Michelle Fairchild, the Chief Dietitian, was being rather vague about the job that was supposed to be available, I was baffled, but fortunately patient. The job turned out to be Michelle's job as Chief Dietitian. She was leaving to take a position at Memorial Sloan Kettering Medical Center. Having been there as a student, I was concerned about coming in as the Chief Dietitian. In fact, I was older than the other dietitians, but, unquestionably less experienced in dietetics. They were great. We worked together overcame some difficulties, but all in all I look back at an extraordinary first job. In addition to being the Chief Dietitian, I was the Renal Nutritionist and the Home Care Dietitian. I will always remember Florence Hauck the Home Care Administrator for her unending support of the role and importance of the dietitian on the Home Care team.

In 1978 after some years of exploration there was talk in New York, in dietetics circles, of serious pursuit of professional licensure. Those of us who were interested were advised that "The American Dietetic Association (ADA) leaders were opposed to licensure." The message was clear if you wanted to go anywhere within the professional organization, licensure was on the wrong side of the fence. It pleases me no end to have been part of the change that on October 6, 1985 saw the ADA House of Delegates approve the policy of the ADA which "is to endorse strongly the licensure of dietitian/nutritionist as a means of protecting the health and welfare of the public.

There is a long list of dietitians who brought us from "no go" in 1977 to "go" in 1985. The late Alene Vaden was instrumental in making the case to the House. Dietitians in New York worked tirelessly for years, Ruth Harmon, Sylvia Berger, Susan

Braverman, and countless others across the country since those early attempts. In 1983 the NYSDA published "in Pursuit of Licensure," a guide for states interested in looking at state regulation. Susan Braverman and I wrote it together (to my knowledge it was the first document of its type for dietitians). By 1987, Licensure was a hot topic and Ross Laboratories invited me to write a Dietetic Currents issue. I wrote it with Lynne M. Oudekerk, M.A., R.D., and published in the fall of 1987, interestingly, seventeen states had regulation at that time while at this writing twenty-five states have some form of regulation. The HOD has a Licensure Advisory Committee, for which I was lucky enough to be the first Chairman; it is active and productive. I have been fortunate to have had the opportunity to speak on the subject of professional regulation from Oahu to Providence, and from Miami to Detroit encouraging dietitians to become politically active. As part of the Long Range Plan of the Licensure Advisory Committee we submitted a goal which stated "Dietitians/Nutritionists will have an increased role in state political and policy making processes and positions." This seemed to make some people uncomfortable, but the goal stood. Political clout will enfranchise us as a force to be reckoned with.

In 1980, I left the New York Infirmary Hospital to teach at NYU and in 1981 I became a teaching fellow within the Department of Home Economics and Nutrition. I love to teach and miss it.

I have taught Nutrition II, Nutrition Assessment, and Advanced Medical Nutrition. Students keep you on your toes they make you think all the time. I am a great believer in clinical subjects being taught by clinicians. Working and teaching allowed me to bring my daily experiences to class, made dietetics real for the students. The further I got away from being a clinician the less good a teacher I believe I became.

For a time in the late seventies I did some contract work for the world famous Milton Glaser. He is the artist, designer, and illustrator who invented I [Love] New York. He was redesigning the Grand Union Supermarkets and needed a nutritionist to look at products while he looked at the packaging, store layout and Grand Union image. It was great fun.

Christmas of 1981 my life changed forever, most people do not get to middle age my current status without a few bumps and bruises. I had the rug pulled out from beneath me. My only daughter, Donna, aged 17 emerged from major surgery in a coma. The story would take a long time to tell and is not happy reading. She is only ever so slightly, better today, here with us at home, now 25 years old. I do not believe that this was part of some grand master plan, nor do I accept that some good must come from all this. Rather I subscribe to the notion that we live in an imperfect world, inhabited by imperfect people. God, did not intend this to be the life for my beautiful, talented, bright and comedic child who will never know that she was accepted into her first choice college, on an early decision basis only weeks after this happened.

God was there for me to pray to for strength, wisdom, and guidance. It was difficult to work with Donna hospitalized for 14 months. Bringing her home in February 1983 was a fearsome prospect, but it has all turned out to work very smoothly. With a wonderful staff of nurses and therapists she is in excellent physical condition and she is here with her family.

In January of 1983 I took a part-time job at St. Luke's Hospital (now St. Luke's-Roosevelt Hospital). I was hired as the Dietetic Internship Coordinator. My job was to develop and design a proposal for a Dietetic Internship and to work with the staff on Inservice Training.

I thought it was the best job anyone could have. The opportunity to create a new program. I was there because Dr. Rita Franseze (now Rita Jackson) was the director of the department. We worked very closely to design what we believed to be a comprehensive, challenging, and innovative program which would combine both Clinical and Food Service Systems Management. It took more than a year and a half to develop, working with departments throughout the hospital and many outside affiliations. It was also to give me my most disappointing moment of my professional life. ADA's Commission on Accreditation department did not accept the program. Rather we received an evaluation including three pages of suggested changes. It was a bitter pill to swallow. Worse yet was that Rita Franseze left and the administration that followed was no longer interested in an internship. The good news is that I recently met the newest Director, an R.D. who has expressed some interest in looking again at the possibility, perhaps one day there will be an internship there after all.

Today, I am learning my family business, Real Estate. We build, develop and manage properties from small shopping centers to 500,000 square foot buildings. I still do nutrition consulting. This year I worked for the Italian Trade Commission. We traveled to three cities, Philadelphia, Chicago, and Washington, D.C. to present a luncheon and seminar to media representatives discussing Monounsaturated Fatty Acids, like those found in Italian olive oil. This gave me the opportunity to work with Chef Giuliano Bugialli, with whom my husband, T. Grant and I have taken cooking classes.

I understand that articles from some of the syndicated columnists appeared in as distant places as California and Florida.

My greatest passion has become my professional involvement at ADA. I have long supported the notion that if you are not part of the solution you are part of the problem. I have been part of District, State and National Dietetic Association activities since I began to work in the profession. I have served on nominating committees, on Licensure committees, as New York State Dietetic Association Secretary (NYSDA) and I have served for 5 years in the House of Delegates as a representative from New York.

In the time that I have served in the ADA House of Delegates, I have seen a great deal of maturity within the house and it's processes. Dietetic professionals need to work closely with there delegates to get there felt needs expressed and represented. The best delegates have well developed channels of communication and work diligently to represent their constituencies within the house as well as to bring back and interpret ADA activities to their members. I am a great supporter of Jack Bellick's belief in working at the district level. This keeps you in touch with what is going on at the grass roots level.

In addition, many of the most exciting and vital ideas begin among those who bring a fresh perspective to the field.

Currently, dietitians in our area are concerned about professional recruitment and retention and all the attendant issues which surround these topics. Judith Gilbride and I are about to introduce a resolution that the house conduct a hearing in 1990 on these topics with the hope that representatives from all regions of the country can bring relevant experiences ideas and concerns to the discussion. This way we can become more proactive in dealing with these knotty problems.

My greatest commitment is to see that the National Center for Nutrition and Dietetics (NCND) becomes a reality. As a member of the Board of Directors of The American Dietetic Association Foundation (ADAF) I see the Center as a unique contribution our profession can make to the nutritional well being of people. Who would ever imagine that the distinct fields of Real Estate and Nutrition could merge. It did for me when as a member of the ADAF Board and as the representative of both ADA and ADAF Boards I participated in all phases of the negotiations for the Real Estate Deal which brought ADA/ADAF to its new headquarters at 216 West Jackson Boulevard and gave the National Center for Nutrition and Dietetics a home. I was privileged to be able to have the opportunity to help make it happen. It has been people like the extraordinary Edna Langholz, Susan Braverman, and Mary Abbott Hess who helped me to be in the right place at the right time.

I have not had a long and illustrious career in dietetics and I wondered, why ask me to write about my professional experience? I have been lucky in many ways. I have had special teachers, extraordinary mentors and made countless friends through dietetics. Former students still come up to speak to me at meetings and I remain the NYSDA delegate to the Westchester Dietetic Association.

The ADA has a newly approved Strategic Plan for the Profession. It cannot possibly move from a vision to a reality without the support of its 57,000 plus members. Dietitians need to look at this plan, respond to the long range and action plans which emerge. This is a plan written on paper not etched in stone. It can be altered; it can be revised. A major component is constant evaluation both retrospective and prospective.

My personal view is one of cautious optimism. We must continue to be proactive. Education of dietetics professionals needs to match the market. ADA needs to continually assess the needs of members and provide appropriately. A member's obligations is to make those needs felt through their delegates and all other available channels of communication. Dietetics never had difficulty in attracting the best and the brightest. However, today many educational programs see a decreasing number of applicants in a marketplace of ever increasing career options. Few are comfortable discussing salary levels, but it needs to be addressed and soon. I spoke to a frustrated dietitian several weeks ago. She was offered a job in a pediatric intensive care until in a large medical center. She has 15 years of experience and holds a master's degree. The salary was $10/hour. After deducting for child care expenses and travel costs, she knew she could not afford to take that job.

The good news is that I see ADA as growing in its ability to respond effectively to important issues. It has demonstrated this over and over in the recent past. The establishment of the Washington, D.C. office, the Wats line service there, the streamlined position paper process and the issuance of timely statements are powerful indicators. Perhaps no where is this more evident than in the creation of the National Center for Nutrition and Dietetics. Programs on the drawing board include a library, information center, and research endowments. The Center will serve ordinary citizens, dietetic and health professionals and corporations. It is a special experience to be part of the birth of the Center.

Risk taking carries the possibility of resounding failures and exhilarating successes, I have had my share. I trust there will be more risks ahead for me to take.

Elaine Ranker Monsen

Elaine R. Monsen, PhD, RD is Professor of Nutrition
at the University of Washington, Seattle, WA
and Editor, Journal of The American Dietetic Association

Elaine R. Monsen is an illustrious researcher and academician who also makes time for the awesome responsibility of editing the Journal of The American Dietetic Association. Her studies on iron metabolism and absorption are known world-wide. She devised a model that allows available dietary iron to be estimated from various dietary patterns. Expertise in this area led to invited positions on review panels for the Surgeon General's Report on Nutrition and Health and the 10th edition of the Recommended Dietary Allowances, as well as numerous international speaking engagements. In addition to her busy professional schedule, Dr. Monsen derives pleasure from being involved in her community. She has been active with the Santa Fe Chamber Music Festival and Contemporary Theater in Seattle. She is also Chairman of the Seattle Foundation, a community philanthropic organization.

Elaine R. Monsen

At the beginning of seminar courses, I often ask my students to prepare their resumes and add two questions: "What are your goals for the course" and "What are your goals for life." The nobility of their comments impresses me. I have learned a great deal from my students and value my association with each one. The request to prepare an autobiographical sketch is rather similar, i.e., a resume and analysis of one's life.

In thinking about dietetics and my activities in the field, I find that four factors have guided my career: 1) selecting something I enjoyed doing, 2) developing strong research interests, 3) specializing, and 4) participating actively in team efforts. Without my fully realizing it at the time, I now find that those four ideas have focused my career and made it both exciting and stimulating. The beginning was conventional: a solid education. The timing, however, was unconventional: the second decade after World War II.

Educational Background

Grade school and high school for me were in Lafayette, California, then a countryside farm-like suburb east of San Francisco. It was not until later that I realized what an idyllic setting this had been. The orchards still stretched across the hills, and we would hop on yellow school buses to go to school. As a fourth generation Californian, it is hard for me to see how that countryside has changed into freeways and subdivisions.

I attended the University of Utah, where my mother had received her bachelor's degree. One morning, while preparing for a mid-term, I started querying myself about the future. I knew that I wanted a strong scientific field with a wide range of applications. Food and nutrition was the logical choice. I was very surprised and delighted, many years later, to be named by my department at Utah as their first Distinguished Alumnus. I have never regretted my choice of majors.

Upon graduation I entered the dietetic internship program at Massachusetts General Hospital (MGH) in Boston. The 12 month experience there was an excellent one that offered depth and breadth in the practice of dietetics. I particularly found the clinical research unit to be provocative and stimulating. We worked 5 1/2 days each week, frequently on "split shifts" from 7:00 a.m. to 12:30 p.m. and 4:00 p.m. to 7:00 p.m., with lectures scheduled between shifts. (Despite the arduous schedule, I was still able to arrange two three-day trips to New York City, both times taking a night train to New York, seeing four plays, and taking a night train back to Boston.) I still vividly the numerous large quantity foodservice and clinical experiences. I had the opportunity of working with one of the first patients diagnosed with PKU. We had excellent field trips, still fresh in my memory, where I could see entire processes from planning through production to delivery. Despite the long hours, this was an important and exciting phase in my education and made me want to continue graduate work.

Unfortunately my father, a physician and surgeon died suddenly. I came home briefly before returning to MGH to complete my internship. While in California I interviewed at the University of California at Berkeley (UCB) and decided to apply there for graduate work. I was accepted into the program in nutritional biochemistry at Berkeley and was awarded a teaching assistantship, which allowed me to teach two different year-long courses over a two-year period. I found that serving as a teaching assistant was challenging. It required a level of knowledge far beyond that required as a student. The year at Berkeley I was awarded a research assistantship and worked on several laboratory research projects. During the time at Berkeley, I was fortunate to receive a Mead Johnson Scholarship and a National Science Foundation Graduate Fellowship. These two fellowships were beneficial; they allowed me to complete my graduate work and encouraged me to do so.

Although my formal education, i.e., undergraduate years at Utah, dietetic internship at MGH, and the doctoral program at Berkeley, was behind me I was able to augment it twice, once on the East Coast and once on the West Coast. The first was an enjoyable productive year at Harvard University, where I worked with Dr. Mark Hegsted in the Nutrition Department of the School of Public Health. I was again indebted to the National Science Foundation for awarding me a Post-doctorate Fellowship. A few years later, I had a second post-doctoral year as a visiting scholar at the Food Research Institute at Stanford University. Staffed by economists and demographers, the Food Research Institute focused on global problems of food supply, demand, distribution, and economics. I came across the ideas of societal food choices, the starchy staple, and price elasticity.

Research Interests

The two major research interests I have had are iron metabolism and absorption and lipid metabolism. My lifelong interest in lipid metabolism began first, spurred by my father's recent death from a heart attack. During my graduate work at Berkeley, I had the opportunity of working with excellent lipid researchers. I decided to look at the question of dietary effects on red blood cell composition. To do this, I studied the effects of the level of dietary saturated fatty acids on red blood cell lipids. It was fascinating to see that exchange occurred between fatty acids of the plasma and red blood cell membranes. Diet, which we knew had an impact on plasma lipids, appeared to influence red blood cell lipids as well. My husband dubbed my research "the study in red."

I continued my research in lipid metabolism when I began teaching at the University of Washington. Because equipment and laboratory space were extremely limited, I decided to devise an experiment that did not require elaborate facilities. To do that, I used a factorial design of two different levels of exercise and two different diets. Serial samples were obtained so that it was possible to obtain more data from the same subjects.

Early in my career at the University of Washington, I became curious about the increase in the RDA for iron: 18 mg. iron/day for women during their reproductive years. It was clear that this level was beyond the amount that would be consumed in the usual diet. I wrote to the chair of the RDA committee, who recommended that I talk with a well known researcher at the University of Washington, Dr. Clement Finch, who was also head of the Division of Hematology. We began a long, very productive and pleasurable collaboration. His view was that the RDA for iron was too low; mine was that the new RDA level was too high. In trying to resolve this question we both came to respect each other's scientific orientations and reached a median ground. I have continued my interest in iron metabolism and iron absorption with Drs. Finch and James Cook and have completed several studies of how different food combinations and nutrient combinations affect non-heme iron absorption.

Through collaboration, we devised a model that allows one to estimate available dietary iron from various dietary patterns. Our studies indicate that homeostatic mechanisms within human beings are very strong. It appears that at the point of deficient erythropoieses, iron absorption markedly expands in an effort to maintain homeostatic balance. Once erythropoiesis is able to continue at a normal rate, absorption modulates to a point at which the body in usual circumstances will retain only the amount of iron that is physiologically appropriate. The studies on iron bioavailability, particularly the influence of one food on the absorption of iron from another food, have been important in the field of trace element research.

The area of lipids has continued to be a second strong area of interest for me throughout my career. I have recently completed a collaboration study on the lipid components of seafood: i.e., fatty acids and sterols. In addition, through my lipid interests, I am the coordinator of our postdoctoral training program on lipid metabolism, arteriosclerosis and nutrition, working closely with Dr. Edwin Bierman in the Medical School at the University of Washington.

I have found that my strong interests in research in lipids and in iron have given focus to my career. They give a center from which to read and interpret the scientific literature. They allow connections to be made that relate numerous areas of interests. To have strong research interests enhances one's professional life and stimulates one's thinking. Further, I have found that just being curious, as I was about iron requirements, or personally concerned, as I was about lipids, can open up and focus a whole research career.

Expertise and Specialization

Because of my experience as a researcher, an author, and a reviewer, I was asked to be the Editor of the *Journal of The American Dietetic Association*. I will discuss this highly specialized activity in the next section as I have discovered that my effectiveness as an editor is related strongly to team efforts.

Expertise within the broad field of nutrition has brought me invitations to work on several committees for the American Institute of Nutrition, the American Society of Clinical Nutrition, and The American Dietetic Association. Recently, I was elected for a three-year term as Secretary of the American Society for Clinical Nutrition.

Because of my specialization in iron metabolism I have had the opportunity to be on many review panels, most recently for the Surgeon General's recent report on "Nutrition and Health" and for the 10th edition of the Recommended Dietary Allowances, a publication of the Food and Nutrition Board, Institute of Medicine's National Academy of Sciences. My interest in iron has also involved me with the Pan American Health Organization as a Scientific Advisor for Iron Fortification of Foods and the Food Fortification Committee of the National Nutrition Consortium, Inc.

One of the most exciting and pleasurable honors I have received was being selected to present the Frances Fischer Lecture at the International Congress of Dietetics in Paris in 1988. Pleasurable because I was asked to speak of my research on iron metabolism and absorption. Exciting because the meetings allowed an opportunity to meet with colleagues from all over the world. The lecture itself, which I presented in English, was translated simultaneously into French. I have found it to be a highly enriching experience to visit with colleagues in America and abroad; I hope to have many more opportunities to discuss with others the new issues and research in dietetics and nutrition.

The issues involved in professional and scientific ethics are a new area of keen interest to me. Ethics are an integral part of the research, data interpretation (both one's own data and the data of others) and publication. I have recently been appointed as Chair of the Subcommittee on Scientific Misconduct of the Intersociety Ethics Committee. Four societies are involved actively in this concern: the American Society of Clinical Nutrition, the American Institute of Nutrition, the American Society of Parenteral and Enteral Nutrition, and the Canadian Society for Nutritional Sciences. In the last few years, I have been active in the Council of Biology editors and recently participated in the First Instructional Congress in Peer Review, in which ethics was a dominant theme. Increasingly, ethics are discussed in our professional work. National politics are not alone in their interest in this topic.

Team Effort

Throughout my career, I have been helped immensely by colleagues, friends, and family. The interest and continuous support of my husband and daughter have been great strengths for me. We have enjoyed our community and received much pleasure from being involved in it. My husband has been on the boards of the Seattle Art Museum and the University of Washington Art Gallery as well as being a founder of the Seattle Opera. I have served on the board of A Contemporary Theater and have been the President of the Santa Fe Chamber Music Festival in Seattle. For the past decade, I have been an active board member of the Seattle Foundation, a community philanthropic foundation, and will be Chairman for the 1991–1993 term. Being an active participant in my community has increased my enjoyment of Seattle substantially.

When I returned to the University of Washington from sabbatical years at Harvard and Stanford universities, I missed the many seminars from visiting scientists. I organized an interdisciplinary group called the Nutrition Studies Committee. Established by the Graduate School, it allowed scientists across the campus to meet together to sponsor seminars, to communicate their interest in nutrition, and to allow scientific interaction. Many collaborative projects were started by the individuals who attended these seminars and the campus was enriched by the many seminars from visitors passing through the Northwest. Certainly, in my research, the interaction of many collaborators, primarily at the University of Washington but also at other campuses, has provided opportunities to study the problems of iron absorption and of lipids. Currently at the University of Washington there is an excellent team of individuals interested in nutrition and dietetics, led the last few years by energetic, productive Dr. Bonnie Worthington-Roberts.

The team with which I work most closely now is associated with bringing out monthly the *Journal of The American Dietetic Association*. We have a close collaboration between the staff in Seattle and the Chicago staff. The group in Seattle is composed of myself; Deborah Shattuck, Assistant to the Editor; and the many colleagues whose counsel I frequently seek and whose friendship I hope not to strain. Joan Karkeck is an especially able and ready counselor on whom I often impose. The *Journal* staff at ADA headquarters in Chicago is composed of Deborah McBride, Administrator of Publications; Chris Bouey, Managing Editor; and Vicky Guinta, Advertising Sales Manager. Dolores Henning, Managing Editor through 1989, was a great guide and tutor in helping me get started with the many tasks associated with the *Journal*. The 21 members of the Board of Editors, located throughout America and Canada, provide valued expertise and viewpoints. In addition, several hundred reviewers willingly and competently review articles submitted to the *Journal*. It is the skilled researchers and authors who form the backbone of the *Journal*. Perhaps the reason I find being an editor so stimulating, despite the immense workload and constant deadlines that must be met, is that it allows me to keep abreast of the most current research and to feel, vicariously, involved.

As I look to the future and consider the history and goals of our profession, I see the field of dietetics becoming increasing exciting and pertinent. Entrepreneurial activity in the field has blossomed. In multiple new ways, dietitians in foodservice and clinical dietetics are meeting the needs of the public. Dietitians are administrators, managers, program directors, counselors, teachers, researchers, and authors. As we continue to be experts in the area and are increasingly recognized as leaders in nutrition and dietetics, the field of dietetics will continue to grow and expand and offer satisfying and stimulating career opportunities.

Aimee N. Moore

Aimee N. Moore, PhD, RD
is Professor Emeritus of the School of Health
Related Professions, College of Medicine
University of Missouri–Columbia

From smoking "rabbit" tobacco in corncob pipes to earning a bachelor's degree from the University of North Carolina at Greensboro, from her induction into the U.S. Army Medical Corps on the very day dietitians were first commissioned to turning around a $100,000 MESS debt into a surplus of $80,000, from receiving the Mary Swartz Rose Fellowship on two occasions to receiving the prestigious Marjorie Hulsizer Copher Award, Aimee N. Moore graciously credits those around her with helping her make choices in her personal and professional life. The impact of her family, friends, and colleagues, on her personal and professional achievements is threaded throughout her story. The name Aimee N. Moore is synonymous with computers in food service management, but her autobiography paints a portrait of a woman with a zest for actively participating in life. Retirement, it would appear, has provided her with more time to pursue another great love: travel. "I hope my good health continues because there are many places I still want to visit."

Aimee N. Moore

Early Years

Both my father and mother were descended from French Huguenot families who had settled in South Carolina before the revolution. They lived in antebellum homes on large farms, and while they did not have much money, they were well educated, solid citizens, who had inherited their land for many generations. That means a lot in South Carolina—it guarantees social acceptance.

My father was an officer in World War I, and was in France when I was born. He had studied dairy husbandry at Clemson before the war, and worked on a dairy farm for several years upon his return from France. But he had always wanted to be an Episcopal minister, and, when I was in the second grade, he received a scholarship to go to the seminary for three years. I had two brothers by that time. We lived with my mother's aunt in the Trezevant family home, a mile from my grandfather in a rural community populated mostly by relatives, or so it seemed to me. My grandfather was one of six children, all of whom had established homes in the area. Much of the land had belonged to his father.

I went to school on a school bus and carried my lunch with me. My aunt's home had electricity and running water, supplied by a Delco generator—this was before rural electrification—but when the generator broke down we used kerosene lamps and drew water from a well. The rooms we lived in were heated by fireplaces. The bedroom my family used was 25' x 25' with 16' ceilings, so you can imagine that it was hard to keep it warm. My brothers and I loved living there.

We moved to North Carolina when I was ten, the first of our extended family to leave "home." Weldon was a small town and it did not take long to settle in. The rectory was not next to the church, thank heavens, and we lived in a neighborhood on the edge of town. All of our neighbors had several children and we roamed in packs. Always something interesting to do, like building a boat out of packing boxes to use on the creek (which was about two feet deep) to fighting the Crusades using garbage can lids as shields and bamboo spears. We smoked "rabbit" tobacco in corncob pipes, took unsuspecting friends on "snipe" hunts, played tricks on Halloween, in other words, lived a very normal life.

I loved to read, as did my brother and the boy next door. Since the librarian would let us take out only two books at a time, we went together and each took two. We had a one-room library, and I think each of us read every book in the library before we graduated from high school.

When I was in the eighth grade, at the height of the depression, the School Board decided to shorten the school year by one month. My mother and the mothers of three of my friends decided that instead of letting us run free, they would take turns each morning to teach us some skill, like sewing, dancing, marketing, cooking. One day each week we prepared lunch for our families. We were given a set amount of money and shopped to get the best bargains. I showed great aptitude, and one of the mothers told me I should consider dietetics as a career. I didn't know what a dietitian did at that time, but I decided to find out. I never changed my mind about what career I would follow.

One of the projects for making money to go to camp was to solicit orders for mayonnaise each week. My best friend and I drummed up quite a business, and we had a surplus of egg whites since we used yolks only for the mayonnaise. So we started making angel food cakes. I'm sure our families had to help with expenses, but we did get to camp.

College/Internship

There was never a question about whether I should go to college, even though it would require a sacrifice from my family to scrape together the money. Nor was there a question about which college I would attend. The state-supported university for women in Greensboro had an excellent scholastic reputation and the cost was subsidized by the State. If I remember correctly it cost about $500 per year for room, board, laundry and incidental fees—there was no tuition.

I went there from a very small high school (28 in our graduating class) and eleven years total instead of twelve, so the competition was rough. I started making average grades, but steadily improved so that I was on the honor roll by my junior year.

The summer after my junior year I was selected by the faculty to receive the Danforth Scholarship, given by the founder of Ralston Purina to a home economics student from each Land Grant University. We spent two weeks in St. Louis, staying at Barnes Hospital with the dietetic interns, whom we did not get to know because we were too busy. Then we went by chartered bus to a camp on the shore of Lake Michigan for two weeks. It was a leadership camp and we had classes each morning, sports in the afternoon, campfire in the evening. Mr. Danforth scheduled each of us for a visit while we were there, and it was very inspirational to meet him.

In my senior year the faculty member who taught Institutional Management was on sabbatic leave. The visiting professor who took her place was Lucille McMackin, on leave from Western Reserve University Hospital. She was the best teacher I ever had and from her I learned what a dietitian should be. When I applied for an internship at the end of the year, I wanted to go to Western Reserve. I was accepted there and at the University of Michigan. Lucille prepared me to select Michigan, since most dietitians considered it to be the best at that time. I was not disappointed, but I was sorry not to be with Lucille for another year. I did go to Western Reserve to visit her and I met several of her friends. Lucille died of spinal meningitis the following year.

My year at the University of Michigan was one of intensified learning. The other interns and I worked hard, and played hard. There were 16 of us, and one had also been a Danforth Fellow. We have had several mini-reunions throughout the years. I see a few of my classmates regularly at ADA.

Pre-War Years

My first job after graduation was in Mississippi. The Dean of my college recommended me, and I was among the first in my class to get a job. I worked in the Mississippi State Sanatorium with two other dietitians. At that time I was told there were only six ADA members in Mississippi, and three of us worked in one small institution. After one year, I wanted to be nearer my family in North Carolina, so I moved to Virginia. Shortly after that, my father also moved to Virginia, and I could spend weekends with them. That is the only time in my career that I lived near my parents.

Soon after Pearl Harbor, I tried to enlist in a hospital that was forming in Richmond to go overseas. I was turned down because I wore glasses! A year later when I again applied, I was eagerly accepted.

Army Experiences

I was inducted into the U. S. Army Medical Corps on February 1, 1943, the day dietitians were first commissioned. My serial number was 7. Since I outranked the dietitians already there, I was made Head Dietitian at the Army Hospital at Camp Pickett, VA, a 2200 bed one-story unit which covered a lot of territory. It was just a few miles from where my parents were living. I had no uniform and received no basic training.

The day I reported to the Commanding Officer, I was told that the Mess Officer had been ill for two months, and his replacement had gotten the Mess into debt—about $100,000. I was told that my first responsibility was to erase the debt ASAP! I WAS FLABBERGASTED! At 23, I was the youngest as well as the newest dietitian in the unit. Fortunately, the task was not impossible, and before I was transferred to be sent overseas six months later, we had accrued a surplus of $80,000. I rewrote the menu, closed the back door, stood by the garbage cans to observe waste, reduced serving portions, etc., etc. And the Mess Officer and other dietitians were my friends.

I did not receive any uniforms, except the seersucker wrap-arounds that we wore on duty, until I went to the Port of Embarkation. We were issued bedrolls, into which we stuffed all the "essentials" like toilet paper, sanitary napkins, tooth paste, etc. which probably would not be readily available overseas. The rumors were not accurate, but I never ran out. Our clothes and the rest of our gear, which included mess gear, steel helmets and helmet liners, a webbed belt from which to hang much of the gear, and a shelter-half (half of a two-man tent with poles and stakes), were stuffed into a duffel bag.

When we went aboard our ship, we found that there were 35 women and about 3,000 men on board. The ship had been a British luxury liner, and the women were assigned the honeymoon suite—two rooms and bath equipped with triple decker bunks. You could not sit up in your bunk. Since the ship was faster than the other trooper carriers, we did not go in convoy. We zigzagged across the Atlantic, and did not know our destination until the day before we arrived in Casablanca. Because batteries of guns had been installed on the deck, the ship tended to roll in an exaggerated manner. Add to that the fact that all portholes were permanently locked, and blacked out, and we ran into bad weather the first day out, most of us were seasick. For three days I ate nothing but crackers and oranges. Fortunately, the weather cleared and I got my sea-legs, so I survived the 12 day trip.

There were 15 dietitians and 20 physical therapists in our group, but the orders we received in Casablanca were reversed, and none of us had the right assignment. So we stayed in Casablanca for a month waiting for our assignments. We saw a lot of Casablanca! Saw the movie "Casablanca" while we were there.

When I finally got to Tunis, I found that the hospital to which I was assigned was in Bizerte, but they did not expect me. So I had to spend the night in Tunis. After I had returned a third time to the billeting office, because the places assigned me were already occupied, it was getting dark. The British Lance Corporal, who was assisting me, and I were standing in the lobby of an apartment house discussing what to do next, when a young girl approached and invited me to stay with her family. So we talked with her mother and decided it was probably as safe as any alternative. The corporal left, promising to come back to check on me, and that began a very interesting friendship for both of us. The family spoke French only, and my French was very poor, but we had a great time. Several aunts, uncles and cousins were invited to dinner that night to meet their American guest. I had cous cous for the first time, and found that everyone was waiting for me to start first. Teaching me broke the ice, and we had an animated, if disconnected, conversation. I returned to visit them several times, bringing chocolate and other goodies from the PX. The corporal joined me a couple of times.

The Station Hospital to which I was assigned was a tent hospital. The kitchen was constructed with telephone poles to raise the roof which was covered with the canvas. This leaked when it rained, and it rained a lot at that time of year. We used field ranges for cooking and baking. I had never seen a field range before then, but I figured out that we needed a heavy iron sheet above the burner to spread the heat more evenly. This did help. What we needed most of all were umbrellas, but we couldn't make those, so we just shifted the ranges to get away from the drips.

We were issued a powdered form of citric acid to provide Vitamin C, but it was not very palatable, and very few would touch the "lemonade" we made with it. Therefore, the Army purchased truckloads of lemons for a while, and issued them to us. But we had no lemon squeezers, no extra sugar, no ice; we just couldn't use many of them. The citric acid did do a good job of cleaning the aluminum stoves.

The turkeys issued to us for Thanksgiving dinner did not arrive until late Wednesday afternoon, and they were frozen solid. As soon as supper was over, we lined them up on the mess hall tables, and borrowed all the fans in camp to try to defrost them enough to get the giblets out of the cavities. The cooks had an all night party, and by supper on Thanksgiving we had a feast.

We never knew until the ration truck arrived what we had been issued for the next day, so there was little we could do to plan ahead. We had lots of C-rations on hand, because they always issued more than anyone would eat, but fresh meat was always preferred. The only people who really ate C-rations with an appetite were the newly arrived casualties who had been in the field and had had little hot food for several weeks. Even they quickly tired of them. We tried to disguise them by making up new recipes incorporating them in unusual ways. Dried eggs were also hard to sell. We made French toast and pancakes with lots of egg in them, and cooked them on the line, and this helped. But the margarine or butter was the consistency of axle grease, to prevent it from melting in the hot sun at the ration dumps, so we had to serve it already melted. We didn't have syrup or brown sugar, and apple butter and orange marmalade got very boring. They always threw in enough of those to bring the calories up to par. We did get a lot of peanut butter, and that was always welcomed. One day we were supposed to have spaghetti, but they had none so they sent us flour as a substitute. Another time we were supposed to get 200 pounds of raisins (too much to begin with), and we received 2000 pounds. I couldn't believe my eyes as the men toted in box after box.

By the way, I finally found a use for the shelter half—it made a good bedspread because my tent also leaked. And I used the helmet as a wash basin for my clothes.

The hospital was transferred to Italy to be set up near Naples in time to receive casualties from the battle from Monte Casino. But the equipment and other supplies were sent to the wrong port, and when they were finally located and delivered to us, the attack had already begun. We stayed up all night putting together the hospital and the next day we had 750 badly injured patients. We were set up in an old army barracks and the Mess was assigned space which in the past had been the stables. Thank goodness, we had several days before the equipment arrived to scrub it down.

The barracks were built around a parade ground and this was filled with men on litters awaiting triage under a blazing sun. We went from one to another with water, fruit juice and soup until they were all finally taken to the wards. Many of that batch of wounded were Arabs from Morocco, and I knew they didn't eat pork. But Spam is what we had so we disguised it as best we could and called it something else. I decided that if they had never eaten pork, they wouldn't know how it tasted, and I was right.

That place had been built to last. It was constructed of stone and the walls were about 18 inches thick. We were closer to the fighting there and the area was frequently bombed by the Germans. One night the bombs fell close enough to shatter the glass in my bedroom window.

It wasn't all work and no play, though. Almost every Saturday I was able to go to Naples to the opera, and I thoroughly enjoyed that. We met some Air Force officers who invited us to a dance. They were stationed in Bari on the East coast of Italy. They flew a B19 bomber over to pick us up. Of course, it was forbidden and we did not ask permission—we sneaked out by lowering our musette bags from a balcony to the street below, and sauntered out quite innocently. The party was great fun. When we ran out of cold beer, a couple of pilots loaded several cases of beer into a plane, took it up to 10,000 feet long enough to cool it off, and the party continued most of the night. On our return trip we flew over Mt. Vesuvius which was beginning to erupt, and tipped the wing into the cone so that we had a bird's-eye view. They also let us take turns piloting that hugh bomber. We flew over the massed fleet which was preparing for the invasion of Southern France. Once we spent a few days in Sorrento, visited Pompeii, and went for a swim in the Blue Grotto on the Isle of Capri.

When I was in Italy there were about a dozen hospitals near Naples, so we established a local dietetic association. Since I was the only dietitian in my hospital, I enjoyed meeting other dietitians.

Shortly after the invasion of Southern France our hospital was transferred to St. Tropez. The women were transported on one ship, the men and equipment on another. We arrived before the beaches and paths had been cleared of mines, so our movements were severely limited. After about a week, we set up the hospital in a hotel. The women were quartered on the two top floors, and we had to walk up and down most of the time since the one elevator was reserved for movement of patients. I was on the eighth floor, and the kitchen was in the basement.

Because we were one of the first units to set up Southern France, the Field Bakery had not yet been activated. The bakers in my hospital and I decided to bake fresh bread every day. We had no mixers, and the ovens were heated by coal, so we had quite a time learning how to control the temperature. But the bread, which was baked directly on the hearth, was wonderful. We were almost sorry when the Field Bakery was opened.

After about two months in St. Tropez, it was decided to move our hospital to Grasse, just north of Cannes. We moved into a modern hospital which had been occupied by the Germans. They had destroyed much of the machinery when they left, but it was gradually repaired.

We moved the hospital from St. Tropez to Cannes in one day—patients, staff, enlisted men and equipment. It was quite a logistical problem, but everyone just worked hard to accomplish it successfully. We had been together for over a year by that time.

The kitchen had a lot of steam equipment and electric ovens, but we were never able to get the ovens repaired. And there was a Hobart mixer! One of the steam kettles had a direct steam inlet. It was designed as a soup kettle. I had never seen one like it, and neither had the cooks. One morning one of the cooks chose that kettle to cook the scrambled eggs. Of course, the liquid eggs filled up the steam inlet until the pressure built up enough to blow it out. We had scrambled eggs all over that kitchen.

That really was a lovely hospital. We had German POW's who kept the kitchen immaculate, and French cooks for the Officers Mess. That had a separate kitchen and dining room. We had linen table cloths, waiters to serve us, and that created a very nice ambience.

The Officers Club was in a villa right on the Mediterranean. We had an Olympic-size swimming pool, an institutional-size kitchen and it was furnished beautifully. We occasionally went to the beaches in Cannes, but the Club was more fun. Since Cannes was a recreational area for the Allied Forces, we could stay in any of the hotels free, and we did that several times.

One of my friends was an official of the Red Cross, and had been in the French underground. He had lived in Cannes before the war and was captured by the Germans. He was important enough to be exchanged for a German prisoner and could not be in the Armed Services subsequently. He was an architect and had built many of the lovely villas on the Cote d'Azur. Barry knew many of the wealthy French families, and was invited to lunch, cocktail parties, dinners. Frequently he invited me and my roommate to go with him, so I saw the inside of many of the villas. Barry was the grandson of the Steinway piano founder, and was an accomplished pianist. One weekend he persuaded me and my roommate to go with him to Monte Carlo to visit a friend, who just happened to be the daughter of Rimsky-Korsakov. Monte Carlo was off limits, so we had to go in civvies. We took a lunch, which I prepared, and had such a good time that we missed an appointment with the Princess of Monaco, whom Barry knew well.

There was a hepatitis epidemic that summer, and it was decided to send all hepatitis patients to our hospital. No one knew much about hepatitis then, and, by segregating the patients, we hoped to cut down the spread of the disease. At one time, we had 750 patients with hepatitis.

After VE Day, it was decided to send our Station Hospital to the Philippines. Since I had accrued too many points to be sent there, I was transferred to a General Hospital in Aix-en-Provence. That hospital was scheduled to be sent back to the States, but when the prisoners were released from the concentration camps, many of them were transferred to our hospital until they could be rehabilitated sufficiently to be sent elsewhere.

Finally, about mid-September, it was our turn to be sent home. The ship was loaded to the gills. The men had to sleep in shifts, and we were each served two meals a day. The galley served meals 24 hours a day. We landed in Boston, and we were royally welcomed into Boston Harbor. Our first meal was a steak dinner with all the trimmings, apple pie and ice cream, and all the milk anyone wanted. Then we all stood in line to call home. I was discharged from Fort Jackson and my mother and father picked me up during a flash flood. But nothing could dampen our spirits.

Graduate School

I had never seriously thought of going to Graduate School because it cost too much. But the GI Bill took care of that. I applied to Teachers College, Columbia University shortly after I returned home, and was accepted. The Fall Semester had already begun, so I started the Winter Semester 1946. Because I was out of sync, I was told that I could not take one of the required courses in accounting. But I petitioned to take the exam from the first semester, and I crammed accounting and passed. By doing that, I could graduate in one year. Mary deGarmo Bryan and Orpha Mae Thomas were my primary professors, both of them excellent teachers.

During my first semester, one of our visiting lecturers was Dorothy Proud from Cornell University. She had been on the staff at Western Reserve, and was a friend of Lucille McMackin. After class I introduced myself, and she remembered meeting me. When she went back to Cornell, she told Katherine Harris, the Chairman of Institutional

Management, about me. I met Miss Harris a few weeks later when she came to New York. I was invited to go to Ithaca to be interviewed by the faculty and was offered a summer job in Extension to work with Dorothy Proud.

During the Fall Semester, when most students entered the graduate program, I was one of the few already acquainted with Dr. Bryan. I became her protege and general factotum. I took a special project for three hours credit, and I EARNED those credits and more. But it was very good experience. Among the many things I did for her that semester was to edit a book that she was writing with several other authors (including Katherine Harris) to try to make the styles of the different authors similar. I had to really tread lightly because I did not know exactly which parts Dr. Bryan had written. I also prepared drafts of letters to answer questions from school food service directors who requested lists of small equipment, critiques of floor plans, etc.

Just before the semester began, Dr. Bryan had an urgent plea from Brooklyn College for someone to teach a course in Institution Management. I was selected by Dr. Bryan, and I dared not refuse. She thought I should consider teaching as a career, and that would be good experience. It really stretched me to take on that responsibility in addition to a full academic schedule (18 hrs), but I was glad that I had when later in the semester I was offered a position to teach in the undergraduate program at Cornell. I began teaching at Cornell in February 1947.

Cornell University

I worked harder and learned more the first few years I taught at Cornell than in any comparable period of time in my whole career. The standards were very high, and the students were very bright. Because the College of Home Economics was a Land Grant college, the tuition was much lower than for Cornell University which was not state supported. Cornell was considered one of the best universities in the country, and the competition to get into Home Economics was intense. All students were personally interviewed, and most of those who were accepted ranked in the 90th percentile of their high school classes. I taught Quantity Food Preparation to dietetic majors and Food Purchasing to dietetic and hotel students for the entire time I was at Cornell.

Each entering class was assigned an official counselor from the Dean's office who advised a class of students all four years. I was the unofficial adviser for all dietetic majors, and I got to know those students very well. I helped them select internships, and wrote letters of recommendation, listened to their tales of woe, and celebrated their achievements with them. When I moved to Mizzou, some of them came here to get a graduate degree.

Miss Harris was very active in ADA, and I was sent to ADA meetings every year. She introduced me to her colleagues who taught Institution Management in all the major universities. We had lunch together every year, and I was always the youngest person there. I was honored to be included in that group of outstanding professors such as Bessie Brooks West, Levelle Wood, Margaret Terrill, Beulah Hunzicker, Fern Gleiser, to name a few.

Miss Harris was a very innovative person, and it was a privilege to work with her. She had done research with graduate students for many years, but in the late Forties she established a position for a full-time research program. Then she died in about 1954 and I inherited my first graduate student.

When I was eligible for a sabbatic leave in 1956, I decided to go back to Graduate School to study for a doctoral degree. I was accepted at Michigan State University.

Doctoral Study

I was fortunate to receive the Mary Swartz Rose Fellowship in 1956 and again in 1958. In those days, $1,000 went further than it does now. It helped a great deal to defray my expenses. And I was honored to be selected twice for that prestigious award.

Katherine Hart was my mentor at Michigan State, although I could not get a Ph.D. under her. She steered me to Paul Dressel in the College of Education and I majored in Evaluation in Higher Education. Katherine was on my Committee, and through her influence I was permitted to take most of the management courses in the School of Business.

Margaret Gillam was doing a special project for the Kellogg Foundation, and had an office next to Katherine Hart. I had known her in New York and she befriended me in many ways. When I was writing my dissertation, she was out of town for a few weeks, and "lent" me her secretary. It was much appreciated. She knew Mary de-Garmo Bryan very well, and regaled me with tales of the early years of ADA when she and Dr. Bryan often travelled together. Most of my friends at Michigan State were on the faculty.

Mizzou

When I completed my doctorate in 1959, I fully intended to continue teaching at Cornell ad infinitum. I had been there 12 years and loved my job and Ithaca. But as soon as I received my degree, I was offered the opportunity to interview for positions all over the U.S. I was not interested in most of them, and interviewed to be head of the department at only two prestigious universities. Then I was persuaded to interview at the University of Missouri-Columbia.

The position at Missouri intrigued me because I would have the opportunity to manage the Department of Nutrition and Dietetics at the Medical Center as well as develop an undergraduate dietetic program and a graduate program in Food Systems Management. It was a unique opportunity, and I accepted and moved to Columbia in the fall of 1961.

In 1961, the Medical Center was just completed and some of the patient areas were not yet opened. I reported to the Director of the Hospital, the Deans of the School of Medicine and Home Economics. My salary was paid by Medicine, but my academic appointment was in Home Economics. I was on to the Executive Committee of the hospital and a similar committee in Home Economics.

The first major decision to be made was whether to establish an internship program or a coordinated undergraduate program (CUP) in dietetics. Because there were internship programs at Barnes Hospital and the University of Kansas, we opted for the CUP. But there were many things to be done to develop the department before we could begin to develop the CUP.

In 1961, the food delivery system for the patients was decentralized. Food was delivered in bulk to five pantries and trays were set up, delivered, picked up and the dishes were washed on each floor. This was very labor intensive. In 1965, funds were made available to remodel Main Kitchen and equip it for centralized tray service. This was much more efficient and the quality of food was improved because much of it could be cooked as required for tray service. Food cost could be controlled much more easily because waste could be reduced.

In 1966, the decision was made to build the Mid-Missouri Mental Health Center (MMMHC) adjacent to the University of Missouri Medical Center (UMCMC). Many of the major services such as pharmacy, radiology, pathology, and dietetics were to be contracted. In exchange for providing dietetic services, MMMHC agreed to build a cafeteria for the entire complex in the new building. This freed up the cafeteria space adjacent to Main Kitchen for an enlarged Computer Center. It also meant that food prepared in the Main Kitchen for the cafeteria, which served about 1500 meals at noon, had to be trucked about 1000 feet to the new cafeteria. The space in the new cafeteria was about two-thirds that in the old cafeteria, so that created additional problems. Because the new design was an open square with much self-service, waiting time for patrons was actually reduced, but finding a seat was difficult.

In the mid-sixties, the Medical School was also expanded and a Clinical Research Center was added. This created another satellite cost center, which added urgency to the development of a computer-assisted management system.

Development of Computer-Assisted Management System

In 1962, UMC School of Medicine received a Regional Medical Grant with the primary goal of improving health care and making accessible to providers of care throughout the region the latest in technology and research. It was decided to utilize computer technology to facilitate the process, and in December 1963 an electronic computer of medium capacity was installed.

Each department head and faculty member was urged to utilize this management tool. A two-page single-spaced proposal was submitted by the Department of Nutrition and Dietetics. Basically, this was conceptualized as a foodservice management system which would integrate a patient care system. Each sub-system was planned as an integral part of the total system and an effort was made to determine how subsystems would interact and affect the total system. This plan was subsequently developed in essentially the same order as submitted in the next 15 years.

Our primary goal was to make the Department of Nutrition and Dietetics at UMC more efficient because it was the site for educating dietetic students at the undergraduate and graduate level. Our secondary goal was of almost equal importance—to make computer technology developed at UMC available at cost to other hospitals and educational institutions.

Let's set the stage for this project. No one on staff had had much experience with computers. In 1963, that was not unusual. We were told to use personnel in the Computer Center as technical advisers, and programmers were assigned to each project. No extra funds were alloted to the department. The entire system was developed by department staff and graduate students except for one programmer whom we hired when our project was "bumped" so frequently because the programmer assigned to us was preempted for a project deemed more important. I was concerned that my graduate students would be delayed unreasonably. Eventually we were able to hire our own computer analyst and other supportive personnel through reclassification of positions which was made possible through the greater efficiency achieved by computerization. We were permitted a fair amount of autonomy in planning our budget as long as we did not exceed our allotment. Throughout the years we were given as much computer time as required—not insignificant to our success. Many of our graduate students were full-time dietitians in the department, because we had no funds for research assistants. Twenty graduate students assisted in the development and implementation of the system.

Probably, the fact that from the beginning the development of computer systems at UMC was lodged within the department which would utilize the system contributed significantly to the success of computer utilization at UMCMC. Radiology, Pathology and Dietetics became nationally and internationally recognized for computer applications in their disciplines. Because of this, a very competent staff was assembled and outstanding graduate students were attracted to UMC.

In 1969, a conference on Computer-Assisted Food Management Systems was held at UMC and the Proceedings from that conference received wide distribution. It was used as a text in many universities and had to be reprinted. DIETETIC COM-PAK (DC-P), an educational model designed to teach the concepts of computer assisted management by giving students hands-on experience, was developed by Loretta Hoover as partial fulfillment of the requirements for her doctoral degree. We applied for grants to bring faculty from universities and internships throughout the U.S. to train them to use DC-P. Upon completion of the workshops, the institution was allowed to purchase DC-P at cost. More than 50 universities did purchase the program.

Frankly, I cannot understand how anyone can manage a complex foodservice system efficiently without computer assistance. I fully expected that by 1980 computer assistance would be an integral component of every large foodservice system. Yet, as 1990 approaches, there are few computer systems in any hospital that I know about which approach the scope of the one at UMCMC.

In April 1989, the focus of the Ross Roundtable was on Computers in Dietetics. I was a keynote speaker and almost half of the participants were former graduate students from UMC. The Proceedings of this conference will be published in early 1990. An expanded description of the components of the system developed at UMC will be included.

Graduate Program in Food Systems Management

When I came to UMC in 1961, there was no graduate program in Food Service Management (FSM) in Missouri. As soon as I became a member of the Graduate Faculty, shortly after I arrived, the first graduate student was enrolled. Before I retired in 1983, 38 M.S. and 7 Ph.D. degrees in FSM had been granted. I was the Chairman for most of these, and on the Committee for the others. Most of these former graduates are in leadership positions, and are very active in The American Dietetic Association. They network very effectively.

There were very few assistantships available until 1967 when the Allied Health Professions Advanced Traineeship Grant Program was initiated. I applied for and received grant support for 18 master's degree and 4 Ph.D. degree candidates from September 1967 to June 1974. Approximately half of these students studied nutrition. The students received a stipend plus tuition and fees.

Although it could not be made a requirement for graduation, all of my graduate students were pressured to publish their research, most frequently in the Journal of The American Dietetic Association. Most of them complied and I was coauthor. This did much to enhance the reputation of dietetics at UMC.

Coordinated Undergraduate Program in Dietetics

In 1971, the School of Medicine received a grant from the U.S. Public Health Service (USPHS) to develop a CUP in Dietetics with two areas of emphasis—Food Systems Management and Medical Dietetics. In 1972, another grant was funded to expand the program from 40 to 60 students (15 students in each program per year). The total funding was over one million dollars. This program was designated by USPHS as one of 18 Allied Health Programs of National Significance and each grant was fully funded for five years at a time when funding was truncated at most universities.

The CUP at UMC achieved national acclaim as a model program and was visited frequently by faculty from other universities. The faculty also answered many questions and gave advice by telephone and mail. In 1974, ADA received a grant to present five regional two-week workshops to assist university faculty to develop CUP's; UMC was subcontracted to present one of these workshops and was fully subscribed. Participants came from as far away as Seattle, Rhode Island and Texas, though they could have attended programs much nearer home.

Probably, the initial success of the program could be attributed to the close association with the Department of Nutrition and Dietetics at the Medical Center. I was Director of the department and the CUP was under my jurisdiction. The staff dietitians had part-time faculty appointments in the CUP and the CUP faculty attended department meetings. Staff could attend seminars, etc. and faculty were actively involved in the day to day operation of the department. Because it was a stimulating place to work, we attracted well-qualified dietitians and faculty. Most of the dietitians had master's degrees, and many others were enrolled in graduate school.

Throughout my career at UMC I was active in committee work in the College of Home Economics and the Medical Center. I was elected to serve on the Faculty Council for two terms. I also served on the Intercampus Faculty Council, and on many other University committees.

In 1979, there was a change of administration at all levels—university, campus and hospital. During that period, a management consultant team was hired to evaluate every department in the Medical Center. The Department of Nutrition and Dietetics received glowing commendations with no suggestions for change. Imagine my consternation when I was requested to step down as department head in August 1980, with no explanation given. I became a full time faculty member overnight. It was ironical that I had received the prestigious University Faculty-Alumni Award in 1979.

When I retired in 1983, the FSM program was discontinued because the University was in dire financial straights and it was decided not to replace my position. The program is still strong, but the emphasis has been changed to a generalist program.

Consultations Abroad

In 1967, I was granted a sabbatical leave to go to Hacettepe University in Ankara, Turkey for six months to assist in upgrading the undergraduate dietetic program and internship. I represented the University of Nebraska which had an affiliation with Hacettepe and had received a grant from Rockefeller Foundation for that purpose. I taught a course for graduate students and advised the Director of the Medical Center about the Department of Dietetics in addition. Before I left, I persuaded the President of the University to send four dietitians to the U.S. for two years to learn how to be dietitians American-style. I was their sponsor and I persuaded the directors of internships at Iowa and Kansas to each take one of them for two years, and I kept one at Mizzou. One went to the University of Nebraska and completed a Ph.D. degree there.

In 1968, Rockefeller Foundation sent me to Bangkok, Thailand to assist in planning the Dietetic Department for Ramathibodi Hospital which was being constructed by Rockefeller Foundation funds. I spent a month visiting hospitals and restaurants to learn about food habits and equipment available in Thailand before making my recommendations. In turn, Rockefeller Foundation sent the Director of the Dietetic Department to UMC for a year to study and work in our department.

In 1975, under the auspices of Pan American Health Organization, I was a consultant to the Caribbean Food and Nutrition Institute. I presented a week-long workshop for administrative dietitians in Port of Spain, Trinidad, spoke at the Annual Meeting of the Caribbean Association of Dietitians and Nutritionists, and visited hospitals and school foodservices in Barbados and Jamaica.

In 1979, I was consultant to the Title VII program in the U.S. Virgin Islands. I visited programs in St. Croix and St. Thomas and presented a week-long workshop for site managers.

Professional Association Activities

Shortly after going to Cornell, I was instrumental in establishing the Cayuga Dietetic Association. I was elected to be the first President, and became a member of the Executive Board of the New York State Dietetic Association. I served on that Board in many capacities until I left Cornell. I also served on several ADA committees during that time.

When I moved to Missouri, I helped to form the Central Missouri Dietetic Association. I served on the Executive Board of the Missouri Dietetic Association in many capacities, most notably as Delegate for ten years. One of the most important assignments I had as Delegate was to chair the Ad Hoc Committee on Specialty Board Certification for four years. I served on innumerable other ADA committees, most recently on the Strategic Planning Committee. I have been Area II coordinator for the ADA Foundation Planning Committee. I have been Area II Coordinator for the ADA Foundation to raise funds for the National Center for Nutrition and Dietetics.

Throughout the years I have spoken frequently at ADA Annual Meetings, at state dietetic association meetings all over the U.S., and the Canadian Dietetic Association. One year, when ADA met in Denver, ten of my former graduate students were on the program presenting their research findings.

I have also taken a leadership role in the Foodservice Systems Management Education Council, serving progressively as Treasurer, Secretary, Chairman-elect, and Chairman. This is a national association of college and university faculty with the primary goal of improving undergraduate instruction and promoting research. Proceedings are published and have become valuable tools for curriculum development and evaluation.

Although I have not participated as significantly in the American Home Economics Association, I was formerly Chairman of the Institution Management Section. I presented papers at several Annual Meetings and at Missouri and Arizona state meetings.

My activities in these professional organizations have been richly rewarded. In 1976, I received the Medallion Award from The American Dietetic Association. In 1983, I was named the Outstanding Dietitian of Missouri. In 1986, I received the most prestigious award of ADA, the Marjorie Hulsizer Copher Award. None of these honors would have been awarded had it not been for the loyal support of my staff and former students who nominated me. To them and to my colleagues throughout the country I give my heartfelt thanks.

Retirement has been great fun. I now have time to travel extensively, and I purchased Eastern Airlines Get-Up-and-Go passports for several years which allowed almost unlimited trips throughout the U.S. I also spent a month with my niece and her husband in Japan, led a group of dietitians on a month-long Scientific Exchange to China in 1985, then returned to China in 1988 for another month. That time I had an opportunity to visit the families of several men who had studied at Mizzou and had worked for me. On two occasions, I've spent a month in Honduras visiting another niece and her family. They have moved to Guatemala, so that is next on my list. My most recent major trip was to Tahiti, Australia, New Zealand and Fiji. I hope my good health continues because there are many places I still want to visit.

Anita L. Owen

Anita L. Owen, MA, RD
is Senior Vice President,
Nutrition Education and Research,
National Dairy Council, Rosemont, IL

Among her vast and varied accomplishments, Anita Owen is probably most well known as co-author of the classic community nutrition textbook, *Nutrition in the Community: The Art of Delivering Services*. Innovation and optimism are the hallmarks of her dynamic professional style. Her early work in public health led to the development of the first statewide WIC program in the nation. One of her initial contributions to ADA was the development of the first National Nutrition Week (now month). She was chosen to be a consultant to the U.S. Senate Select Committee on Nutrition and Human Needs. Public health administration became a springboard to an academic position at the University of Michigan and then on to the private sector for this 61st President of ADA. She has worked extensively in the Philippines as well as Taipai, Taiwan, and Bangkok. From debating with the Diamonds on national television to promoting the National Center for Nutrition and Dietetics, this leader's effective communication style has greatly advanced the image of our profession.

Anita L. Owen

As the only child of supportive parents, I grew up in Jessup, a small Pennsylvania coal mining town on a friendly street in which the neighboring houses were occupied by various aunts, uncles, cousins and grandparents of a close knit Italian family. That early environment bred in me the confidence and security that has helped me during the loops and turns of my extremely varied, occasionally glamorous, and always eventful 30 year career in nutrition. I've enjoyed every aspect of the field. I've tackled a whole list full of jobs in institutional, governmental, academic, business and entrepreneurial environments and have traveled tens of thousands of miles working with health professionals.

When it was time for me to embark on a college career, my mother suggested that I speak with Carolyn Sebastianelli, who was born and raised in Jessup, attended Marywood College in Scranton, and became a dietitian. Carolyn attended high school with my mother and she was greatly admired in the town for the work she was doing. Although I had no idea what a Dietitian did, it sounded interesting. I spoke to Carolyn and from there I applied to Marywood College where I received a Bachelor of Science Degree in Dietetics and Education. Thank goodness for Carolyn. I probably would not have been here today had it not been for her guidance.

Despite the casual and naive manner in which I followed Carolyn Sebastianelli's footsteps into dietetics, I must admit that it was a very good choice. I was impressed with all the options the field offered when I was in college. I felt it was a career in which there would be many opportunities.

After Marywood, I completed a dietetic internship at Grasslands Hospital in Valhalla, NY where I was employed as a Clinical, and then Teaching Dietitian at Westchester County Medical Center for about five years after my internship. Interestingly enough, after 30 years I returned to Grasslands as an Adjunct Associate Professor to teach Community Nutrition in the Department of Community Medicine, New York Medical College.

Columbia University Teacher's College was the next stop in my educational career, where I received a master's degree in 1962. Over the years, though, I have enjoyed various aspects of education. I continued to be a student pursuing graduate studies in biochemistry and anthropology at the University of Arizona; in Management at the University of California, Berkeley; University of North Carolina at Chapel Hill; and the University of Michigan, Ann Arbor.

Throughout my career I have always enjoyed developing and pioneering new territory and new areas; these activities were always very exciting and stimulating.

A move westward to Arizona in 1963 placed me in the field of Public Health Nutrition. As a County Nutritionist I developed the first nutrition component for the nursing home program and acted as nutrition consultant to nursing home facilities to upgrade dietary services. After that position I became the Nutritionist for the Migrant Health Program and developed the nutrition component for this program.

In 1966 I became the first Chief Nutritionist for the State of Arizona. Despite funding and other limitations, we approached the task of building an effective nutrition program with confidence and skill. We made nutrition an integral part of a number of state agency programs as a result of some creative programming and networking with the private, as well as the public sector. Within two years, working with groups and individuals we became the driving force in the expansion of the Nutrition Council of Arizona to 80 agencies in the field of government, health and business. The Council worked to make better use of available funds in the state and to develop programs needed by the people of Arizona.

One accomplishment that I find most rewarding was the work we did in Arizona to deliver nutrition services to rural communities. We developed a nutrition delivery system during the era of hunger and malnutrition in the United States. To do this we utilized the survey data developed by Dr. Arnold Shaefer, Ph.D., Director of the Ten State Nutrition Survey and George M. Owen, M.D., Director of the Preschool Nutrition Survey. My first grant proposal was written to the Center for Disease Control (CDC) to develop an innovative model for a nutrition delivery system. Our first grant was funded; as a result we embarked upon the task of developing a nutrition delivery system for low income groups in Arizona.

These were exciting times in the field of public health, since we had the opportunity to be a part of the development of the Supplemental Feeding Program for Women, Infants and Children (WIC Program). In our efforts to lay a solid foundation for nutrition, we developed the first statewide WIC Program in the nation. Writing in the June, 1974 Good Housekeeping magazine, Joe Bell, reporter for the magazine, said, and I quote "the first statewide WIC operation was in Arizona where the need was urgent and the machinery had long been readied by a dynamic young State Nutrition Director with snapping eyes and a no nonsense approach named Anita Yanochik Owen." At that time we had developed a newsletter called "Keep WIC lit." We published this newsletter to facilitate legislative action throughout the country on WIC legislation. Every time it was published, thousands of letters of support reached congressmen urging them to pass this important legislation. I was happy to be involved as one of the major architects of the WIC program working with Senator Hubert H. Humphrey, Alan Stone of the Senate Select Committee, and several other members of Congress to develop the medical, nutrition and feeding program for low income pregnant women, infants and children.

There are many fascinating stories to tell about the development of the WIC program, one example that demonstrates the tenacity we had in developing the program and our commitment to getting things done involved the Navajo Indian tribe. We were very anxious to develop the WIC program on the Navajo reservation, because of their health and nutrition problems. I was informed by the Department of Agriculture that we had 48 hours to develop this program or funding could not be obtained for another year. In view of the fact that it takes approximately 7 hours to get to the reservation from Phoenix, let alone starting the system, our task was formidable. This would have been a major setback for most people, but not for us. Undaunted, we worked with the Governor's Office to charter a plane. It worked—we airlifted six nutritionists on dirt runways on the reservation and issued the first voucher within 40 hours. The Department of Agriculture could not believe it. A USDA official, Harold T. McLean, Administrator of the Northeast Regional office, who was the first Director of the WIC program for USDA said "Anita Owen was the major force in the early founding and development of the WIC program. Her tireless efforts on behalf of the needy have made a significant contribution to the structure and integrity of the program today."

We also gained public policy skills at the state level by leading the movement to obtain an enrichment bill for Arizona which we accomplished in a one year period. This was done by working with both the private and public sector.

Working in Arizona was one of the highlights of my career as a young professional. When I left the Arizona State Department of Health in 1976, we had developed a nutrition program from a one member staff operation with a $15,000 budget, to a $9,000,000 program with 20 nutritionists and a network of more than 125 nutrition aids. Indeed, those were exciting times. Because of our work in Arizona, I became a consultant to the Senate Select Committee on Nutrition and Human Needs, I was privileged to present testimony on national nutrition policy and other aspects of health care.

Another enjoyable aspect of the Arizona State Department of Health experience was our working with students. We considered it a wonderful opportunity to have students from all over the country work with us. Students found the public health nutrition program in Arizona a dynamic one. One student stated, and I quote "Classroom subjects came alive, community diagnosis, community assessment, nutrition surveillance and evaluation techniques. Our discussions were spirited."

After my work as Chief Nutritionist, I was selected to become the Assistant Commissioner of Health for Arizona with 500 employees. I administered the statewide program of health services which included the State Laboratory, Communicable Diseases, Dental, Nutrition, Health Education, Nursing, and local Health Services Programs. I happened to be the first female non physician to hold such a position in Arizona.

In 1966, with Reva Frankle, Director of Nutrition for Weight Watchers, we began writing a textbook on Public Health Nutrition. The book, *Nutrition in the Community the Art of the Delivering Services*, was completed in 1978 and is now in it's second edition. Today this is considered a classic textbook and is used extensively throughout the United States and many foreign countries. Reva and I felt that from our experiences in public health, Reva's in New York and mine in the southwest, that it was important to have a practitioner's approach to delivering nutrition services. We committed to paper the experiences that we had in delivery services in our many wonderful years in public health.

A move to the midwest in 1977 brought me into the academic field as Assistant Professor of Nutrition in the School of Public Health at the University of Michigan, Ann Arbor. I thoroughly enjoyed working with students at the University. Jean M. Bogdanski, MPH, RD, class of 1979, University of Michigan, made the following statements in a recent publication about the courses at U. of Michigan. "I have been lucky in life. I have been especially fortunate to have attended the U. of Michigan School of Public Health and there to have met Anita and Dr. George Owen. Anita was and has been a motivational and inspirational person in my academic, professional and personal life. Anita captivated her students by her enthusiasm, energy and leadership. She touched a part of us that made us want to excel to produce 110 percent. Upon graduation we knew we had an excellent education taught by a professional who had worked in and developed a model nutrition delivery system. Our aspiration was to become as good a practitioner as the Assistant Professor who taught us."

Still yearning for Public Health activities similar to the Arizona experience, I acted as a consultant to the Detroit Health Department where we initiated the Nutrition Surveillance System with the nutrition staff and attracted funds for the first sentinel site clinic developing the initial project for the nation.

After leaving Michigan in 1980 I tried my hand at private business and developed Owen Associates, Inc., consultants in nutrition and health care. In the business world I worked in many diverse areas. In the domestic area I developed a series of handbooks on nutrition information for physicians for a nationally known company. I developed a guide for planning nutrition services in primary health care for the Federal Government also. In addition, I completed work such as a supplement on community nutrition for the new Manual for Clinical Nutrition and provided consultation and workshops on nutrition education to several private and public groups throughout the country.

Internationally, traveling extensively with my husband, George Owen, M.D., who is Vice President, Medical Director, Bristol Myers International Company, I did many exciting nutrition programs. In our travels I developed a series of nutrition and management workshops for dietitians and nutritionists in Manila, and wrote a column called "Mom's Nutrition Corner" for the Manila Sunday paper, over a four year period. In February, 1985, I was made an honorary member of the Nutritionists and Dietitians Associations of the Philippines at its Pearl Anniversary ceremony in Manila. I certainly cherish this award. In addition to my work in the Philippines, I developed workshops in Taipai, Taiwan, and Bangkok and Stockholm. This was a very exciting part of my business, since there was great interest in nutrition and management in those countries.

Being involved in one's professional associations has many rewards, benefits and opportunities. I began my work with The American Dietetic Association as Public Relations Chairman in the early 70's after going through the chairs in the Arizona Dietetic Association, including President. I was ready for a National position and Public Relations was the first one. At that time we developed the first National Nutrition Week as part of ADA's Public Affairs program. The ADA leadership role gets into your blood. I then moved on to Delegate at Large, Speaker-elect, Speaker, and then finally, President-elect and President of The American Dietetic Association, which was one of the most rewarding experiences I have ever had. Being the 61st President of The American Dietetic Association gave me an opportunity to meet many of the dietitians throughout the country. I chose as my role, to develop a stronger, more effective communications network with the media and industry. I travelled to at least 37 states in the one year I was President. I completed several innovative projects for the Association, attracting several million dollars for various work with industry and government.

I enjoyed setting up the first leadership workshop in the House of Delegates as Speaker and developing the first newsletter for the House. These were communication pieces that were necessary during my era and indeed we followed through and helped with the communications process within the organization.

Visibility for the dietitian was another major area that I pursued as President. During that time we developed brief statements that could be turned around in 48 hours for quick response to the media. We also handled the Board of Directors in a different way. We set up work groups whereby each member of the Board of Directors was on a team with the staff, developing the objectives that needed to be accomplished.

One of the most terrifying experiences as President was to debate the Diamonds' on television reviewing their book, *Fit for Life*, with Bryant Gumble as host. It was an experience that we should all have once in a lifetime, nevertheless, it was worth it because ADA was seen throughout the country, as a group willing to take on misinformation and attempt to set the record straight.

One of the most exhilarating experiences was our work with the committee to develop The National Center for Nutrition and Dietetics. We were able to take our dreams and goals, and aspirations for the profession and develop the National Center. It was a worthwhile activity. It is really the future for the young members of our Association and we are moving along on this effort. I am happy to say that I will be, in 1989, the President of the ADA Foundation. Soliciting funding from the corporate world will be our major thrust. I believe the Center is the wave of the future for dietetics. I firmly believe that the development of the Center is one of the most important steps that the Association can take to advance the profession in the 21st century. I was proud to be part of the steering committee to develop the State program for fund raising. It was a successful venture and continues to have members work and contribute to make the Center a reality.

My most recent challenge, Manager of Nutrition for Nabisco Brands, Inc. has been another exciting position where I have learned a great deal about economics, marketing and the corporate world. Dietitians have a major contribution to make in the area with an applied knowledge of nutrition and health in addition to food.

I have enjoyed speaking to members on future trends for dietitians in the 21st century. It has been a rewarding experience because we, as dietitians, must look at our fast paced society and where we are going. As I speak to dietitians about the future, I urge us to confront changes with innovative thinking. In this era of rapid technological change, dietitians will need to do more than just keep pace, we will need to stay ahead, exploit technology aggressively and imaginatively and apply it experimentally to new ideas.

It is important for society that dietitians become the nutrition experts for the country in the 21st century.

Sara Clemen Parks

*Sara C. Parks, MBA, RD is Associate Dean
for Commonwealth Educational System Programs,
College of Health and Human Development,
Pennsylvania State University, State College, PA*

Sara Parks writes of the love, support, and guidance she received from her parents who placed high value on education. She was only one of two women from a high school graduating class of 56 students to attend college. Her story seems to be the reverse of Loyal Horton's: being a woman in the man's kingdom of business. However, she admits that there was a silver lining to the cloud—being a woman has helped her to beat a few traffic tickets! She was able to reverse a decision and entered graduate school as one of two women in a class of over 200. Her love of teaching is revealed through her words and deeds and has been recognized by several prestigious awards. In a delightful writing style, Sara Parks reminds us that her profile is neither her eulogy or obituary, but perhaps a map of possible routes to take along a career highway with some of the sights to be seen along the way.

Sara Clemen Parks

It is less than original and more than obvious to credit one's parents for any success in life one achieves.* Nevertheless, I happily start this personal narrative with my father and mother, both of whom guided me toward a career in service and education. My father's influence was strong but subtle. A man without much in the way of formal education, he valued education highly and encouraged all of his children to follow its path as far as that path might lead. Meanwhile, he exuded an informal warmth and neighborliness that revealed for me the worth of friendship, social objectivity, and a concern for others. The local grocer in our small Iowa town, my father was the sort of man who would carry his customers on the books until they could afford to pay their bills. Not only have I had marvelous parents, I have always enjoyed the love and support of an older brother, John, and two sisters, Susan and Sharon. Always we were a family team.

My mother's influence was more direct and probably even stronger than my father's. As a girl growing up in Dyersville, Iowa, I always dreamed of becoming a career woman like my mother. In fact, at first I wanted to be exactly like her: a Registered Nurse and a Director of Nursing somewhere in a midwestern hospital. But my mother, with the wisdom to match her considerable skills, somehow knew that nursing and I would never be compatible. I recall that after several requests, she finally escorted me through her hospital, taking the time to show me her sickest patients, the more troubling procedures, and the dullest of nursing routines; and she was absolutely right, I cringed at the mere thought of taking blood and I instantly sensed that my professional dream was much too specific for a little girl who had yet to complete junior high school.

But that same day, my mother also took me down (it's always "down," isn't it) to the hospital's dietary department where I met a large, jolly nun clearly and abundantly in love with her work as a nutritionist. The picture of that contented woman remains vivid in my mind, a model that immediately replaced the image of my mother's caregiving career and a model I still emulate.

I often refer to nursing as my "road not taken," but I also like to think of dietetics less as a substitute profession and more as my ideal profession, the place in life where I felt most comfortable and effective performing a service. I would confirm this attitude much later when I discovered to my surprise and delight that I could combine two services—dietetics and education—so as to build a career notable enough that at this moment I find myself describing it for the benefit of others who might one day like to do what I do.

When I was a girl in Dyersville, tradition discouraged women from aspiring to higher education, and only two women of the 56 students in my high school graduating class went on to college. But both my mother and father saw intelligence and initiative

*I acknowledge with gratitude the help of my colleague, John Swinton, an editorial specialist at The Pennsylvania State University, who helped me prepare this profile.

in me, and luckily I had an aunt and uncle in Lincoln who could keep an eye on me as I worked my way through the University of Nebraska. By this time, I knew that I wanted a career in therapeutic dietetics, and I matriculated at Nebraska as a nutrition major. But insightful as ever, my mother urged me to augment my studies with business courses, and I took a minor in business administration—even though, as I recall, my adviser considered business "too easy" for a science-based dietetics student, and even though I often found myself the only woman amid dozens of college boys.

Grass-green from college but having served a rigorous dietetic internship at Henry Ford Hospital in Detroit, I took my first job as a dietitian in St. Mary's Hospital in Grand Rapids, Michigan. The Dietary Department at St. Mary's was then in flux; a steady stream of supervisors flowed into and out of the work there; and within six months, I had become the boss of a two-person staff while being supervised and mentored by Lorraine Jacoby, herself a superb manager busily building a dietetics staff to complement our 425-bed hospital. But no sooner had Lorraine rounded out her staff than she received an irresistible job offer in Boston and left me in the Director of Dietetics position. Only a couple of years before, I had been a college student. Now I had a profession, a career, responsibilities I could hardly comprehend, and supervisory control over 110 employees—to say nothing of the practical managing, budgeting, and health care liaison work the hospital expected of me.

Few youngsters could successfully carry out a sudden challenge of this magnitude without the encouragement and help of colleagues, and two of St. Mary's administrators, Dan Vaughn and John Baumgartner, seemed to know my capabilities and seemed to know, as well, exactly when I needed personal friendship and professional support.

As I grew into my work as Director of Dietetics at St. Mary's, Dan and John learned of my interest in business and encouraged me to apply for the MBA program at Michigan State, 70 miles to our east. I liked the idea, I applied, and I got summarily rejected. To tell the truth, I could not, for the life of me, understand why, and it annoyed me. My record at Nebraska had been sound, my work at St. Mary's was exemplary, and I had a demonstrated interest in the business field. My response to the form-letter rejection was to jump into my car, drive Interstate 96 over to East Lansing, and schedule an appointment with the dean. He asked to see my credentials, he agreed that they far exceeded the School's admission requirements, and during our conversation, he led me to believe that my being a woman had somehow played a part in the initial rejection. But he reversed that decision and admitted me as a "provisional" student, one of six women in a class of more than 200.

My return to the classroom complicated an already complicated life, and the next four years, though happy and rewarding, were also among the most hectic of my career. I commuted from Grand Rapids to East Lansing continually, fitting in classes whenever I could and trying to keep them from interfering with my hospital responsibilities. I admit to a heavy foot, and I must confess that I quickly got to know every state trooper between Grand Rapids and East Lansing on a first-name basis. Having alluded to the

219

possibility of latent sexism in the Michigan State Business School's admission policies back in the late sixties, I should balance the account here by suggesting that, as a young woman with a pretty face and an ingratiating smile, I may have escaped a few speeding tickets in those days that should have been mine.

I had begun my MBA program in 1967, I managed a leave from St. Mary's for the one semester of residency on campus Michigan State required, and I was well on my way toward my graduate degree when, early one evening, I received an excited telephone call from a professor in Michigan State's hotel and restaurant school. That call would soon change my life profoundly and alter my career expectations, pulling me away from dietetics toward a career in education based on my dietetics background.

The call came from Dr. Thomas F. Powers, engaged at that moment in presenting a "Management Careers for Women" panel discussion. One of his panelists had been forced to cancel, and somehow Ted had learned about my dual career as hospital dietitian and business graduate student. (It was hard in those days at Michigan State for a woman to hide.) Tom marshaled every ounce of his persuasive Irish blarney and blandishment and convinced me to step in for the absent panelist. There I stood in my dormitory, in my blue jeans, in hair curlers, and without makeup, and I asked him when he needed me.

"Would you believe," he replied, "tonight. In fact, within the hour."

As you can imagine, I had all kinds of doubts and misgivings, but I recalled then something my mother had always said: "You're just as good as anyone else. Just don't get too sold on the idea that you're a lot better."

I appeared with the panel, apparently acquitted myself with poise, and received my MBA shortly thereafter, in the spring of 1970. Tom Powers, meanwhile, is not the sort of person who forgets either a favor or a good performance. He traveled east that summer to interview for the recently vacated directorship of Penn State's Food Service and Housing Administration (FSHA) program; he received the appointment; and one of his first decisions was to invite me to head the program's Administrative Dietetics unit. I met the faculty members and liked them immediately. To this day, I am grateful for two administrators, Ray Studer and Ted Vallance, who immediately put me at ease. More generously still, my long-time colleague Jim Keiser and his wife Jo welcomed me into their home and in a real sense became my surrogate family while their own three teenagers whirled around us keeping my mind from thoughts of loneliness.

Tom Powers was, and still is, energetic and forward-looking, and he saw his Administrative Dietetics unit as a link to Great Society programs and government funding in the same way that academic food service and hotel units had always counted on industry. Suddenly my role became professor and academic researcher and someone in need of a background and a dossier that would attract and hold the confidence of those who underwrite and otherwise support allied health programs on university campuses.

At first I was overwhelmed and even a bit terrified. Pennsylvania was, for all my new friends, unfamiliar and far from my home and former work. I had come from an "industry model" so to speak, where my work received daily evaluations, into an academic model, where I had to work toward general goals more or less on my own. Powers gave me constant encouragement—my success, after all, would be his success as well—as did the dean in Penn State's College of Human Development, Donald Ford, who literally took me aside one weekend and helped me draft and polish my *curriculum vita*.

Then something new and wonderful happened to me to drive away the doubts and despair forever and to let great floods of enthusiasm rush in: Like so many professors before me, I discovered students. Looking back, I can see that my profession had already become part of my baggage; I could take my dietetics skills wherever I went. But I have remained content and happy at Penn State for 19 years because of my friends here, my colleagues, and most of all my students.

I still wonder whether Tom Powers noticed my love of teaching right from the start. In any event, he certainly made it easy for me to enter the classroom, and he involved me almost immediately in curriculum planning, where I have an aptitude and a solid reputation for success. Specifically, I helped design FSHA's "capstone" course, the course that "brings the whole curriculum together" for our students, forcing them in their senior year to draw upon all their previous work—in accounting and finance, marketing, cost control, layout and design, computer science, foods, personnel management, written communications, and so forth—in order to design an actual hospitality or health care operation for the year 2010.

I have taught that course—FSHA (now Hotel, Restaurant and Institutional Management, or HR&IM) 490—twice a year, every year for my 19 years at Penn State. Asked just this year to serve as an Associate Dean in Penn State's College of Health and Human Development, I stipulated that I be allowed to continue teaching that vital 490 course that gives me so much pleasure.

But Tom Powers' challenges and programmatic aspirations reached far beyond the Penn State campus. My original letter of offer required that I write a series of correspondence courses designed to lead an "extended" associate degree for the newly defined "dietetic technician" profession. Powers saw, with his usual acuity, the need dietary employees everywhere have to advance in their work, and the logistical problems they face when it comes time for them to complete their course work on campus. It was an insight that I, with three years of lengthy commutations between Grand Rapids and East Lansing, fully understood. In fact, the extended degree idea came, in a sense, right out of my St. Mary's experience working among bright supervisors with family responsibilities that kept them from returning to college. "Gee," I would hear them say, "if we could just find a degree program for people off campus."

Powers hired a small staff to help with the research, writing and editing, and I began to produce the series of courses that, eventually, made up Penn State's "Diet Tech" extended degree program.

Meanwhile, he pushed me still harder. "Sara," he told me soon after my arrival in University Park, "get on the phone and call the President or Executive Director of The American Dietetic Association and volunteer your services." He had anticipated clearly the need we would have to work with our professional association, but he did not yet understand my reluctance to confront important people in lofty positions. I braced myself, reached an administrative assistant somewhere in ADA's Chicago office, gave her my name, and quickly hung up with a huge sigh of relief.

The ineffectual first effort did not satisfy Tom. "Go higher," he ordered, and as tense as I was, I placed repeated calls until I finally reached the highest realms of ADA. I received, as you might guess, quite a warm reception—volunteers usually do—and thus began a long, cordial and mutually beneficial association.

To its credit, I think The American Dietetic Association immediately recognized the value of the work we proposed to do out of our cramped basement offices back in Penn State's Food Service and Housing Administrative program. And the ADA saw as well potential value in a young professional with a degree in dietetics and her RD certification, both complemented by a master,s degree in business administration, and I became an early member of the ADA Foundation's Board of Directors precisely because Audrey Wright, an administrator of Father Walter's Child Care Center in Montgomery, Alabama, recognized that need. Audrey had been the ADA's first Chair-elect of its Council on Practice; I had been the first Chair-elect of its Committee on Educational Preparation; and we worked closely enough for me to discover that Audrey—a fine, sensitive, dedicated woman—was fully cognizant of the ADA's need, then, to welcome a professional educator like me onto the Foundation Board.

(Before I proceed, please let me parenthetically acknowledge the women who, besides Audrey Wright, helped establish me firmly within the ADA's councils: Edna Langholz, who appointed me to the Task Force on Education; Mary Lou Smith, who appointed me to the Conceptual Framework Committee; and Janice Neville, who appointed me to the ADA's Strategic Planning Committee. Edna Langholz also became the first executive director of the Foundation and the National Center for Nutrition and Dietetics—a hectic time for all of us—but a most cherished period of professional and personal collegiality. Last, but not least, was Anita Owen—she was President of ADA the same year I became President of its Foundation. Together we made a beautiful team and developed a friendship I will treasure forever! As you have no doubt noticed but I am proud to point out, all three committees have strategically influenced the direction the profession of dietetics has taken in recent years.)

You may remember my mentioning the hectic schedule I once pursued, speeding back and forth over Interstate 96 between St. Mary's Hospital in Grand Rapids and my business program at Michigan State. Apparently I am someone who thrives on travel because my progression through the ADA's various committee assignments, the many conference appearances as I cleared Penn State's various academic hurdles, and (recall with sadness) poor and declining health in my family all forced me into a close and continual association with highways and airline terminals.

Though I referred to Penn State's "academic hurdles," the highest of which is almost always the attainment of tenure, I must say I had little trouble gaining job security at the University. I attribute my expeditiously granted tenure, once again, to

Tom Powers' foresight. Remember that my original letter of offer clearly stipulated my need to produce—from scratch, really—the Diet Tech curriculum. It sounded like a forbidding challenge at the time, but as I would later learn, specific objectives like these lead to success a lot quicker than grandly nebulous goals. The establishment and operation of Penn State's Diet Tech curriculum led directly to my academic tenure, and in no small measure, to the reputation I now enjoy for administrative effectiveness.

As those in The American Dietetic Association know, our Diet Tech courses succeed both because they meet a need in the market (marketing is a facet of business administration that has always attracted and fascinated me) and because they are innovative and unique. Taken together, they comprise a one-of-a-kind, award-winning college-credit course for non-traditional students. The 1987 Huddleson Award I won for the outstanding publication in the Journal of The American Dietetic Association underlines this predilection of mine for the innovative.

Let me refer again to my mother's influence to explain why I lean instinctively toward innovation and uniqueness within the service context. In our house, I could request a toy, or clothing, or a treat of some kind, and the outcome of that request would usually depend on my reason for making it. If I asked for a pair of saddle shoes ''because all the other girls have them,'' I was pretty much doomed to go without. If, however, my reason had something to do with genuine curiosity or experimentation, my chances improved enormously. I have succeeded within The American Dietetic Association at least partly because I am continually curious about what our ''markets'' need, and I recently became an Associate Dean in Penn State's new College of Health and Human Development at least partly because our bright young dean, Anne C. Petersen, wanted some marketing expertise behind the courses the College offers on Penn State's branch campuses.

Your editors have asked me to describe the ''struggles'' I contended with through the course of my career so far, and I notice in retrospect that all of them—occasional sexism (including the overly solicitous professors and a temporary inability to borrow money for school in my own name), a low grade now and then, the need to work 40 hours a week to get through the University of Nebraska, and the dispiriting times when both my father and mother were stricken with serious illnesses—occurred early and at a time when I probably needed some steeling, some beneficial tempering in the flames of adversity.

As this narrative of mine shows, I have become increasingly freer to practice my dietetics training within an academic framework. I have become ''free'' (and I use the word in something like a spiritual sense) to serve a broad but amorphous society with my dietetics expertise and to serve my students concretely and directly. The profession exhilarates me precisely because it encourages—it demands—problem-solving of me and my students and because it remains my professional motivator.

Nevertheless, I expect more from the dietetics profession, and from those who teach and study it, than I have yet seen. I would welcome less memorization and a much heavier emphasis on problem-solving. Rote strategies simply do not become a profession that must increasingly respond to individual needs. Dietitians must be technologically astute: We must welcome those methods and processes that free us from routine thinking and practice so we can liberate ourselves professionally. We should, moreover, be less bound by science than we are and much more interested in strategies that blend the more reliable scientific insights with a specific consumer's lifestyle.

I see a great capacity within the ADA to embrace these innovative attitudes and strategies. The Association is, after all, stronger now than it has been at any other time in its history. But we must keep our social responsibilities in mind, including the uncomfortable fact that those who need us most cannot always afford to pay us fairly. We exist only because we answer a need, and as much as I welcome the idea of entrepreneurialism within the profession, we need to keep the needy in mind.

As a girl, I remember my curiosity and skepticism when my mother gathered me up and packed me off with her to watch a regional production of some Shakespearean play in Dubuque. I would watch those plays, with all their archaic phrasing and stylized poses, and then I would re-read their plots in a children's book I kept at home. All the while I wondered what the relevance might be—until, that is, I found that I needed, and found that I had somehow acquired, an emphatic understanding of a great variety of personality types. Dietetics presents us with this wonderful personality spectrum, and campus life fills in its subtlest shades. Both careers have encouraged me to focus continually on my responsibility to others.

This sense of responsibility to and interest in others might have led me in a different direction, and there is one direction I occasionally regret ignoring. Early in my Penn State career, I received an attractive offer to become a vice president of a large food service company, and I must say I would have liked to have tried that work, at least for a while. But I was not ready then, and I am disinclined now, to give up my teaching or my commitment to providing dietary employees with a second chance at higher education.

My interest in teaching, a recurring theme in this profile, has produced tangible recognition. In 1978, I won an Amoco Award here at Penn State for my innovative classroom work, and I am most proud of a strictly local honor, The Evelyn Saubel Award, my College bestows annually (in my case, 1987) on the faculty member judged by students to have had the greatest and most positive impact on their college careers. Mrs. Saubel, a retired professor, remains our College's link with its home economics heritage, and she is one of those lovely and gracious old-school mentoring types who raises the tone of things around her and improves appearances wherever she goes.

My references to an early need to cover long distances in short periods would lead you to suspect that I have enjoyed the constant travel throughout my career, and you would be mostly right. On Penn State and ADA business, I have visited most of the country and a good deal of Canada as well; and frankly, I look forward to travel abroad, which has so far been only an unfulfilled prospect. I hope one day to visit as much of Europe as I can absorb and especially the Scandanavian countries.

To relax around the house between trips, I like to cook and to read popular novels—and Agatha Christie mysteries in particular. I take occasional quilting lessons, and by way of professional enrichment, I have been working my way toward a doctorate in higher education with an outside emphasis in marketing.

Glancing back over these remarks and attempting now to sum up what I have said that might help those just beginning their careers in dietetics, I see that I picture myself, paradoxically, as an independent-minded, fully committed career woman who, nevertheless, owes a great deal to a great many relatives and friends. My learning has come steadily, like my experience, and I hope to know a lot more tomorrow than I know right now. One thing I know for certain, and that is one cannot accomplish much by one's self alone. Dietetics provides a perfect example of what I mean: Its attendant information is both profuse and diffused, and the solo practitioner begs for failure. I, for one, could not have accomplished a fraction of what I have listed here without those I credit here and many more besides; I make it a point to ask for help whenever I need it; and having received the help I need, I feel a greater obligation to give it back.

Having asserted my frequent need for help and the debt I owe family and friends, I will say without intending to be trite or facetious that my best "career move" came in the spring of 1975 when I married Henry Parks, a businessman here in State College, Pennsylvania. All my love for Henry aside, he is my best friend, my most constructive critic, and the mellowing agent in my life. He continues the gentle prodding I once received from my mother and then Tom Powers. But even better, Henry understands and appreciates the fact that he has married a career woman. He will watch me to see if I grow too comfortable, too complacent; and if I do, he will chuckle a little, lean over and say, "Come on, Sara, you've got more to give than that."

It may not be quite grammatical, but we allow what Henry calls a "you-me-we" philosophy to govern our major decisions. We sit down together and try to determine how each decision will affect me, and Henry, and our life together. It seems to work just fine.

Also, I have so far been unusually fortunate in my choice of bosses. Tom Powers has already received the ample credit he deserves, and Tom was succeeded as HRIM Program Head at Penn State by our close mutual friend from Michigan State, Leo Renaghan, now a professor of hospitality marketing at Cornell. My boss since 1982 has been H.A. ("Andy") Devine, and it is no doubt a good thing that Andy and I share a mutual respect. My recent promotion to Associate Dean means that I have moved forward on some academic fronts, while the role as teacher and HR&IM faculty member I gratefully and cheerfully retain means that Andy still serves as my superior much of the time. (Such, on occasion, are the amusing ambiguities and ironies of college life.)

Finally, and still in the context of my helpful friends and colleagues, let me tell you that I work every day with two wonderful women and accomplished academic dietitians—RDs both of them—in the office where we administrate our Dietetic Technician Extended Degree program: Jan Raytek and Ellen Barbrow, my close colleagues for the last 15 years. Just as accomplished in her way and a critical member of our team, Joyce Wilusz manages our secretarial and clerical work.

In my writing, as in my career, I much prefer to focus on the future than to dwell in the past; I enjoy an agenda far more than a history. Please, therefore, accept these remarks as though they were directional signals or road signs pointing out possible routes to take and suggesting some of the sights to see along the way. I am, in fact, only slightly ahead of you on the highway. This is not a eulogy or my obituary. It is a summary in mid-career and—who knows?—perhaps the start of something new.

Corinne H. Robinson

Corinne H. Robinson, MS, DSc(Hon), RD
is Professor Emeritus, Department of Nutrition and Food,
Drexel University, Philadelphia, PA

Most dietitians and many other health professionals recognize the name of Corinne Robinson from her famous textbooks, *Normal and Therapeutic Nutrition* and *Basic Nutrition and Diet Therapy*. With over a million copies in print, including several foreign language translations, her books have been a primary vehicle for promoting nutrition education. When asked to describe her career in one word, she replies "EDUCATOR." This Copher Award winner was Professor of Nutrition and Food, Drexel University. Over three decades she taught several thousand undergraduate students as well as graduate and medical students. She has served as Chairman of ADA's Diet Therapy Section and the Dietetic Internship Board. She also represented the Association as liaison to the National League for Nursing to identify the goals for nutrition education in nursing curricula. Since her retirement in 1967, Corinne Robinson has been actively involved in efforts to assist older Americans as well as continuing with an assortment of ADA projects.

Corinne H. Robinson

Having now lived over four score years, I can look back on almost 60 years in dietetics. And what a varied career it has been: from the hospital internship to the research laboratory; from clinical dietetics to the university classroom; from writing textbooks that have now sold over a million copies to guiding graduate students through the awkward stages of writing their theses; from lecturing far and wide at dietetic meetings to engaging in the politics accompanying county programs for older Americans.

Finding My Identity

Things might have turned out quite differently. When I registered and paid my $221.65 in tuition, room and board fees at St. Olaf College in the fall of 1926, I was determined to pursue a music major. But rather like Jay Gatsby, the central character in Scott Fitzgerald's classic novel, whose short time at St. Olaf left him "dismayed at its ferocious indifference to the drums of his destiny, and despising the janitor's work with which he had to pay his way through"*, I too became disillusioned with music and the liberal arts. Money worries seemed overwhelming. My part-time jobs, from washing dishes in the school infirmary at twenty cents an hour to housekeeping for the family of the athletic coach, cut into my piano practice, but also left me feeling, in that era where few students at the college had to work, something of a social outcast. With no foreseeable prospects of marriage after college, with parents who could not genteely support a spinster piano teacher, what was I to do? I thought I could become a missionary, a nurse, a teacher—none of which appealed to me. Maybe I was too shy to ask for advice, but it seemed that my two years at St. Olaf were leading, not to destiny, but to a dead end.

It required only a modest nudge from the first of several mentors to resolve my predicament, as I came to appreciate a quite different career. I suppose you can all it the practical side of me, and here the story begins well before college. The 1915 Smith-Lever Act first authorized the 4-H movement to develop among young people skills in homemaking. In 1923 when I was 14, a 4-H club was finally organized in Ettrick, Wisconsin, the small town of 400 people in which I grew up. I plunged into its activities. For example, during 1925 when I was 16, I baked 55 loaves bread, 24 dozen fancy breads, 16 cakes, 19 pies, as well as cookies, doughnuts, popovers, and waffles. I canned 93 pints vegetables, 244 pints fruit, 62 pints pickles, and 38 jars jams and jellies. Beyond the skills developed, 4-H provided two quite material rewards: money and exposure. My prize monies at the county and state fairs, the fruits of a month's work, averaged about $400 in today's economy, giving me income for college that would otherwise have been unobtainable in my small farming community. My success also meant trips as a teenager to the state fair at Milwaukee and to the National 4-H Congress in Chicago. At trips sponsored by the Congress I was exposed to the stench and violence in slaughtering animals at the Armour plant, to the kitchen and home furnish-

---

*From *Scott Fitzgerald, The Great Gatsby*, Macmillan Publishing Company, 1987 [1925].

ings departments at Marshall Field, and to the other parts of the rapidly urbanizing world to which people in farm communities weren't exposed. And it brought me to the attention of Elizabeth Salter, State 4-H Club Leader for Girls in the Wisconsin Cooperative Extension Service. In 1928 she convinced me of the opportunities in dietetics, arranged for my transfer to the University of Wisconsin, and found a home where I could work for room and board. Looking back, Salter got me back on the track, dietetics, to which I was destined.

Becoming a Dietitian

Home economics and dietetics under that umbrella were relatively new fields when I enrolled at Wisconsin in 1928, and their reputations were often undervalued. The liberal arts "on the hill" looked down on home economics as the "bride's course," although in practice things were quite different. The home economics pioneers were part of the same reform movement that placed American agriculture on a scientific basis, and they contended that the average household did not practice healthy and sound home management. Thus they were educating reformers and educators who would bring effective techniques into the home. To me, these practicum courses, such as foods laboratory or clothing construction, weren't satisfying, as I had already mastered the skills and their underlying principles at home and through my 4-H activities. I found them to be atheoretic. But Wisconsin's program was also anchored in science and as a dietetic major I enjoyed two semesters of organic chemistry, physiology, physics, biochemistry, bacteriology, and agricultural chemistry. During my sophomore year I discovered that I enjoyed chemistry, and this enjoyment was confirmed at Wisconsin. With proper advisement, I might have pursued a chemistry major and a quite different career, but this did not occur to me at the time.

I suppose I could call Helen Parsons, my advisor at Wisconsin, a mentor. I often found myself at odds with her absorption in research, and I also felt that she lacked comprehension of the practicalities of dietetic practice. I rather disliked the tedium of performing adrenalectomies on rats and taking blood samples from rat tails to determine glucose levels for my senior thesis. Parsons, however, viewed such experience as the very core of what the science of nutrition was all about. But I also gained substantially from her. Parsons was an exemplar of the scholar-researcher who taught me the value of keeping up with current research, a skill of vast importance for each of my textbook revisions, in developing good practices in the laboratory and in establishing the scientific rationale for dietary regimens. As my mentor she acknowledged my scientific ability and encouraged me to seek a career in research. She alerted me to the job opening in Cincinnati in research that comprised my life in the thirties.

My differences with Helen Parsons came to a head in my choice of dietetic internships. Parsons strongly recommended the Mayo Clinic Hospitals as she believed the experience in therapeutic nutrition was especially good there. Abby Marlatt, Dean of the School of Home Economics, favored the administrative experience to be gained at the University of Michigan Hospital. I chose Michigan.

229

My first assignment at Michigan was to the main kitchen. In the eyes of the staff dietitian I had much to learn about menu planning: too much chocolate, and how could the bakers find time to press graham cracker crusts into so many pie tins? Yet, of all my experiences at Michigan I enjoyed the administrative assignment most. I could also be motivated by cutting-edge research and its applications. Michigan clinicians and others had found that patients with pernicious anemia responded favorably when they ate a pound of liver daily. Patients naturally rebelled, and our task was to design recipes incorporating raw or slightly seared liver into beverages, soups, and entrees. By the mid 1930s with the development of liver extract containing the effective principle, the herculean task of feeding a pound of liver to patients had now become history.

My admiration for Margaret Gillam, Director of the Dietary Department at Michigan, remained unwavering over the years. I appreciated her remarkable administrative skills, her leadership in our new profession, her graciousness and equanimity even under stress, and above all her ethical standards whether in professional services of in business dealings.

The Research Years: 1931–1941

With the onslaught of the Depression, I took Helen Parsons' advice and applied for a research position at the Childrens Hospital Research Foundation in Cincinnati. The foundation was a gift of William C. Proctor, the President of the Proctor and Gamble Company, and was endowed to undertake comprehensive pediatric research. The stellar staff assembled included Graeme Mitchell and Waldo Nelson, the authors of the classic text in pediatrics, Josef Warkany who established a reputation for his work on congenital anomalies resulting from vitamin deficiencies, Albert Sabin well into his work on poliomyelitis, and Glenn Cullen (for whom my son is named) and Howard Robinson (my future husband) doing their fundamental work in acid-base balance.

As a country girl from rural Wisconsin, Cincinnati was a cultural awakening. At work I encountered internationally renowned scientists. After work I went to symphony concerts, to the theater, to the summer opera with stars from the Metropolitan, to picnics in easily accessible Ohio and Kentucky parks. As the Depression deepened, salaries were reduced, research monies were tenuous, and the gay times of the Jazz Age largely eluded us. But they were good years.

For the first four years I worked under Dr. Chi Che Wang. As she lacked confidence in the accuracy of commercially marked glassware, I spent the first six months calibrating pipettes and volumetric flasks—a task as tedious as had been the rat studies at Wisconsin, but motivated by the monthly paycheck. Wang's research focused on the nutritional requirements of normal teenage girls and on children with nephrosis. My specific responsibility was to calculate the diets and supervise the food preparation for each individual as well as to collect all food samples and excretions for the later analyses. I was also responsible for all analyses of nitrogen, creatinine, and fat. This research yielded co-authorship on four papers published in the American Journal of Diseases of Children.

When Wang's grant ran out, I joined a group in physiological chemistry under Howard Robinson. Our studies on hemoglobin, total serum proteins, protein fractionations, and acid-base balance yielded seven papers in the Journal of Biological Chemistry.

Encouraged by the Foundation I completed a master's degree in biochemistry at the Cincinnati College of Medicine in 1934. My assignment in the required course on Biochemical Preparations was to prepare glutamic acid from wheat flour and cystine from hair clippings that I collected from a nearby barber shop. Another feature of my graduate studies was a Friday afternoon tea where students presented papers on assigned topics, a unique requirement of which was that the paper must be based solely on the French or German scientific literature.

Hospital Dietetics

Having spent the thirties as a researcher, rather removed from the practicalities of dietetic practice, I next took a job in New York City spending half of my time as supervisor of ward dietary services at Presbyterian Hospital and the other half as instructor in nutrition and diet therapy in the Columbia University-Presbyterian School of Nursing. In Nelda Ross Larsson, I found a true mentor who cultivated talents I had not recognized in myself: in lecturing to professional groups; in writing, for Larsson recommended me to the Macmillan Company editor thus opening my extensive writing career; in honing my skills as an educator and professional dietitian; and in establishing a friendship that would endure until her death.

My hospital experiences were anything but routine, for World War II intervened. Two days after was declared an unidentified plane flew over the city and the sirens blasted off. I led my nursing students from the laboratory where they were preparing breakfasts to a "safe area." The plane proved to be friendly but the muffins in the turned off oven were a soggy mess.

In the dietary department we employed more black women for the first time, fearfully acknowledging that this could provoke an explosive incident. We coped with "meatless" Tuesdays and Fridays, and "paper days" without pantry maids while we braved patients' complaints of cold food, not to mention mountains of trash. We developed recipes for high-protein beverages as we worked with physicians to improve the protein status of severely burned casualties of the war. We also went on rounds with physicians and made notations in patient's records—uncommon practices at that time. We taught dietetic interns and supervised interns and nursing students in the day-to-day meal services.

The Lean Years

In 1944 I married my fellow researcher and coauthor, Howard Robinson. Soon thereafter I was pregnant with my only son. Today, with improved practices in obstetrics, a career path with women bearing children in their thirties, following a decade of career advances, is taken for granted. That was less so in my generation. For while I gave birth in September 1945 to a healthy son, I myself was felled by a ruptured ovarian cyst with its accompanying peritonitis and a threat to my life. At home, I had a new son and a blind and increasingly incapacitated mother-in-law. The outlook for the next two years was bleak.

I believed my role as wife and mother took priority over my professional career but I also heeded the advice of Margaret Gillam, at Michigan, to keep up my membership in The American Dietetic Association and to keep active in the profession. In the later 1940's I resumed teaching nurses at three Philadelphia schools of nursing and was a lecturer in nutrition to medical students at the Temple University School of Medicine. I participated in some of the diet therapy projects of ADA as well as those of the Philadelphia Dietetic Association.

Periodic hassles with my babysitters led to occasional embarrassments when I had to take my son with me on some of my forays. How I remember the time when I brought Glenn with me to a local TV station for an interview. Four-year-old Glenn gluttonously viewed a blueberry pie, occasioning the broadcast host to assure a piece of pie to my son, and entirely disregarding the point of the interview. Not only was my educative mission thwarted, but Glenn never got his pie, a fact he remembers after 40 years!

The Book

Most dietitians know me because of my books, the nine editions of *Normal and Therapeutic Nutrition*, six editions of *Basic Nutrition and Diet Therapy*, the three editions of *Fundamentals of Normal Nutrition*, and two editions of *Case Studies in Clinical Nutrition*. The "big book," *Normal and Therapeutic Nutrition*, has been reprinted as a subsidized text in India and in the Philippines, while *Basic Nutrition and Diet Therapy* and *Fundamentals of Normal Nutrition* have been translated as Spanish-language editions for Latin America. To date, over 1.2 million copies have been sold. While I am proud of my 58 research and review articles published in professional journals and books with other authors, my books have been the primary vehicle for promoting nutrition education and my reckonings about dietetics.

In 1943 I was recruited to coauthor the ninth edition of *Nutrition and Diet Therapy* with Fairfax T. Proudfit. Proudfit, then in her seventies, was a southern gentlewomen with a name that "stood well in Memphis." She was a pioneer in hospital dietetics, a teacher of hundreds of nurses and medical students, and a dynamic leader in the dietetic profession. Her book, *Nutrition for Nurses*, first published in 1918, was a forerunner of other texts, and acquired a significant following throughout the eight editions. The eighth edition had grown to 1069 pages, and the Macmillan editor strongly recommended that the ninth edition be sharply reduced in size. Not surprisingly, this edition, the first on which I worked, required extensive revision.

The ninth edition was finally published in 1948. Through successive editions of my books one can trace the expanding knowledge of nutrition science as well as the changing emphases in nutrition education. The ninth edition reduced by 300 pages from the eighth, still included 158 pages describing food groups and including recipes that the nurse might be expected to use in the home care of patients. The foods section of the ninth edition has long since given way to topics in current vogue and representing the latest findings in nutrition research and in dietetic practice: for example, nutrition assessment; dietary counseling; dietary guides to prevent chronic diseases; nutrient-drug interactions; computers in dietary evaluation; and so on.

As I've aged, I've acquired splendid coauthors—Marilyn Lawler, Wanda Chenoweth, and Ann Garwick on *Normal* and *Therapeutic Nutrition*; Emma Weigley on *Basic Nutrition and Diet Therapy*. With each edition the content has become, scientifically, more technical. Also, with each new edition there is greater emphasis of the blending of nutritional science in the clinical application with the psychologic, social, economic, and cultural factors that influence food behavior. Each edition becomes bigger and more extensive, and, of course, more expensive—a commentary that applies to the works of many authors. I am not sure that bigger is better, nor that undergraduate students require the all encompassing coverage presented in today's books. Perhaps authors and publishers alike are trying to include too wide an audience of users.

Textbook writing is the sublime and undervalued vocation of the generalist. Unlike the research in which I engaged during the thirties, textbook writing requires an extensive survey of a much wider literature. And thus, with each edition of my books, I spent countless hours in the library bringing myself up-to-speed. By the same token, it was not enough to master the research findings. My earlier years as a hospital dietitian and my continuing classroom experience with nursing students and dietetic majors helped to incorporate these findings into dietary practice. I became, I think, a voice of moderation, unwilling to promote marginally tested regimens. But if my textbooks recommended sound rationales, they also radically adapted to the times. Early on I insisted that text photographs show women and minorities in executive positions since such pictures would serve as examples of a rising generation. With a sympathetic editor, I introduced pictures of situations that a nurse or dietitian would likely confront, rather than those so readily available from the food industry but of limited teaching value. In keeping with the times and in demonstrating relevance, I can't say that the effort was fully successful. Today's women, as nurses and dietitians, still haven't assumed full equality with the male physician who, too often, provides inadequate and sometimes incorrect nutritional advice to clients.

Subtly, I hope that my books have influenced the character of the profession. Directly, they have provided the first academic exposure of hundreds of thousands of future nurses and dietitians into the field of nutrition and diet therapy. Providing that exposure is clearly my most professional accomplishment.

The Education Years—Drexel University, 1953–1967

When I am asked to describe my dietetic career with one word I reply: EDUCATOR. This is in direct contradiction to my plans during college years when the last thing I wanted to do was to teach! My ten-year research experience in Cincinnati had given me a strong background in nutrition science while my clinical experience at

Columbia-Presbyterian helped me to bridge the gap that too often exists between nutritional science and its practical applications in the real world of people's needs.

In the spring of 1953 I was appointed Professor of Nutrition and Chairman of the Department of Nutrition and Food at Drexel Institute of Technology (now Drexel University). That summer I began a 14-year juggling act that—more often than not—required 60 to 80 hours a week—teaching, writing, and participating in a variety of committee assignments of The American Dietetic Association. Somehow my personal drive to succeed and my ability to carefully discipline my use of time for these tasks made it possible to accomplish what I set out to do. However, there were times that I was so consumed by professional responsibility that I had far too little time left over for my family. Today, many career women have similar conflicts between their professional and personal lives and need to identify their priorities.

Over three decades I have taught several thousand undergraduate students in nursing, dietetics, and other majors in home economics as well as a smaller number of dietetic interns, graduate students, and medical students. I also regard some 200 lectures to local, state, and national dietetic groups as well as to lay groups as another expression of education.

Undergraduate Program. When I began my work at Drexel I was dismayed to find no course outlines in the files. From the two or three-line description in the college catalog I had to develop each course from scratch. In retrospect, this experience enabled me to develop eight undergraduate courses without any prior restraints and to fashion them into a sequential correlated package to fit into the curriculum as a whole.

Courses and curricula are constantly being revised—often at the suggestion of a new dean, a new department head, or a new faculty member. Revising curricula and initiating new ones become time consuming but essential to the educational process. In the Department of Nutrition and Food we needed some patchwork from time to time for our generally well accepted curriculum in dietetics. We were more concerned with the widely held stereotype that women found it difficult to master scientific courses. Not infrequently, science faculty helped to perpetuate this stereotype. We were also aware that some graduate students experienced some difficulty in mastering advanced courses in biochemistry and nutritional science. After much study we developed an alternate curriculum in Nutrition Science that meets all the academic requirements for membership in The American Dietetic Association, and that also includes the chemistry, physics, and mathematics courses that improve the qualifications for graduate study in nutrition science.

Graduate Program. About half of my time was taken up by my responsibility as Chairman of the Graduate Committee of the college—from reviewing credentials for all students of the college, to advising students on their program of study, to endless meetings of the committee for the approval of student research proposals and completed theses.

In 1953 the graduate program in nutrition was in a catch-22 situation. There were too few graduate level courses to attract students, and too few students to justify adding courses! Over the next few years I added seven graduate level courses so that eventually we could require each student to complete three courses in nutritional science, and could also offer choice of courses on the life cycle, public health nutrition, and therapeutic nutrition.

The thesis requirement was the single greatest challenge to the graduate student. Laboratory facilities were limited, and financial support for research was lacking. Most of the 58 nutrition students that I directed found the thesis experience to be, by far, the most challenging, time consuming, frustrating, and satisfying of anything that they had attempted in graduate study.

We began to question whether every student should be required to write a thesis. For some students there is indeed no good substitute. Others, for example teachers in secondary schools who wished to update their credentials, might benefit more by additional courses and a research report of much more limited scope than the thesis. With such rationale we developed two options: Nutrition Science with a thesis requirement and Nutrition Education with additional course work and a research report.

Some Reflections on Being an Educator. Through the many positive experiences provided by mentors such as Nora Solum, English teacher at St. Olaf, Dean Abby Marlatt and others at Wisconsin, and Nelda Ross Larsson at Columbia-Presbyterian I was convinced that interaction between faculty and students in and out of the classroom was a vital ingredient in education. In my own college experience I had also been disillusioned by professors who delivered their lectures from last year's notes, and other professors who reluctantly rushed from the research laboratory to the classroom, and somehow succeeded in making students feel that they were less important than the research. I am convinced that teaching is at least as important as the number of research papers published.

In the 1950's I was fortunate that the primary emphasis at Drexel was on teaching and that I could devote time and energy to the preparation for each course. Unlike the department in a large university with many instructors, four to six of us had responsibility for the total teaching load. By my retirement I had taught 8 undergraduate and 12 graduate courses.

In my preparation for each class I relied, first of all and perhaps most important, on my own mastery of the topic, and spent countless hours in study. I also tried to avoid slavish dependence upon the text, believing it to be my function to expand upon the topic, sometimes to look at it in a new way, or to raise questions. To use a new approach to the course each time I taught it was as important to me as to the students. But no matter how hard I tried, I found it difficult always to give a dynamic appraoch to the Junior level course in normal nutrition that I taught for 24 times!

Although I used some of the many teaching aids so readily available, I tried to avoid letting them become a crutch! I took advantage, whenever possible, of the immediate present to enrich the day's lecture—perhaps a relevant article from a current nutrition journal, or a TV commercial, or an observation of an incident in a supermarket, or a case study of personal experience, and so on. Few gimmicks can rival the use of snippets of nutrition history, if they are properly dramatized; for example, within two short decades research had taken therapy from the pound of liver a day to the more acceptable injection of liver extract, and then to the purified crystals of vitamin B-12 in microgram quantities!

I believe that my informal encounters with students were as important as the classroom experience. Students knew that they could come to see me, even without appointment, whether they needed the answer to a question, or to discuss a career option, or sometimes simply to have someone to lean upon with a personal problem. An open door policy doesn't always result in the most efficient use of time and interruptions can be frustrating when a desk is piled high with work that needs to be done. But my own feeling of frustration when I was a college student needing advice not readily obtained, had taught me that paper work can usually wait, while a human problem may be immediately pressing for solution.

The primary regard of any teacher, of course, is the achievement of one's students. Whether a note at Christmas or a chance encounter at a dietetic meetings, I always enjoy learning about the careers of my former students. It is satisfying to learn about their promotions, to read papers that they have written, to know that they have earned their doctorates, or that they have been recognized by the profession and the community for their achievements. Once in awhile, too, I learn that a daughter or a son is studying for the profession, and then I know that the mother, or father, has been a great role model!

Drexel has been generous in its recognition of my efforts: the Lindbach Award for Distinguished Teaching (1962), the Service Award of the Drexel Chapter of the American Association of University Professors (1967); and the honorary Doctor of Science awarded at the commencement exercises in June 1976.

Dietetics, ADA, and Me—OH, How We Have Changed!

Dietitians of my generation have lived through almost all of the history of nutrition beginning with the early discoveries of vitamins. We have learned to adapt to the rapid advances in nutrition and food science, and the technology derived therefrom. We have seen the concept of *Prevention* take a new directional emphasis—from prevention of deficiency diseases resulting from *too little* of nutrients, especially vitamins, in the 1930s, to prevention of chronic diseases from which *too much* fats, cholesterol, sugar, salt, and excessive dietary refinement are the villains. We have seen public apathy to nutrition education change to keen public interest. And since I joined The American Dietetic Association in 1931 the membership has grown from about 2,500 to nearly 60,000!

As a registered dietitian I have a responsibility to my lifetime profession and its Association. I have had the privilege and honor to serve for about three decades on a number of important ADA projects and committees: as Chairman of the Diet Therapy Section, the Internship Board, the Program Committee for two Annual Meetings held in

Philadelphia. My membership on the Journal Board gave me the opportunity to review many books and articles submitted for publication.

The liaison that ADA maintains with professional and political groups is essential to the recognition in the community. I represented the Association on the Liaison Committee with the National League for Nursing to define the role of nurses in nutritional care of patients and to identify the goals for nutrition education in the nursing curriculum.

In the 1950s I participated in several projects pertaining to the sodium-restricted diet including the report of the ad hoc Committee on Sodium-Restricted Diets of the Food and Nutrition Board, National Research Council (1954), and the booklets for patient education sponsored jointly by The American Dietetic Association, the American Heart Association, the American Medical Association, the Nutrition Foundation, and the U.S. Public Health Service (1957).

Through 12 papers published in our Journal I have enjoyed a forum for my views on various aspects of normal and therapeutic nutrition, including dietary nomenclature, prescribing diets by dietitians, diet therapy consultation in small institutions, sodium-restricted diets, the Recommended Dietary Allowances in dietetic practice, some historical developments in diet therapy, and nutrition education.

Our profession is constantly being challenged by new research and new issues. Today's Association of almost 60,000 members can be an important force for influencing public policy pertaining to nutrition. We have earned the reputation as experts in providing nutritional care and in the education of professionals and the public. I refer briefly to four areas of opportunity as I see them.

Through testimony at hearings and by communication with legislators, dietitians have contributed significantly to the content of existing laws related to the nutritional welfare of the population. Yet, I sense an apathy on the part of many dietitians to actively promote needed changes in our laws. We often say "Why doesn't ADA do this or that?" We are ADA! Only if we are vigilant in alerting legislators to the need for new legislation pertaining to nutritional health can we expect to be in the forefront for improving the health of our people.

I am sometimes dismayed when I hear an individual complain about the food he or she received during a hospital stay, or when in a TV drama, an actor refers to hospital food as "awful" or "inedible." I suspect these stereotypes, for a number of reasons will always persist, but perhaps they can be minimized. In our quest for specialization in dietetics, or perhaps for status, are we sometimes forgetting that a major responsibility is to assure quality food service whether in the hospital, college dining room, nursing home, or any other institution with which we are affiliated?

Registration of dietitians with the concomitant requirement for continuing education stands as one of the most important initiatives ever taken by our association. How well this education is being put into practice remains a somewhat elusive issue. In the years ahead, it is essential that we establish that continuing education is pertinent to the needs of practitioners in a wide diversity of situations.

Finally, today's public interest in health and nutrition provides an exceptional opportunity for dietitians to provide nutrition education. However, this heightened interest also brings a number of health professional into direct competition for our educational services: physicians, nurses, home economists, sports directors, dentists, health educators, as well as hundreds of unqualified individuals who too often call themselves "nutritionists." We must look to our own capabilities to address this problem. It is not enough to give lectures to a few interested groups. We need to make effective use of the media—television, newspapers and magazines, newsletters, and books. This requires skills in communication and understanding of the socioeconomic, psychologic, and cultural influences that modify behavior.

Retirement Years, 1967–

Retirement can open up a new opportunity in life, or it can be a resignation from everything that makes life worthwhile. One day one is in charge, and the next day someone else has taken over. The special parties with the presentation of the gold watch or luggage help to ease the separation, but not for long. Then the lonely and depressing days set in—unless one has planned as carefully for retirement as for one's career.

Filling the additional 2000 hours given to me annually upon retirement was no problem since I continued to revise my books with my coauthors. The death of my husband in 1970 meant, however, that I had to actively seek outlets in the community to avoid isolation. I was attracted in three directions: in programs to assist older Americans, an assortment of ADA projects, and a commitment to my church.

My interest in aging goes back to the 1940s when I began the care of my elderly mother-in-law. By the early 1950s I had introduced one of the first courses on Nutrition in Later Maturity, and in 1961 I represented ADA at the first White House Conference on Aging. For a community project of the American Association of Retired Persons I chose to assist older Americans in the preparation of their federal and state tax returns. Through this program I became increasingly aware of the many problems confronting older Americans in the community—ranging from inadequate financial resources to isolation in their homes or apartments. Thus, when federal funding for nutrition programs became available, I assisted in the development of the proposal for funds, leading in 1974 to the opening of four nutrition sites. The County Office for Services to the Aging was organized in 1975 and I worked with staff closely as new centers were opened and as programs increased in scope as well as size. As a member of the Advisory Council for six years and its president for one, I learned to listen to vocal, sometimes contentious, older Americans, and to convey their concerns to county politicians. I participated in hearings held throughout the county and justified our proposals to politicians at the county level as well as our representatives in Congress. My insistence that a registered dietitian be employed to direct the nutrition program was, perhaps, my single most important contribution, for it placed the program at a superior level of achievement.

The Lecture Circuit! Many invitations to speak on any one of several current issues in nutrition came from dietetic and lay groups. Some of these have given me very special memories. Imagine, for example, lecturing in 1986 to a group of 35 dietitians seated in a natural amphitheater in Kenya while zebras and giraffes paraded along the crest of the hill just across from the river below. Maybe the lecture was soon forgotten, but the setting was great!

With education as my own career focus, I suppose it was logical that I be selected to present memorial lectures to honor distinguished educators in the profession. The first of these lectures was to memorialize Dr. Mary Schwartz Rose, a pioneer researcher, dynamic teacher, and author from Columbia University and is sponsored each year by the Greater New York Dietetic Association.

In 1976 I presented the Anna dePlanter Bowes Memorial Lecture to the meeting of the Pennsylvania Dietetic Association at Valley Forge. Anna dePlanter Bowes was a Distinguished Woman of Pennsylvania, a nationally recognized educator and public health nutritionist, and my friend.

I had met Lenna Cooper in the 1940s during my years in New York, and always admired her for her pioneering role in organizing our national Association. Lenna's book and mine in the 1940s and 1950s were usually running "neck to neck" in competition, and the two of us would compare notes and visit at Annual Meetings. So I shall never forget the balmy evening in San Antonio in 1975 when I faced more than a thousand Association. members and loyal friends to present the Lenna F. Cooper Memorial Lecture. After being introduced by my good friend, Louise Hamilton, I stood at the podium for a long moment with adrenaline flowing before I began speaking on "Nutrition Education—What Comes Next?"

Travel to Many Points. Blessed with good health, I have enjoyed travel to many European countries, Japan, China, Kenya, Australia, New Zealand, and Russia. These trips have been in the company of my dietitian friends—Doris Johnson, Alberta Hughes, Jean Beeman, and Evelyn Carpenter. From time to time I refresh my memory by looking at slides and scrapbooks and relive special moments such as

- seeing the morning rays of the sun gradually creep over the crest of snow-capped Mt. Kilimanjoro

- standing in awe on the bridge of our ship as it glided ever so slowly into Milford Sound to view the incomparably beautiful Southern Alps

- racing up the Great Wall to have my picture taken with Evelyn Carpenter, and marvelling at the beauty of the mist shrouded limestone hills that border the Li River on the way to Guilin

- cruising on the Volga River as an American and a Soviet professor of political science engage in lively political debate about their respective political systems. And so many others!

Two Special Honors. In 1976 the Executive Board of the Pennsylvania Dietetic Association organized a fund raising campaign to establish the Corinne H. Robinson Scholarship in Clinical Nutrition. The $20,000 goal for a permanently funded scholarship was reached in 1981 with a generous gift from the Hershey Foods Corporation. The scholarship is administered by the ADA Foundation which also selected one or two recipients each year. I treasure the letters that I receive each year from the holders of the scholarship as they write about their past careers, their families, and their goals for graduate study. Today these recipients are appearing on national programs and their articles appear from time to time in the Journal.

The Marjorie Hulsizer Copher Award is the highest honor that The American Dietetic Association can confer on a member. At the banquet of the Association in New Orleans in 1978 it was my great privilege to accept this honor in the presence of my son and editor, and to join that distinguished company of earlier recipients.

My Religious Orientation. My parents raised me in a Christian home, provided me with Christian education, and instilled Christian values for my life. I have tried to balance my secular and my religious activities. For many years I have taught in the Sunday School and Vacation Bible School of my church and have served on a number of committees. In the Synod I have served on committees on aging and on Christian education and have contributed to workshops on Christian education, on retirement planning, and on problems that the "sandwich generation" faces while raising their children as they also care for their parents.

I now serve as president of the council and congregation of Messiah Lutheran Church in Newtown Square. In this role I have set two precedents: as the first woman to ever hold this post in the congregation, and as the oldest individual to serve in this capacity.

Recently I led two short Bible studies for a group of women at the lifecare community where I am now living: "Foods of the Bible," and "Women of the Bible." That I chose to do this says something about me and about some of the driving forces in my life. Even now at 80 years I enjoy teaching. The Biblical writings on food provided a new perspective for Bible study to this group. Moreover, the Biblical writings remind us of humanity's concern about food throughout history. Feast and famine, food as an expression of hospitality, laws pertaining to the use of food, food as symbol—all are recorded with some detail in the Bible.

In my early career I was aware of the inequities experienced by women in pay and in career opportunities. Even today I am frustrated and angry as I see groups of men—sometimes with a single woman—deciding our fate in business, politics, academia, and even the church. So I seized the opportunity to look at the Biblical record of women: great mothers; women of ill repute but with redeeming qualities; downright wicked women; judges; nation builders; women of great faith. The male oriented writing of the Bible have influenced, sometimes dictated, the secondary role for women in our society. I also contend that the example set by many Biblical women and many of the teachings of the Bible provide a basis for women coming fulling into their own in today's society.

M. Rosita Schiller

M. Rosita Schiller, RSM, PhD, RD, LD is
Professor and Director of the Medical
Dietetics Division, The Ohio State University

Strong religious faith and diligence to the pursuit of high ideals have underlined the life and career of Dr. M. Rosita Schiller. This gifted educator is both a nun with the Sisters of Mercy, and Professor and Director of the Medical Dietetics Division at The Ohio State University. She has been a Visiting Professor at the University of Pretoria, South Africa. Dr. Schiller displays qualities to emulate in leadership, mental discipline, commitment to excellence, and concern for social justice. Her early career was dedicated to dietetics education. She has now switched scholarly focus to develop expertise in nutrition and cancer while continuing her commitment to dietetics education. She has lectured in 43 states and has a goal of visiting all 50 before retiring. Goal delineation has been the basis of her life's plan and the one goal that remains somewhat elusive is making and enjoying leisure time for refreshment and relaxation! She attributes her energy to three sources—daily prayer, regular aerobics, and the memory of her parents.

M. Rosita Schiller

My story as a leader in dietetics must be told in the context of my life as a nun. The direction of my life, my education, my practitioner experiences, and my role as an educator are colored by the fundamental choice to join the Sisters of Mercy at age 16 and to remain a member of the order throughout my career. The Order has a tradition of working in the areas of education, health care, and social services.

Until the late 1960's all members of religious orders were assigned areas of study and work, in keeping with the needs of Catholic institutions staffed by the group. After Vatican Council II (1969) personnel policies changed and assignments in the ministry were modified to better accommodate the interests and needs of individual sisters.

As a young novice in the mid 1950's, I was asked to list three career choices. One could be pretty sure that superiors would go along with the requested preference for education, health care, or social services, even if one's preferred area of specialization was not honored. The majors I selected were home economics, biology, and elementary education. Classroom teaching seemed right for me.

Those in charge agreed that I should prepare for home economics education. I had all the qualifications. As a child of 8 or 9 I received fabric and sewing scissors for Christmas; I made doll clothes. Later I joined 4H and entered sewing projects in the county fair. As a farm girl and one of seven children, I knew a lot about both food production and preparation. Making dinner for a thrashing crew of 20 men was certainly quantity cookery! The art of home management seemed second nature to me. Throughout college I did well in home economics education. The highlight of student teaching was an invitation to appear on local television demonstrating proper preparation of oatmeal. Neither public relations nor oat bran were popular at the time, but the experience helped develop skills that would come in handy later on.

One day during my senior year in college the Mother Superior called me to her office. She was a round woman, a former hospital administrator. "Dear," she said, "How would you like to be a dietitian?" I replied, "Oh, yes, Mother." She described how much I was needed to work in one of the 22 hospitals we operated. I had no idea what dietitians did, but I didn't have the courage to ask. Immediately after leaving the office I looked up "dietitian" in a dictionary. My future looked very promising. I was destined to be "an expert in dietetics."

Academic and Experiential Background

At the time of my enrollment, Mercy College of Detroit had about 1200 students, all women. The professors not only taught rudiments of their respective fields, but they took pride in developing qualities of leadership, mental discipline, commitment to excellence, and concern for social justice. Graduating "magna cum laude" meant I had strong potential and my professors expected me to have an outstanding career. Expectency theory worked.

As a dietetic intern at Henry Ford Hospital my evaluations were always good. However, I felt most comfortable during my two week rotation teaching nutrition to student nurses. Only many years later did I learn from Sara Parks, Associate Dean at Penn State University and former Henry Ford intern, that I had been held up as a model for other dietetic interns. I started setting professional standards early; at the time I didn't truly appreciate the importance of this characteristic which was second nature to me.

The dietitians at Henry Ford Hospital were special role models for me. The first was Margaret King, internship director. From the time I first met her, I was impressed by Miss King's friendliness. No matter where she walked in that 1000 bed teaching hospital, everyone greeted her by name. She also knew everyone, or so it seemed to me. I wanted to imitate that quality.

The other role model was Sally Jencks. Miss Jencks was hard on interns. She made us stay on duty until the last detail was attended to. She loved working weekends and holidays and expected us to work, too, without complaint. Miss Jencks loved patients and did everything she could to make them feel special. She had a collection of angels. Whenever a patient was having a bad day she would take an angel to them. Her message was, ''I can't stay with you but here is an angel to watch over you. When you're feeling better, the angel goes to someone else who needs strength or courage.'' I liked that display of compassion. It showed me that first rate dietitians went beyond providing technical skills; they also attended to the psychosocial and emotional needs of patients.

After internship I felt ready to tackle any job. I needed that confidence. I was assigned as the only dietitian in a 75 bed community hospital in Manistee, Michigan. There was not another dietitian within 60 miles to whom I could go for counsel if I needed it.

A first job is important for what it can teach. Mine taught me self-sufficiency, independency, team collaboration, and resource management. There were 12 physicians on staff; the one who taught me the most about being a clinical dietitian was a new internist fresh from Henry Ford Hospital who set up practice in the area. He challenged me to use all the skills I had learned during internship. He depended on me to provide high quality nutrition services and I looked to him for medical information and professional stimulation.

After two years at Manistee, I was assigned as head dietitian in a 425 bed Mercy hospital in Lansing, Michigan. One advantage of being ''assigned'' to positions is that superiors recognized the value of professional development and could move nuns from place to place according to the needs of both the Order and the individual. If the task of finding a position had been left to me, I probably could not have selected a better placement.

While working full time, I enrolled in the master's degree program in institution management at Michigan State University. Like many graduate students I objected to conducting a thesis. Were it not for Katherine Hart, my advisor, this would have been a major mistake. In her wisdom, Miss Hart suggested doing a "project" on accidents in residence hall food service operations. The project was simple. Neither calculating the statistics nor writing the report in thesis format were difficult. The project was submitted, exams passed, and degree awarded. A few weeks later I received a package from Miss Hart. It contained a bound document embossed "thesis."

Miss Hart had tricked me into doing a thesis! As I look back this was one of the most poignant of my academic experiences. This was an amazing lesson on what can happen when a professor knows the combination of a student's strengths and fears and leads that student both fearlessly and triumphantly to the desired goal. I'm still struggling to integrate this practice into my own role as advisor.

After completing my master's degree, having spent six years in dietetic practice, I was transferred to Mercy College of Detroit where I taught in the Home Economics Department. This was a challenging assignment because my courses included advanced nutrition, diet therapy, and institution management for dietetic students, as well as nutritional science for nursing students. Despite the range of content, or maybe because of it, I responded well to the college environment. I was active in the faculty senate, elected president of the local dietetic association and served on ADA committees.

Working with the poor in inner city Detroit was strongly advocated by both college administrators and community leaders. I linked up with a mobile health unit. My role was to teach nutrition to mothers in the neighborhood. When the project was introduced, we offered donuts to help attract women to the site. Every transient in the area came to receive a handout!

One day as I was teaching about meat preparation at the mobile health unit, as requested by the class, I was discussing which cuts to broil. One lady asked, "Does my stove have a broiler?" Several weeks later she invited us to her home to make popcorn and I realized why she didn't know if there was a broiler. There were no knobs on either the burner or oven controls. She was using a fork to turn on the flame. She had one pot to cook in. There were eight children in the home. My sophisticated lessons meant little to this woman, or many others like her, who came to the classes. I was not even in the same stratosphere, let along on the same wavelength.

What a hard lesson to learn! I wasn't able to meet the needs of these inner city women. I could teach nutrition all right; but these women needed hope, not facts about vitamins and minerals. This experience provided the basis for my first invited presentation and published article, "Barriers to Accepting our Professional Responsibility." In a self-revealing story, I described my own naivete and disillusionment. It became clear to me that my sophisticated manner, haughty bearing, and sheltered upbringing stood in the way of open communication with the destitute and the despondent. My talents could better serve others, those with backgrounds and experiences more similar to mine.

At Mercy College we had discussed starting a coordinated undergraduate program in dietetics. We made a visit to Martha Nelson Lewis and the Medical Dietetics Program at Ohio State. I was deeply impressed with both the dauntless courage and reckless wisdom of Mrs. Lewis. This woman could teach me a great deal about dietetic education and program administration.

Doctoral Studies

After teaching three years it became clear to me that education was to be my area of specialization. To be successful, I would need a doctoral degree. I started shopping around for the "right" program. In conjunction with our visit to the Medical Dietetics Program at Ohio State, I made an appointment to meet with Dr. Dorothy Scott, Director of the School of Home Economics, to explore the feasibility of enrolling in doctoral studies in human nutrition and foodservice management. In the course of our conversation Dr. Scott remarked that the University had recently lifted the doctoral requirement for foreign languages. That sold me. At Ohio State I could both matriculate in a doctoral program and learn more about coordinated dietetic education from the pioneer, Mrs. Lewis.

With financial assistance from the ADA Mary Swartz Rose Fellowship, the Kappa Omicron Phi Hettie Margaret Anthony Fellowship, and the OSU Hazel Williams Lapp Research Fellowship, I was able to devote all my energies to study. I finished the program in two years.

The doctoral program meshed well with all my previous experiences. My baccalaureate work was in education and dietetics. At the master's level I majored in institution management and minored in nutrition. At Ohio Stated I turned things around: I majored in human nutrition and took minors in business administration, physiology and biochemistry. This general background could not have prepared me for subsequent teaching and dietetic program administration.

Virginia Vivian was my major professor at Ohio State. Besides academic rigor, I learned two important lessons from Dr. Vivian. First, she taught me how to write with greater spontaneity and lucidity. Her composition seemed effortless; the rights words simply flowed from her pen. She could smooth over my constipated narratives, freeing them from constraint and formality.

Dr. Vivian also taught me the importance of friends, leisure, and relaxation. Often during my degree program I would be waiting for her to return a critique of my latest dissertation activity. Informally she would often comment on what a good time she had with friends at the theater or a Junior Court the previous evening. I'd be miffed. "Why wasn't she home reading my paper?", I'd think to myself.

Only later did I truly appreciate that non-work interests and activities are an important dimension of professional life. Some call it stress management, others consider it nurturing the human spirit. Dr. Vivian demonstrated both the value and importance of maintaining a close circle of friends and business associates. I learned the lesson but it seems I'm forever in need of a refresher course. It is still too easy to get caught up in things to be done, without taking time to celebrate accomplishments, go fishing, or take a walk in the Conservatory.

I had no idea what the doctorate would do for me. It gave me confidence to write for publication. One of my biggest thrills was having my dissertation research published, then noting that others quoted the work. They considered it a "significant" contribution to dietetics. This recognition only increased my desire to pursue further research and writing.

The doctorate also gave me credibility in the field. When I spoke, people listened more closely than in the past. They believed what I said. The credential, in addition to previous experience and well-honed skills, opened the doors to invitations to conduct workshops, deliver presentations, provide consultation, assume leadership positions, and mentor others in the process.

Life as a Professor

Upon completion of doctoral studies I returned to Mercy College of Detroit where I implemented a career mobility program in dietetics and served as its director for six years. The career mobility program was unique, in the tradition of Mrs. Lewis. We offered an ADA approved two-year associate degree dietetic technician program during the first two years of college. Students could enter the workforce as technicians or they could enroll in the second phase of the program: a coordinated undergraduate program in dietetics. Some took a job, saved money, and later returned to complete the baccalaureate degree.

There were several challenges at Mercy College. First, we had to convince the ADA Commission on Accreditation that the program was sound and that our graduates were indeed prepared for entry level dietetic practice. That we did, and the program was granted full accreditation. Another challenge was convincing the dietetic community that a small Catholic college, with the assistance of several local hospitals, could offer a first-rate educational program. Our success was verified by the publication of several articles describing the program philosophy and curriculum. The continuing challenge was to offer a high quality program with only three faculty, limited resources, and little institutional emphasis on research and program enhancement. The task became boring.

When there was a prolonged vacancy at Ohio State for a Director of Medical Dietetics, I was invited to become a candidate for the job. Personnel policies in the Order had changed; individual sisters were encouraged to seek positions primarily in keeping with their own interests, while secondarily taking into account needs of the Order. Recognizing my desire for a new challenge, superiors were quick to give their approval for me to interview at Ohio State, and to take the position when it was offered.

For the past eleven years my life has been marked by one significant event or achievement after the other. My biggest thrill, as it is for many university faculty, was being promoted to full professor. Such an accomplishment is both a reward for past work, and an outward expression of expectations for future contributions.

This position is more rewarding than I ever dreamed. Highlights can be categorized in the University's triumvirate mission of teaching, research, and service.

Teaching is not dull. With the total overhaul of our curriculum in 1988, all courses were revised. New content was introduced, course schedules were changed, and different teaching methods were employed. We maintained full accreditation of our coordinated undergraduate program. With the help of all faculty, we planned and implemented an Approved Preprofessional Practice Program, making dual use of supervised practice in the coordinated program. Such achievements for innovative programs are personally rewarding.

My regular class load is diverse, as it has always been. Courses include Management of Hospital Departments, Principles of Nutrition Education, Nutrition Care Process, Advanced Foodservice Management, and clinical supervision. My graduate teaching is primarily through seminars and advisement.

My biggest thrill as a teacher was being invited to serve as visiting professor at University of Pretoria, South Africa. During the five weeks in South Africa I gave workshops and presentations to both home economists and licensed dietitians on accreditation, marketing, professional image, and diet and cancer. Although home base was Pretoria, my itinerary included Cape Town, Durban, Johannesburg, and the Kruger National Park where I observed exotic animals in their natural habitat. While I was in the country the Association of Dietitians of South Africa was founded. I also met many dietitians who completed internships and degrees in this country including University of Iowa, Cornell University, and University of North Carolina. Despite extreme personnel shortages, dietitians in South Africa gave me many lessons in dedication, innovativeness, compassion, and altruism.

The focus of my research and scholarly productivity has changed over the years. At first, much of my work related to isolated problems of clinical practice or dietetic education. Publications included such diverse topics as quality assurance, team teaching, career mobility, hospital dietetic practice, marketing, research skills, computer simulations, and dietetic education.

During the 1980's expectations at universities changed. Project and training grants, although important, became less valuable than research grants. Nearly everyone on university campuses scrambled to reorient themselves to contribute to new priorities. I took a six month sabbatical.

The purpose of my sabbatical was to become a "specialist" in diet and cancer. During those six months I visited numerous cancer centers, spent long hours in medical libraries studying the latest research findings, prepared and gave presentations on diet and cancer, and talked with several physicians and dietitians about unanswered questions related to nutrition care of cancer patients.

The culmination of my sabbatical was submission of a research proposal to explore the relationship between dietary intakes and weight gain among women on adjuvant chemotherapy following mastectomy. That study, as well as several subsequent and related proposals have been funded. In addition, I joined the American Cancer Society Speakers Bureau and frequently am invited to give presentations on nutrition and cancer to both lay and professional audiences.

Although I now have a defined area of clinical investigation, I still maintain active research in leadership styles, dietetic education, and clinical nutrition management. Perhaps once a generalist, always a generalist!

Committee work is an integral part of life for faculty members. The most enjoyable of these service commitments were the University Senate and its Steering Committee, ADA Commission on Accreditation, ADA House of Delegates (Ohio), and ADA Long Range Task Force. Through these opportunities I was able to establish a strong network of contacts around the country.

Many service activities fringe on teaching and scholarship. For example, I have been privileged to serve as manuscript reviewer for the Journal of Parenteral and Enteral Nutrition, and to sit on the Editorial Board for both the Journal of The American Dietetic Association and the Journal of Allied Health. It is both fulfilling and intellectually rewarding to evaluate manuscripts to determine suitability for publication. I get similar enjoyment from reviewing book manuscripts, consulting for academic programs, and evaluating research proposals for potential funding. These exercises call for both critical and conceptual thinking, attributes instilled in my academic pursuits.

Another favorite service activity is delivery of continuing education workshops and conferences for dietitians and other health professionals. Thanks to the sponsorship of Ross Laboratories, I have had many opportunities to help advance dietetics in Europe and South Africa as well as throughout the United States. Through invitations from numerous dietetic associations and other societies, my travels have included 43 states. My goal is to visit all 50 before I retire.

Looking back over my accomplishments, I marvel at the outcomes. Who would have thought that a farm girl, educated kindergarten through eighth grade in a one-room country school, could achieve such heights in the profession. Only God, to whom I have dedicated my life, could accomplish these things through me. God's favor leaves me both humble and grateful, both energized and motivated for further opportunities.

A Glimpse Within

Strong faith and a delineation of life goals keeps me on target. While faith has always been an important part of my individuality, I reached middle age before I defined my life's purpose and put in writing my life goals. Generally my goals outline a quest for knowing and fulfilling God's plan in my life; being challenged by the work I do; making and enjoying leisure time for refreshment and relaxation; experiencing inner peace; and having a few close friends as well as family, to share my joys, struggles, pain and success. When making major decisions, it helps me to test alternatives against these fundamental guidelines. Will the proposed activity contribute to, or deter from, movement toward my ultimate desires.

My philosophy of life flows from or perhaps lead to, my statement of life goals. For me it has always seemed unrealistic to target one specific position or achievement, such as Dean of New Era University or a million dollar NIH grant, and direct all energies to it. Rather, I like to be more flexible. My five year goals are structured around my present situation and direct me toward greater fulfillment in major dimensions of my life: career, profession, psychosocial, spiritual, travel, family, living situation, wholistic health, intellectual growth, and personal development. This philosophy has, no doubt, diverted me from pursuit of high offices or given insufficient impetus to forge a path toward prestigious awards. Even with this somewhat amorphous life plan, I still spend too much time working and save too little time for personal interests.

How do I maintain interest and enthusiasm for my life's work? I attribute my energy to three sources. The first is daily prayer. This keeps me in tune with God; in prayer I find guidance for major decisions, serenity during difficult times, creative inspiration for new initiatives, and the confidence to take on expanded responsibilities. The second source of energy is a program of exercise and physical health. Regular aerobic workouts and rigorous discipline for weight control help keep me both physically and mentally fit. Having weighed 180 pounds at one time, I resolved that if I was going to be a dietitian, I would be a walking specimen of what I preached. This resolve motivates me to diet and exercise, even when it means getting up earlier in the morning or not always giving in to my craving for a chocolate bar. My third source of strength is the memory of my parents, disciplined German folk, who taught me that diligent pursuit of high ideals would lead to personal satisfaction and self-fulfillment.

A Look Ahead

Health care in general, and the dietetic profession in particular, are in the midst of dynamic change. Leaders in The American Dietetic Association have charted a course which I believe will lead to open waters and clear sailing ahead. Our strategic plan calls for competent practice, political adovcacy and quality services.

As an individual dietitian I can, and I urge all my readers to, help implement the Association's strategic plan while striving to achieve personal goals and realizing the fullness of personal potential. As we look ahead to the next century, I believe particular efforts are needed in four key areas.

First, dietetics needs to be recognized as both exciting and rewarding, offering numerous opportunities for growth, advancement, creativity, service, and self-fulfillment. Only by instilling this perception will we be able to attract first-rate recruits, and retain competent practitioners in the field.

Second, the National Center for Nutrition and Dietetics needs to be both utilized and supported. The profession needs to take an even stronger proactive stance as recognized experts in the field of nutrition. We need to have a public presence which outshines all other groups on issues dealing with the interface between food, nutrition and health.

Third, greater emphasis needs to be placed on research to justify current dietetic practice and to explore new directions for the future. Some of this work can take place in classrooms and laboratories. However, dedicated dietitians, with the help of seasoned investigators, need to conduct more studies in hospitals, clinics, and community settings.

Furthermore, practitioners must interpret research findings and apply them, as appropriate, in diverse work situations.

Lastly, our basic and continuing education programs need to prepare both entry level and advanced practitioners to cope effectively with dynamic changes in practice settings. To deal with such things as technological complexities, ethical issues, personal shortages, clinical specialization, and managerial skills, dietitians must have a strong theoretical base. Both critical and conceptual thinking are also necessary to solve intricate problems and initiate innovative approaches to contemporary situations.

As teacher I offer these reflections for your inspiration. My hope is that you will use my example to gain insights into your personal life, and that these musings will stimulate widespread inner motivation and dedication to excellence.

Sarah Harvey Short

Sarah Harvey Short, PhD, EdD, RD is Professor of Nutrition, Syracuse (NY) University

Stop any student on the Syracuse University campus to ask about the professor who dresses in a blond wig, silver jacket, exotic beads, and who rides a motorcycle into class and he will quickly name Sally Short! Her own students know to be on time for class—just to be sure to get a seat. A showman? Yes. A respected scientist, teacher summa cum laude? Definitely. Obstacles never daunted her. She has had more than her fair share of discrimination against females. Encouragement and support from her family and close colleagues all helped her as she earned two doctoral degrees while working full time and never missing a beat as wife and mother. If she is not teaching nutrition, she is writing or speaking about it. She has lectured in almost every state and in many countries abroad.

Sarah Harvey Short

The Beginning

"The lecture style of a typical professor can be rather routine.. Now and then a professor will make an extraordinary effort to arouse the class to a point where learning can occur spontaneously. . . . Sarah Short, professor of nutrition at Syracuse, explains her unorthodox teaching methods by simply stating, 'If I don't get their attention, I can't teach them.' And she does get their attention. What student could ignore a professor who, dressed in a blond wig, silver jacket, and exotic beads, rides a motorcycle into the classroom? Or a teacher who turns a lecture into a multimedia event complete with flashing lights, slide shows, and rock music? Or someone who presents herself as a living blackboard with chemical formulas painted on her arms and legs? But Short's lectures are more than just showmanship, they include substance as well. For her teaching excellence, Professor Short has been designated one of Syracuse's outstanding faculty members and honored with a teacher/scholar award."

Little did I dream when I started out that I would become a teacher (Never!), would travel and speak around the world (I had never been outside New York State) and would be interviewed on TV, radio and in print (I was so shy I blushed when doing any public speaking).

My entry into the profession of dietetics was not planned. Ever since I was a very young girl, I had wanted to be a chemist. My mother was a chemist and I did well in sciences in school, so I thought that this was a perfectly reasonable profession for me. It was very unusual for women to be chemists when my mother was employed and it still wasn't all that common when I became a chemist. My mother and father certainly encouraged me to go to college. Since Syracuse University was only about a mile and a half from our house, that is where I went along with most of my friends from high school. The girls went to Home Economics College at the University and I did also since I remembered that my mother had majored in Home Economics at a different college and still taken enough science to become a chemist.

Undergraduate Life

At Syracuse, my advisor was Dr. Edith Nason who had a degree in chemistry from Yale. She was most understanding of my desire to be a research chemist and let me take more than half of my courses in chemistry, other sciences and math. Of course I still had to take nutrition, food science and dietetic subjects which meant that I was taking 21 credit hours per semester and going to labs morning, afternoon, and night. I was going to graduate in two years and be a chemist!

What about social life, what about working to help pay tuition, what about exercise?? Students now would think that I had no social life compared with theirs. I had friends but I didn't really date since my future husband was at a university in another

*Excerpted from *Alma Mater: Unusual Stories and Little-Known Facts from America's Colleges Campuses* by Don Betterton Peterson's Guides, Inc., 1988.

city. I did work most summers in a chemistry lab either at Continental Can Company or a Borden's. During Christmas vacation, I worked on the assembly line at Continental Can lugging steel into a machine that stamped out cans. As for exercise, I ran to school for dinner and back to attend another lab. My high school friends and I would walk out to Drumlins (a recreational area several miles from campus) to ski (we didn't have lifts) and ice skate. Of course we would all go swimming in the summer if it ever warmed up enough to go in the lake.

In my junior year, companies manufacturing airplane engines came to campus to recruit, and offered me a job as an engineer. It was tempting, but I refused because I wanted to graduate and be a chemist! At that point, Dr. Nason asked me to help teach food chemistry including a lab to the incoming freshmen students. High school students were graduating in January and attending college after the university term had started. It was my job to lecture so that students could get caught-up enough to attend the regular lectures. This was an awesome task for me—I almost failed public speaking because I was shy and blushed and hated to speak in front of people, but I did it because I was going to be paid 50 cents an hour. I graduated in three years, but then I had to make another decision.

First Graduate School Experience

I was offered a chemistry teaching fellowship at Yale, a biochemistry research fellowship at the University of Wisconsin–Madison or I could go to work. Yale I turned down because I certainly did not want to become a professor. Wisconsin sounded far away and I had never been far away. Besides I would be working in a laboratory for the most famous (at that time) living biochemist, Professor Conrad Elvehjem, a pioneer in niacin research. I left the day after graduation for the University of Wisconsin in Madison.

My luggage did not arrive with me on the train, it was raining, I didn't know anyone within a thousand miles, the campus was HUGE, I was 20 years old and homesick (it was about the first time that I had really been away from home). Was I crazy to come to a place that was colder than Syracuse, New York? Soon the other graduate students arrived, my luggage arrived and the social life started at the university (WOW). The best part of the whole thing was that I could work in a marvelous big lab with people I had read about and admired from afar—people who had published in prestigious research journals. I was very impressed with the whole place. It soon became evident that although I had graduated magna cum laude, so had everyone else in my classes. I had to study as well as work in the lab every spare minute in order to keep my research fellowship. Soon there were more decision points in my life: go to medical school, stay in biochemistry at Wisconsin, or go to work.

Although I could have transferred to medical school rather easily at that time, I did not see how I ever could finance four more years and there were no fellowships available. I felt that I had already asked for too much financial assistance from my parents and I was economizing as much as I could. One day it was 20 below zero, colder if you counted the wind blowing across the lake, when it was time to go back to where I lived (over a mile and a half) down the lake. Should I take the bus or walk and save the five cents it cost. I walked. I wasn't starving but I did count the pennies. My fellowship was sponsored by Armour Meat Co., and therefore I was working with amino acids (actually phenylalanine) in meat. I must say that the rats were eating better than most of the graduate students. I had been taught not to borrow so I thought of my other options. Actually rational thought went out the window because my true love kept calling me to ask me to come back to Syracuse. We had known each other since we were five years old and lived two doors apart. I went back to Syracuse and a job as research chemist at Bristol Laboratories.

The Working Woman

I loved the job and stayed for four years. It was so exciting and just what I had always wanted to do. At first, I was the only person in the department directed by a brilliant man whose innovative discoveries kept Bristol in the forefront of antibiotic production. Everyday, there was something new (and sometimes dangerous) to work on. No more rats or chimps just good old chemical experiments. I was even allowed to take some of my results to the Food and Drug Administration labs in Washington.

Homemaker

My childhood sweetheart and I were married and time marched happily on. After our first child was born, I became a homemaker par excellence with only a small break to lecture part time at Syracuse University. We moved around the Northeast and had two more children. Wherever we moved, we explored the area and went to museums, historical spots, and cultural events. We set up a full scale chemistry lab, electronic lab and microbiology lab in the basement and the children entered every science fair. It is a wonder they didn't rebel, but the whole family had fun together. I firmly believe that husband and children come first, way before your profession. I am very proud of my family.

Our final move was back to Syracuse. By the time our youngest was in school, we realized that all three children were going to need, and want, expensive educations.

Second Graduate School Experience

Looking at the bank account, I decided it was time for me to go back to work. However, no one wanted a chemist who had been home scrubbing floors and washing diapers. How would I overcome this obstacle? Go back to school, but would anyone accept me in graduate school after all this time? Unlikely as it seemed, the medical school (Upstate Medical Center, State University of New York) wanted me because I had once taught chemistry. The Allied Health Department (part of the medical center) had nurses, medical technologists, and other technicians taught by the same professors teaching biochemistry to the medical students. The nurses and technicians were not doing well. Therefore the medical school would accept me in the biochemistry graduate program if I would teach their undergraduate students some chemistry.

I was so excited—I would be going back to school and I would receive my tuition plus $1000 a year to teach general, organic and biochemistry to all the students who had to take these courses plus of course, run the laboratories plus do my own research plus take care of my family and house. There followed three years of sheer terror. Looking back at it all, I don't know how I did it. Actually, it was only with the great help of my husband, three marvelous children, and my parents, and a wonderful neighbor that I survived. The medical school threw me into biochemistry class with the medical students, a course in radioactive isotopes, and a course in physical chemistry. Competing with medical students just out of college was a cutthroat semester; in the next course, I didn't know an isotope from a hole in the ground; and in physical chemistry (which combines the hardest of chemistry, physics and math), I once passed a test, but not too many other students did better than that. I lived through the semester, barely. Every time there was an exam, one of my children was sick or some other calamity took place. Thank goodness, I could take sick children to my mother for the day. Every once in a while, I would have hysteria but mostly we all coped. Obviously the social life was cut back although I still did entertain, clean (the family all helped on weekends), sewed all my clothes plus some of the children's clothes. I always felt driven, pushed, under stress because there was more to do than there was time. I found the only way to make more hours was to cut. back on sleep (sometimes to two hours a night).

There was no time to be sick, but no one told my body this and I had a reoccurrence of the rheumatic fever I had originally while moving so much. At this point, I couldn't stop—I hadn't even started to reach the goal of full employment, so I kept on going.

It was hard learning to study again. Every once in awhile when sitting in the big biochem lecture hall with all the young medical students, a little tear would run down my face, but then I said, "Darn it (actually I said something else), I'm not going to let them get the best of me." Other circumstances didn't help either—the medical school stated that they were less than enthusiastic about giving masters degrees and we were lead to believe that in order to win that degree, we would have to publish in approved research journals, save lives and do everything except walk on water (which was left to the future MD's). So my research started in thyroid biochemistry. My advisor was a patient and erudite gentleman. We started and finished three years of work with thyroid derivatives. I took care of a total of 2000 rats which meant feeding, watering, cleaning and injecting them everyday including Christmas, holidays and when I was sick or well. I hated those rats and they hated me. I could take care of 132 at a time and my family helped. Our older son, who already wanted to be a physician, helped me inject all the rats on the weekends. Our younger son and my husband helped weigh and feed while our daughter helped give water to the rats.

I did publish in an approved medical journal. We did save lives since I discovered that one of the thyroid derivatives being given to those with high serum cholesterol levels was more active fed than injected. This would have meant that a risk of heart problems would have been higher, not lower, for these people. I did graduate with all my family watching and I certainly was proud of my new master's degree. I was also touched because all of my students stood up during the graduation ceremonies and applauded when I received my degree.

First Doctorate

Now what should I do? I still wasn't making enough money to help out very much and my children were getting closer and closer to college age. I probably could stay at the medical school and take more courses hopefully toward a doctorate. Opportunities opened up in industry now with a new chemistry degree, but that would mean 9 to 5 hours every day with short vacations. I wanted to be able to spend more time with my husband and children.

Professor Marjorie Dibble and I had been friends during the year I was a part time lecturer in the nutrition department at Syracuse University. This was before our family had started moving from place to place. Professor Dibble was now department chairperson and needed someone to teach nutrition. She asked, I said "yes" if I could keep my job teaching chemistry at the medical school and work on my doctorate at Syracuse. It was agreed. I must have been crazy because now I was teaching three courses plus overseeing labs at the medical school, teaching three courses plus food science labs at Syracuse, AND taking courses toward my doctorate AND taking care of husband, three children and house including all the cleaning, ironing and sewing.

The first year was trauma—organizing three new courses when I had been away from nutrition and food science for SO long. Although the campus of the Upstate Medical Center and that of Syracuse University adjoin, most of the time I was running up and down the hills trying to be on time. It seemed that SOMEONE up there was watching over me because one day I just happened to drop in to check up on the chemistry lab at Upstate. There was a lab instructor present but I found a student who had just spilled concentrated acid down the front of her. After quickly dumping water all over her, I ran her through the tunnel to the emergency room yelling ahead for an MD. Fortunately we were in time to save her from disfiguring and painful burns. I, however, was a wreck and asked myself "What am I doing?" My answer was still, "trying to contribute toward the education of three children."

Since I was a lowly instructor at Syracuse, I wasn't making much money but I did receive free tuition. My prospects for getting promoted and perhaps making more money looked slim until I earned my doctorate. If I continued doing what I called "hard-nosed" research in a lab, it would have to be at the medical school almost on my own, since the laboratories in the nutrition department did not have any of the equipment that I had been using. This would mean more running up and down the hill with no backup personnel to help. Another decision point in my life.

Learning Laboratory

While I had been teaching at Syracuse, I found a new interest. I liked to teach nutrition and I liked to try new ways of holding student attention. First a bit about teaching food science. The basic food science course had been taught by lecturing to 20 students at a time (100 students total), demonstrating and then having them do their food lab experiments (which sometimes they could eat). This meant saying the same thing four or five times a week. When you do this week after week, your eyes sort of spin around in your head and you forget whether you have covered this subject at all or four or five different times. It was decided that the demonstration part would be put on film (at least the baking, batters and doughs). After this was done I became interested in self-instruction methods of teaching basic information. I had read about what Dr. Samuel Postlethwait was doing at Purdue in botany and biology and decided that it sounded great to have students proceed at their own pace to achieve mastery of the topic.

It was decided that I should produce audio tapes and a workbook to go with the films that had been made and that I should develop slides for the units that were not covered in the films. This, of course, should be done in my spare time and with little (mostly no) money. I discovered that the audio department in the School of Communications was throwing away tape. I went, emptied their wastebaskets, brought the tape home, erased it with a magnet and used it to tape the lessons. Then I learned to make slides on the copystand which was trauma because I did not know the first thing about photography. Worse was yet to come, because I was told that I needed objectives. What were objectives? A sweet, dear faculty member in consumer education attempted to teach me—a frustrating experience, but she finally taught me enough to write a workbook for students.

Discovery of Computers

At this same time, I was supposed to be learning two languages for my doctoral exams. I am definitely not good in languages so I begged to take computer language for one of my requirements. A major language on the mainframe computer at that time was APL (A Programming Language) which was put there for the engineers to do their homework. The author of the language, speaking at an IBM meeting, stated that this language was a high powered mathematical language and was not for such things as words. However, since it was all I had, I decided that if you could put numbers together and add them, you could put letters together to make words. My son, Bill (the future ScD. in electrical engineering) was very interested in computers. I persuaded the Syracuse University academic computing center to let us bring a terminal home for the weekends so we could work on programming. Perhaps, I should add that terminals at that time weighed 100 pounds and to use them you had to tie into the mainframe on your telephone lines. The first time we worked on a program and requested a printout, both of us jumped into the car and drove way over to Syracuse University to see if it had really printed out our commands miles away. It had—WOW, a whole new world

257

opening up. Bill learned faster than I did and he programmed a big testbank of questions so the student could take quizzes anytime they were ready on terminals we had set up in the learning lab.

More Educational Experiences

The whole course evolved slowly and painfully into 23 learning modules using slides, films, computer assisted instruction (I did that), and computer testing (Bill did that) all tied together with a workbook for each student. Students could come to the learning lab (an unused classroom) that was set up with old library carrels and tape recorders, movie loop projectors and slide projectors I borrowed from Audiovisual Services on campus. We were in business—the campus newspaper even carried a story titled "Home Economics teacher USES computer" as if nutrition teachers did not have enough brains to do this. This whole concept was fairly new at the time in the area of nutrition and food science and we may have had the very first course taught completely by self-paced audiovisual methods. Naturally being a doctoral student, I published and the speaking requests started coming in from state and even national conventions.

How could I learn to speak to audiences (not students) and not blush? "Learn by doing," I said to myself and started speaking at every church group, grade school, high school, community service group that needed a speaker. Sometimes the conditions were a little extraordinary. As the mother of three children whom I breast-fed, I found it challenging to speak to a LaLeche League meeting where all members of the audience were breast-feeding their children. However, I learned to speak and hold the attention of an audience.

Time marched on, I was still teaching chemistry at the medical school, many courses at Syracuse University, speaking, writing, taking care of family and house, but I finally earned my doctorate four years after I started. Meanwhile my children had grown and the oldest went to college. I was able to help some because Syracuse had reciprocal tuition arrangements with Cornell where he wanted to attend. So we had one in college. Our next son won a full tuition scholarship to Massachusetts Institute of Technology and we had two in college. Our daughter was still in high school.

Second Doctorate

After I had my Ph.D. in nutrition, I thought about what I had been through learning to study and becoming current in biochemistry and nutrition information. I decided that I would never put myself in that position again—I would keep on going to school forever.

I started my second doctorate. You would think that it would be easy to start a second doctorate with the ink still wet on the first degree. Oh, no. They wanted me to take tests. "Why?", I said. "To prove I was capable of doing graduate work," they said. "Here is my Ph.D. diploma to prove that," I said. Their answer was still "no" since no one had gotten a Ph.D. and then wanted a doctorate in education. I thought I should have some formal courses in education if I were going to go wandering about the country talking about nutrition and food science education methods. I received a letter telling me that they would not accept me. I made a few phone calls implying that their graduate students would no longer be welcome in my learning lab to do research. My letter of acceptance came in the next mail. Blackmail? Probably.

Registered Dietitian

We have yet to say anything about becoming a dietitian (registered, that is). At about this time, The American Dietetic Association announced exams would be given to qualified candidates in order to become a registered dietitian. I had never done a hospital internship so how could I qualify? Oh happiness, they announced there would be a grandfather clause so that those graduating long ago with proper credentials, necessary courses, and a doctorate in nutrition/dietetics would be able to qualify. Thanks to Professor Marjorie Dibble, who pushed me into applying. And that is how I became a registered dietitian. However, although I had the proper academic credentials and I certainly knew my way around a hospital after working in one for many years, I still feel there is a hole in my background because I did not do a hospital internship.

My Media Start and Educational Methods

On January 25, 1975, something happened which changed my whole academic life. I received a phone call from the Syracuse University news bureau asking me if I had seen the New York Times. Rarely did I have time to read anything but scientific journals so I was surprised to hear that my name had appeared in print. I dashed out to purchase a paper thinking that I would be in small print on the back page. Oh no, there was a half page about my teaching methods including a picture of me in costume on a motorcycle. That changed my life. Letters, phone calls, offers to appear on TV, radio, in newsprint poured in from almost all over the world. It was astounding what a half page in the New York Times does to your life. Perhaps I should explain why a picture on a motorcycle should be published?

A few years after I started teaching the basic nutrition course, it became larger and larger. Attendance was no longer mandatory at Syracuse and I found it very difficult to teach students who were not in class. I had to find a way of making nutrition classes fun, interesting, exciting while providing current nutrition information. It was the time of "Laugh-in" a television show with quick costume changes, flashing colors, rock music and one-liners. It if works for the TV audience, why not in nutrition? My son, Bill put together an audio tape with me talking about nutrition and one-liners from popular songs, TV shows or commercials dubbed in after each one of my sentences. We thought it was funny and hoped the students would, too. My daughter and I started sewing little costumes of wild colors and paintings that had something to do with nutrition. My older son and my husband helped us carry all the equipment to the auditorium for our BIG show. Now I had to have a gimmick—we would hear the zoom-zoom of the motorcycles outdoors—well, why not IN the auditorium? The only problem was that the auditorium was two floors underground and it was an amphitheater with many steps down to the front. This auditorium was also the pride of Syracuse University with all kinds of audiovisual equipment hookups and with blue plush carpeting. Stains from motorcycles would not be welcome.

The first show involved six op-art (big splashes of bright colors which we finger-painted) slides, but I put each slide in a separate projector so I had a six-projector slide show plus we had the audio tape preceded by loud rock music. My electronic son also fixed polarized slides, strobe lights, musicvision (lights go up and down with the music). My elder son and my husband helped carry all the equipment over to the auditorium. I had one or two costumes made with the help of my daughter. My legs were painted with nutrition symbols plus the formula for cholesterol in fluorescent paint which was picked up with black lights. I rode into the auditorium and down the stairs on a motorcycle and the show started. It was an overwhelming hit. More students came to class to see what was going to happen next.

Over the years, these "happenings" evolved into a production using six slide projectors all going at once on the walls (now with over 1300 slides), two overhead projectors with moire patterns focused on the ceiling, loud music, audio tape with nutrition information and funny audio clips, strobe lights, black lights, strawberry incense, posters with fluorescent paint, five costume changes plus paint on my legs. Sometimes I entered on a motorcycle, sometimes I popped out of a cake, once I lead the Syracuse University marching band into the auditorium and once I was carried in on a surfboard. I shouldn't forget the time I was carried in on a stretcher and sustained a concussion falling down the steps in the dark. I was then carried back out to the hospital where one intern couldn't understand someone whose legs were a variety of painted colors. The rest of the doctors and nurses in the emergency room had all been in my class at one university or the other and recognized the "crazy" professor.

Of course, there were those in academia who asked if the professor had to put on a three ring circus to teach. I said "well, whatever works," but I decided that I should have some proof. I did pretests and posttests and all that education type of stuff since I was working on a doctorate in education. No one in the room could pass the pretest on the information covered in "the happening" while after the show, everyone received an A or B grade. Ten weeks after the presentation, the retention was way above what would be expected.

Obviously I could not put on a happening every class period. Usually I had one on the first day of class (after which 50 to 80 more students add the course) and when I am teaching a class on weight control. It takes so much time to prepare one of these shows and make the audio tapes. It also takes at least three audiovisual experts who know that all of the audiovisual equipment has to go on all at once. During my other "normal" lectures, I use music when the students are coming in and leaving, many slides that I take when traveling or in grocery stores or copy from magazines and comic strips. I show TV commercials and ask the students if they would buy this product and why. I used to be given the commercials on 16 mm movie film from TV stations but now I can show videotapes on new big projectors in the auditorium. I also try to tape commentaries on nutrition from commercial TV to show to the class for discussion.

I learned to wordprocess on the mainframe so I could have 270 copies of notes printed to hand out after class. The students then were not under pressure to take so many notes and could feel more free to enter into discussions. Now I can wordprocess on a personal computer and interface with the mainframe. I feel fortunate to be able to make use of the fine Syracuse University computer facilities.

Family Recognition

Time kept right on going along and I kept teaching at Syracuse University, and at the Medical Center and working on my education doctorate. At this point the whole family made the local newspapers because our elder son Walter graduated from medical school (and would continue to become an orthopedic surgeon with a second residency in hand surgery), our youngest son William received his masters in electrical engineering at the Massachusetts Institute of Technology (and would go on for his doctorate), our daughter Sarah graduated from high school (and would go on to Denison University to major in mathematics and computer science), I received my second doctorate and my husband supported all of us in so many ways. I can never thank him enough.

More Media Work Plus Computer Diet Analysis

I continued teaching at the medical school until eight years ago, at which point I decided I had enough running up and down the hill. Also I had become very busy speaking to state and national conventions, doing TV, radio and print interviews both national shows (Today Show, Good Morning America and more) plus traveling across the country doing local shows or speaking. Eventually I had traveled in 47 states and six continents. I was also attempting to write journal articles, articles for popular magazines, textbook (never finished) and chapters in books—I hate to write. My younger son and I also had a share of a diet analysis software commercial venture. More about that.

In 1970, Bill developed an interactive (you type in information about your food intake and answer comes back immediately) computer program on the mainframe to analyze diets. This was years and years before diet analysis packages were offered in every journal and it was years before this type of thing could be done on personal computers. The diet analysis information was not yet put on computer tapes by the United States Department of Agriculture so Bill entered the nutrition information by hand—a tedious and time consuming job. At the end we had a program that would provide a diet analysis (calories, protein, carbohydrate, fat, vitamin and mineral content plus more) of your diet for one day or any number of days. Eventually there was an energy program which would give you an idea of energy expended during the day. It was used by my students to analyze their own diets so they could see where problems might develop and change their eating habits. It was also used by graduate students for projects and dissertations. When the food and nutrition information came from the USDA on computer tape, we breathed a sigh of relief since now we had most of the information straight from the authority. We still had to enter information from industry and journal sources plus nutrient information not furnished by the USDA. The commercial venture faded away but Bill has graciously and generously volunteered his time and expertise over the years to keep this huge diet analysis program current.

Third Doctorate?

I had said that I would never stop my formal education so what would I do for my third doctorate? I've tried several fields. Clinical psychology for behavioral modification was one option since I was counseling people about weight control. However, I would have to be a full-time student for at least part of the time and I didn't want to leave nutrition. I took a course and explored physiology of exercise since I was now working in sports nutrition. This is certainly a fantastic world of information, but I found it wasn't for me. They said they would accept me in law school but I would have to go full time the first year. Obviously I haven't found a more exciting field than nutrition. I do still take courses—mostly big and little classes in computer science, but I don't feel driven to complete another degree, yet.

Sports Nutrition

Early in the 70's two quite tall young men came into my office almost dragging a third fairly hefty friend. They were all members of the SU varsity crew. "We are sick of rowing this big crew member around" the two slimmer ones said. "What can you do about taking some of his pounds off?" That was the beginning of sports nutrition research that has lasted to this day and I hope will continue.

By this time, we had the diet analysis program in place and I started working with athletes. Word spread and soon I was consulting with 18 different teams at Syracuse University (not all at once). Coaches send individual athletes to me to "instantaneously" take 20 pounds off or put 20 pounds on. I finally asked the coach of one of the big-money sports on campus "How many hours do you have your athletes see the strength coach? How many hours will you let them see me?" His reply was "I see your point," but that was the end of the conversation. I go along with no grant, no money and no prestige. The athletic department says that I am their sports nutritionist but they do not pay me or give me an office and recognize that nutrition is important. Other places do, however, and I am asked to consult and speak and write. I guess it is true that you are never a prophet in your own hometown.

Interactive Videodisc

What else am I doing at present? For the last eight or nine years, my son Bill has urged me to look into interactive videodisc technology for my learning lab. He gave me the following explanation (plus more) and told me to start! Videodisc is a storage medium like videotape except that it looks like a large audio compact disc. It is indestructible, inexpensive (after the first very expensive one is made), has a huge storage capacity and is interactive. One side of a disc can hold 30 minutes of a movie or videotape with two different sound channels or 54,000 slides (675 carousel slide trays) or a combination of movies and slides. You can look at just one picture or frame at a time, but its potential is that it is interactive. It does not have to be shown from start to finish, but in an order determined by the user's needs and responses to questions. You may have seen examples of this at Disney Epcot Center's information booths. An introduction is given, you are asked the information you need. After your reply, the information becomes more and more specific until you are at a level of looking inside exhibits or at restaurant menus and making dinner reservations.

To use this new technology in my learning lab is taking (and will take) much money, expertise and time. A grateful alumna gave me enough money to buy some beginning equipment and we bought a prepared videodisc on cooking (none available on nutrition). Bill wrote a computer program so that we have several demonstration teaching modules. However in order to put even part of a course into a learning lab we have far to go. We are working on three parts of this project at the same time.

I have to write the food science and nutrition information and do an educational flow chart. This involves writing small pieces of information, asking questions and depending on how the question is answered, branching the student to new information, more information, or starting again. This has to be done for a whole course. Secondly, we have to prepare a video, film, and/or slide presentation to go with the information and have it made into a videodisc. We also have to know which picture is on every frame of the disc so that the computer can find it. Thirdly, a computer program has to be written to present the food science/nutrition information and ask the questions on the screen plus make computer graphics to be used with the whole package. The computer program also has to find the correct visual (video image or slide on the disc) at the right time in the correct sequence to go with the information or the question. The student just touches the screen to answer.

"This is a very powerful method of individualizing instruction" (W.R. Short). I just hope that I can complete even part of this project in my lifetime. It seems overwhelming but exciting.

How Does the Media Find You?

The wonderful department secretaries, my students and I all marvel at the amount of mail and phone calls coming in from around the world and questions from newspapers, magazines and the electronic media. How does all this come about? You need one big media break—mine was the New York Times article about my "wild" teaching methods. Then the advertising and public relations firms in major cities (mostly New York City) call to ask for a quote or for information for a project they are writing or producing. The minute you answer the first question with something quotable, your name is (I think) posted up on Times Square—"for free nutrition information, call Sarah Short." You do not get paid for doing national or local TV shows or radio or newspaper interviews. This astounds my students, but it is true since the media thinks you are selling something and being paid.

If you are not being paid then you do not get rich doing this type of thing. However, I feel that I am trying in my little way to have correct nutrition information reach the public. Usually the public wants to hear and see incorrect information and the promise of instant success, but I try. You are not paid for quotes in popular magazines, either. Be very careful about quotes because I have found that some magazines have people making up quotes who have never spoken to you. That you can't control, but actual quotes you can ask to have read back to you. You do receive money for whole articles if you are asked to be the author. They usually ask for an entire new diet for a month with all needed nutrients and a few calories and they want it tomorrow.

There are advantages and disadvantages in speaking to the media. You must be prepared for any questions. This means much studying and homework. I subscribe to 20 to 25 medical, nutrition and food science research journals plus 8 to 10 newsletters and I receive four more medical journals. Every day, I read, skim, clip and file. If you are going to answer media questions, you also need to know what is news and what people are concerned about. Therefore, I skim the popular press for nutrition issues and I walk through "health food" stores in the malls to see the products people are buying. This is tremendously time consuming, but if you are called and say "I don't know anything about that issue," you probably will not be bothered again. Most people do not realize that the media callers want information from you immediately and they want the information to be current and correct. I try to answer the phone near my files and reference books so I can doublecheck my information while answering. However, if I really do not know about the subject asked, I never hedge. I try to refer them to an authority in the field and tell them I would be happy to answer questions when they have one in my field of expertise.

Philosophy

My personal philosophy of life and work were inherited from my parents who drummed in "finish your work before you play." I now wonder if work ever is finished and when is the play part? Personally, I always look for the options. Is there someway to accomplish what I want to do with little or no money but lots of energy? When I walk around campus or anywhere, I look for things I might be able to use now or later in the learning lab or classroom (one person's trash is another's treasure).

I try to push myself. Children have a little saying when daring themselves to jump in the lake: "one for the money, two for the show, three to get ready, and four to go." Even if I'm tired, do not want to do something; I have a firm rule that on "four," I go. Keep going. Nothing is accomplished sitting around.

Professional Beliefs

I believe that the profession of dietetics/nutrition is a worthwhile one to choose for a lifetime. It incorporates science (chemistry, biological sciences, and math), art (food preparation is an art form), communications skills, business and marketing skills. The humanitarian rewards are great; the monetary gains may not be so good. The salaries in industry and public relations firms are probably better than in all other areas, but it would be sad to lose all the good hospital and community dietitians. Of course, consulting dietitians can make high salaries but it takes time to build up a practice. What is unique about the dietetic profession is that there are so many opportunities—in medical settings, community agencies, academia, industry, advertising and public relations firms with food accounts, writing and communications firms are only some of the options.

I think the profession is only starting on a big upswing. When all states have licensing laws and when more laws are passed to prevent unqualified people from "practicing nutrition," dietitians and qualified nutritionists should have more respect. The actor whose major punch line is "I get no respect" should try being a dietitian. We have to fight. Some days, it seems the unqualified people (translate that into quacks) are winning. In the United States, anyone can publish a book on nutrition even if they have no qualifications whatsoever. When will the libraries and newspapers put these books under the fiction lists?

Products that have no nutritional value or may even be harmful may be sold as "food supplements." If the product is not a food or a drug, it falls between the cracks of the Food and Drug Administration jurisdiction. I used to say that I loved the United States Postal service because if they saw malpractice, they would stop the company's mail. I still like the Postal Service, but those who peddle useless products now have 800 phone numbers, take your credit card number and send the products by private trucking firms. I used to tell young dietitians to go to medical school so we would have more physicians that knew nutritional information. Now I say go to law school so we will have more lawyer/dietitians to fight the unqualified people in our society selling misinformation and useless products.

While I am on my soapbox, we are in a profession where abuse is heaped upon us. Everyone who eats is a nutritionist. Everyone has read about nutrition, seen it on TV, heard it on the radio, and read about it in the newspapers. Therefore, everyone is an expert and thinks "so what is so difficult about being a dietitian?". People don't sit around telling civil engineers how to build a bridge. You don't hear too many telling brain surgeons how to operate. Why does everyone pick on us?? Because the media is attempting to sell the public on the idea that there are easy answers to all health problems—just buy this product and you will never be sick, live to be 99, and still be sexy.

I'm getting apprehensive about telling what profession I am in because once I say the word "nutrition," I have to listen to an hour nutrition lecture from the taxi driver or whoever is sitting next to me on the plane. Even when I am out socially, someone asks a nutrition question and everyone present answers with great authority, but I am never asked (yes, they do know where I work). It isn't that I care about being asked, it is just that everyone thinks they know more about the subject that a full professor of nutrition.

The young dietitians are more assured, more aggressive and I know that they will change things around. You will, won't you???

Discriminations Against Females

We were asked to write about minority struggles, about which I know little. However, if this includes discrimination against females, then I can comment. When I was working as a chemist, it was just assumed that women would receive less pay—they always had and always would since "women are not the main breadwinners," I was told. Men hired after me received more money and better jobs even though I had more education and experience and had produced new products for the company. Actually, I thought I was lucky because my mother told me about her first days on the job as a chemist. The men did not want a women chemist working in their lab and proceeded to spill acid on her. Compared with that, my life in the lab was easy.

Every time I was hired to teach, I did not have too much bargaining room. I needed that job to pay my tuition, so I did not do any salary negotiating. That was a mistake. At both universities, I started at a rock bottom salary. Mostly, universities offer very small raises unless you are funded under a large grant. There are problems with "soft money" because when the grant is over, you may be expected to find another grant quickly or else have no salary. Anyway, I found that 3% raises of a very small salary was still a small salary. Until the last few years, I was never paid the average for my rank at the university and some of the time I was paid the lowest in my rank. Why? I was teaching in a former college of Home Economics (most have new names now) which was (and is) mostly female. Every time the faculty complained, the administration replied that since there were no male counterparts with whom to compare, it would not be discrimination. We probably could have started a class action suit but this takes much money and time. Some years I was earning as much with my part time job teaching at the medical school plus consulting as I was working full time at Syracuse University. Do I sound bitter? Maybe because it is unfair and I hate things that are unfair.

If I felt so strongly, why didn't I go elsewhere? I said it was because my husband had a good job in Syracuse and we couldn't just pull up stakes (especially with three children) and move. Women just never thought of doing such things at that point in time. I thought of myself as a wife, mother, homemaker first and then as a professional person. My solution to not receiving enough money was to take on more jobs. At some points along the way, I was teaching at two universities, acting as nutritionist for the software company, writing for magazines, lecturing around the country, and doing some consulting all at the same time.

Personal Accomplishments

Rarely do I think about my accomplishments, but then when I do, they seem as if they had happened to someone else. There were many decision points along the way. Did I make the right turn? My husband asked me yesterday if starting all over, would I do things differently? No, I don't think so. There have been ups and downs in my life, but mostly I have been happy and very, very fortunate. My husband and I have been friends and in love since we were little. We have three wonderful, talented, loving, and beautiful children and now we have four grandchildren, all of whom we adore.

My husband and I both travel for business and we have become addicted to travel—we have been around the world, but now we want to see the places we missed. At this writing we are on our way to China. A few years ago I was invited to speak in Kenya so my husband and I could see that part of Africa. This is the way to become truly educated about our planet and world-wide nutrition. It was an enlightening experience.

Professional Accomplishments

Recognitions of special significance to me were ones awarded in my hometown. Each year a Syracuse newspaper has a big luncheon to recognize women of achievement. In 1979, I was given the Woman of Achievement award with all my family and friends present. Syracuse University each year has a big convocation with all faculty members attending. At the 1986 convocation, I was presented with the University Scholar/Teacher of the Year Award.

What else have I done? I have taught 14 different courses in nutrition, sports nutrition, nutrition education, biochemistry at Syracuse University; and 8 different courses in chemistry plus nutrition for the medical students at Upstate Medical Center (now Health Science Center), State University of New York. I am a member of 18 national/international professional organizations in areas of nutrition, food science, education, sports nutrition and served as president of one. I was elected to five national honorary societies and Board of Scientific Counselors (U.S. Department of Agriculture). I am listed in American Men and Women of Science, The World Who's Who of Women, Who's Who in America, and Outstanding Educators. I have written three books, three chapters in books and many journal articles. I am a peer reviewer for four research journals and review nutrition textbooks for two publishers. I have been invited to speak at over 200 national or state conventions, medical schools, universities and industrial meetings including The American Dietetic Association, American Medical Association, IBM, National March of Dimes, National Food Editors Conference. I have been interviewed by TV, radio and print media over 1000 times nationally and in major cities across the United States including, The Today Show, Good Morning America, Not For Women Only, Real People, USA national cable network syndicated series of nutrition segments, New York Times, Reader's Digest, Wall Street Journal, Vogue, Mademoiselle, Computerworld, Voice of America. I've traveled on six continents, seen 34 countries and 47 states.

That is probably more than you really wanted to know about me and more than I have ever told anyone.

As you can guess, I like talking about and teaching nutrition. I am not going to retire until I am told to leave and then I'll look for another job teaching nutrition. I like working with athletes and I like learning more about computing. I like to learn and hope I will always be capable of learning more. May all of you have as happy a personal and professional life as I have had.

Grace Severance Shugart

Grace Severance Shugart, MS, RD is Professor Emeritus,
Department of Dietetics, Restaurant and Institution
Management, Kansas State University, Manhattan, KS

Grace Shugart, like many of today's students, was undecided about a career when she entered college in 1927. Although dietetics was suggested to her by guidance counselors, she had visions of being a theater organist. After a frank self-evaluation of her musical abilities at the end of her freshman year, she opted instead for a major in dietetics and institution management. The professional can be thankful she did! This famed co-author of *Food for Fifty* and *Food Service in Institutions* has a unique understanding of people which was nurtured during the Great Depression when she saw patients paying hospital bills with potatoes and men exchanging an hour of work on the hospital grounds for one meal. She was a member of the ADA Executive Board for 10 years and served as President in 1968–69. This Copher Award winner served on Senator Bob Dole's Committee on Human Nutrition and Needs. Grace Shugart was on the faculty of Kansas State University for 24 years and was honored with the establishment of the Grace M. Shugart Lectureship at the time of her retirement. Here she reflects on the many changes which have occurred in the profession since she joined in 1931.

Grace Severance Shugart

Most of my early years were spent in Pullman, Washington, where my father was a faculty member at the State College of Washington (now Washington State University). After graduation from Washington State in 1931 and completion of a dietetic internship at the University of Minnesota Hospitals, I started my professional career as a dietitian at the Northern Pacific Railway Hospital in Glendive, Montana. After three years in that position, I accepted a graduate assistantship in the institution management department at Iowa State University. At the end of a year I became food director of the cooperative dormitories, thus delaying completion of the M.S. degree until 1938. A year later I resigned to be married and was inactive in the profession except for five years as instructor in the institution management department at Iowa State.

In 1951 I joined the institutional management faculty at Kansas State University as coordinator of residence hall foodservices and assistant professor of institutional management. When Mrs. West retired in 1957, I became professor and head of the department, a position I held until I retired in 1975. Since retirement, much of my time has been spent in revisions of the two textbooks of which I am co-author: *Food for Fifty*, now in its eighth edition, and *Food Service Institutions*, in its sixth edition.

Although active in the Iowa Dietetic Association and the Kansas Dietetic Association during the early years, my involvement in The American Dietetic Association did not start until I was elected Delegate from Kansas to the House of Delegates. That was followed by a three-year term as delegate-at-large, then food administrative section chairman. I became a member of the executive board in 1965 when I was elected speaker-elect of the House of Delegates and became Speaker in 1966. I served as President-elect in 1967 and President in 1968. Other major assignments included member of the internship board, Chairman of the Program of Work Committee, Chairman of the Task Force for the 70's, Chairman of the Nominating Committee, consultant to the Bylaws and Structure Committee, chairman of a committee to develop appeals procedures, and the ADA Foundation board.

Although my major efforts were with ADA, I also was a member of the American Home Economics Association, the School Food Service Association, Council on Hotel, Restaurant, and Institutional Education (CHRIE), the Society for Advancement of Food Service Research, and the Food Technologists. Honoraries included Omicron Nu, Phi Upsilon Omicron, Phi Kappa Phi, and Theta Sigma Phi (now Women in Communications).

I was invited to be a panel member for the White House Conference on Food, Nutrition, and Health in 1969 and was a member of Bob Dole's Committee on Human Nutrition and Needs for Kansas that same year. From 1969 to 1972 I represented dietetics on an Allied Health Professions Review Committee, in which grant applications were reviewed for HEW.

I wish I could say that I always had a burning desire to be a dietitian, but I can't. Like many students today, I was undecided about a career when I entered college and knew very little about dietitians, except for an early negative encounter while in high school. During my senior year, a vocational guidance counselor evaluated my interests and qualifications and recommended dietetics as a career choice because it combined my interests in food and also management. At that time, though, I was involved in music and journalism activities and had visions of being a theater organist. Like a typical sixteen-year old, I thought I knew best and decided to major in music. At the end of my freshman year, an advisor pointed out the options that would be open to me as a music graduate, all of which required more talent than I had. This frank evaluation of my musical ability might have been depressing had it not been that I had come to that conclusion myself and had decided to enroll in home economics, with a major in dietetics and institution management. In retrospect, I think my mother probably influenced my decision, too, because of her interest in preparing good food and serving nutritionally balanced meals. As children, the importance of good nutrition was emphasized at home and I remember how adamant she was that we not eat between meals, especially sweets. I can still hear her say that if we were really hungry we could eat an apple or a slice of homemade bread and butter (we didn't know about cholesterol in those days). I was encouraged to participate in cooking at home and was given an opportunity to help with meal planning.

In college, I especially liked the management courses but was also interested in foods and nutrition. At the time of graduation in 1931, I was unsure about the direction I would like to go, so I applied for a hospital internship, which at that time was the most logical route to follow. I completed the internship and I know now that it was a valuable experience, but at the time it was rather traumatic because my knowledge of hospitals was very limited and I had not lived away from home before. I realize now that I was totally unprepared for the types of situations I was to experience. This is no reflection on my college courses because they included excellent practical on-the-job application in college foodservices and adequate nutrition theory. Many students today, through summer experiences or clinical components in their courses, are exposed to the practical application of theory and have developed some communication skills and understanding of people, which help bridge the gap between college and internship and/or the first position.

Still unsure about a career choice after my internship, I quickly accepted a position as dietitian in a 60-bed hospital when it was offered because during the depression one didn't turn down a job. I was in charge of the dietary department, housekeeping, laundry, linen room, and garden, and I hadn't been there a week before I was asked to order the garden seed. I often thought that I must have grown up in a very sheltered environment. While I knew there was a depression (reinforced when my first paycheck, along with the salaries of all other hospital employees was cut 10 percent) I saw some of the devastating effects of the depression for the first time when I saw patients paying their hospital bills with potatoes, eggs, chicken, and other foods. Since this was a railroad hospital, we were asked to feed men who were "riding the rails" in exchange for an hour's work on the hospital grounds during their stopover. Many of these men were well-educated but were unemployed and hoped to find a new location where there might be job opportunities.

My experience there, in which I was totally responsible for the department, helped me to gain confidence and reinforce my belief that my interest was in management. I was happy there and probably would have remained longer than I did were it not for my department head at Washington State who thought it was time for me to start graduate study. She recommended me for an assistantship at Iowa State and suggested I accept it. Later, as food director in the cooperative dormitories there, I found that I liked working with students and that my interest was in foodservices that provided food for well people with healthy appetites.

In 1939 when I was married, I resigned my position because I was expected to. At that time you either had a career or a family, not both. Besides, most foodservice positions required that you be away from home at mealtime. In spite of the absence of married women on the faculty, I was asked to substitute for faculty members who were on leave for various reasons. The first appointment was to be for one quarter but was extended to five years. While this experience aroused an interest in college teaching, the appointments were temporary and did not necessarily contribute to attaining a career goal.

When my husband and I moved to Kansas in 1950, I decided to call on Bessie Brooks West, head of the Department of Institutional Management at Kansas State University. I had never met Mrs. West but of course knew about her. As we visited, I asked her about opportunities in Kansas for dietitians. Fortunately, she was looking for a food service coordinator for their expanding residence hall program. This was a new position, and they needed someone who was interested in teaching also. I accepted the position, and thus began an enjoyable association with a remarkable women and an opportunity to be part of a well-known department and a successful residence hall program.

I must have been a "late bloomer" because it was at this point I decided that if I were going to work I should think in terms of a career rather than just a job and that it should be a position that had potential for professional fulfillment and advancement. I had found that temporary positions lead nowhere and do not give the personal or professional satisfaction that comes for a position with potential for the future. When I was in college, students tended to take life as it came and did not think in terms of lifetime goals. Today, students are advised to look at their entire life span and make flexible plans, recognizing that there may be interruptions for child rearing or changes to accommodate a husband's career goals. Most of today's graduates are more widely traveled and have had more life experiences than graduates of my era. They tend to be more confident, more goal-oriented and seem willing to assume some responsibility for their career development.

Most of us are influenced in some way by one or more mentors during our professional careers; in fact, I have sometimes felt that at the appropriate time someone was always there with an opportunity or some good advice, and even a little "prodding."

Had the head of my department at Washington State not continued her interest in my progress after graduation and urged me to start graduate study, for example, I might have settled in comfortably in my hospital position probably for too long a period. My only regret is that I did not go beyond the M.S. degree, but at the time I should have been working on it, the Ph.D. was not considered necessary for foodservice administration and my career goals were too indefinite.

I was fortunate to have had several mentors during my career who contributed to my professional life. Fern Gleiser, head of the institution management department at Iowa State University, who guided me through graduate studies and offered me the opportunity to remain on the faculty, was an inspiration to me because of her professional integrity and behavior. She, along with Lenore Sullivan who taught quantity cookery and catering in the department's tea room at Iowa State, helped me develop an appreciation for fine food.

Bessie Brooks West at Kansas State, who is well known for her food standards, reinforced my interest in food quality. Through her confidence in me, her helpful suggestions, and her delightful sense of humor, she inspired me to do my best. She was forward-looking and willing to listen to ideas of her staff and students. Her interest in students and her confidence in their ability helped me in turn to realize and encourage the potential in students. In addition, it was Mrs. West who urged me to become more active in the ADA. Doretta Hoffman, Dean of Home Economics at Kansas State, offered me an opportunity for advancement and encouraged my professional growth.

I have observed many changes in the profession since starting in 1931. Just as there are many more career opportunities open to women today, the options in dietetics are more numerous and attractive than was the case when I graduated. When I finished my internship, beginning positions in dietetics, as in other fields, were scarce. The new graduate could become an administrative or therapeutic dietitian if she were fortunate enough to find an opening or, as in my case, the only dietitian in a small hospital. Commercial foodservice and school foodservice (called school lunch then) had very few openings for college educated managers. Consultants were unheard of, and I don't suppose any of us had heard of entrepeneurship. Just as women are gaining entree to professions once not open to them, dietetics is no longer a profession for women only, with many more men becoming dietitians and foodservice managers.

Since retiring, I have watched with interest the expanding range of opportunities available in all areas of dietetics and the degree of specialization, especially in clinical dietetics. Role delineation studies have helped identify responsibilities for the various types of dietetic positions, of which there are many today.

The current interest in nutrition has enhanced the position of the dietitian in the eyes of the public and other professionals and has provided an opportunity to become highly visible in nutrition education. It is exciting to see articles in national magazines by registered dietitians and to see television appearances by attractive, articulate, and knowledgeable dietitians. Perhaps we are at last finding our "place in the sun" and are gradually changing the image of the dietitian. For years, dietitians were criticized for knowing their subject but not being able to present the material in an interesting fashion.

Today's dietitian is provided with technical and clerical assistance, thus providing time to participate in more appropriate professional activities. Relocation of dietitian's offices has increased visibility and availability to other health professionals, and I believe the clinical dietitian has made progress in establishing a place on the medical team. Health care legislation resulted in a need for dietary consultants, and aggressive dietitians are creating opportunities for self-employment. I wonder if I would have had the courage to start my own business.

Not only have opportunities expanded but the duties and required skills of dietetic personnel have changed. Administrators and managers are using a systems approach to foodservice management. There is more emphasis on marketing, financial accountability, and information systems which means that administrative dietitians must know about financial management and should be knowledgeable about the computer and its uses in dietetics and foodservice management. I hope the increased emphasis on systems and management techniques has not detracted from the administrative dietitian's concern with production of quality food, however. Increased involvement in nutrition education for the public requires a knowledge of interpersonal relations. Although there is not general agreement, I believe in a broad, basic dietetics program, followed by specialization through graduate study and/or experience.

Working conditions for dietitians have changed, too. In the 1930's and 40's, board and room were included as part of the salary for many health care workers. The salary in my first position was $80 per month (that was before the salary cut) plus board, room, and laundry. All personnel lived in the hospital, which meant we were on call seven days a week, and it was customary for dietitians to work split shifts and in many cases seven days a week. Board and room were provided in many residence halls positions, too, including my first one. I suppose the provision of room was more economical than addition to the cash salary, but I suspect part of the reason for dietitians to "live in" was for convenience in opening and closing the foodservice. It was customary at that time for the dietitians to personally unlock and lock the kitchens and storerooms. Since then, the addition of qualified supervisors and technicians has eliminated the need for the dietitian to be on duty such long hours and has made these positions more attractive to married dietitians and those with family responsibilities.

I cannot look back on my career without commenting on my professional involvement in the ADA. The opportunity to meet and work with outstanding professionals and to have a part in guiding the association programs and planning for its future was most rewarding. As a member of the first Program of Work Committee, then Chairman of the Task Force for the 70's, it has been gratifying to see the first attempts at delineating a program of work that started as a listing of current programs. develop into a vision of the directions the association and the profession should be taking.

As a member of the coordinating cabinet and executive board for ten years (1959–1969), I saw several major developments that were to affect the profession as well as the Association. Registration, with its built-in continuing education component, was adopted by the members; the Association made its start is legislative activities, officially testifying at a Congressional hearing for the first time, opening a Washington office, and writing our first position paper; an accreditation process for educational programs was established; and restructuring of the Association that included broadening of membership categories was in process during that period. Having a part in all of this was truly a stimulating experience.

The years spent at Kansas State were enjoyable and challenging. I was proud to have a part in the development of one of the early coordinated dietetics programs, and it has been satisfying to see the graduates of that program functioning successfully. The Association with the many outstanding leaders in dietetics while working with the ADA was a learning experience for me, and I hope that I may have passed some of that on to our students. The climax of my 24 years at Kansas State was the establishment of the Grace M. Shugart Lectureship at the time of my retirement. This series of lectures, now in its fifteenth year, was established to continue my interest in introducing students to leaders in our profession.

Throughout my career I was fortunate to have a very supportive husband who has been proud of my accomplishments, even when my travels as ADA President took me away from home frequently. I admire the young women today who successfully manage a home and children and a career with such aplomb. Granted, many men today are willing to share household chores, and the working hours for dietitians have become more realistic. There is also a better understanding of home obligations by associates than there was in earlier years when married women first began to enter the work force. In dealing with my own career and home obligations, I tried to set priorities and found there was a limit to the commitments I could make, and I even learned to say "no" once in a while.

One of the highlights of my career occurred in 1980 when I was given the ADA Copher Award. I was especially pleased with the closing statement on the plaque which says "in appreciation of . . . her unique understanding of people and her ability to maintain a stable balance between heavy professional responsibility and a happy home life." That is what I tried hard to do, and apparently that came through to my peers, who selected me for this award. Other honors of which I am very proud were the Distinguished Kansas Dietitian of the Year in 1977, Distinguished Home Economics Alumnus Award in 1978 and the Alumni Achievement Award in 1982 from Washington State University, and the ADA Medallion in 1978.

The 37 years I was active in the profession were fulfilling and enjoyable, and it is my hope that I may have contributed in some way to the profession.

Mary Lou South

Mary Lou South, MS, RD
is a Licensed Nursing Home Administrator
in the San Francisco, CA area.

Mary Lou South recounts affectionately of the support she has always received from her family. In fact, she writes with a positive and warm outlook on all the experiences of her life and her career. During her dietetic internship she realized a strong interest in administrative dietetics. She functioned in the management area, went on to a successful private consultative practice, and ultimately to managing her own convalescent hospital. She seems to thrive on excitement and challenges. A veteran commercial airline passenger, when Mary Lou South wanted to know more, she earned her pilot's license. She does not shy away from hard work nor stressful situations, earning her master's degree while serving as ADA Speaker of the House and President-elect. Through dedication to her career and commitment to the profession, this 56th ADA President supports her greatest pride—being a registered dietitian.

Mary Lou South

The profession of dietetics has been very good to me and I have given a lot to it in return. I would like to be able to tell you that my interest in dietetics was developed at an early age, but that is not the case. In fact, my career path was fairly uncertain until I entered Iowa State University for my last two years of undergraduate education. Furthermore, I had never even entered a hospital kitchen or worked in any kind of food service until I went to the University of Minnesota for my dietetic internship. It would be truthful of me to say that early on I doubted dietetics was the career for me, but it seemed too late to make a change.

Just like the parents of most of my peers, mine placed a very high value on education, a strong work ethic and high moral standards. It is these three values that I learned early that have given me the ability to make a success of my career and of life too. My parents were certainly my first role models and from their actions and example I developed my strength and character. Unfortunately, my father died when I was in my mid-twenties and he was not here to see me through most of my professional successes and failures. My mother was a Home Economics teacher, which I suppose is one of the reasons that I considered dietetics as a career. However, my mother never worked professionally after she married my father. She was a magnificent woman and those who knew and met her would describe her as awesome and regal. She was a liberated woman before the phrase was even coined and my father always supported her efforts. She was also extremely bright and had an emotional strength that I never saw anyone match. Although I unfortunately did not inherit her mind, I think I did inherit or learn some of her strength.

I was reared in a small college town, Pocatello, Idaho. Very early my parents agreed with my two sisters and me that we would each attend college in our hometown (Idaho State University) for two years and then transfer to the college of our choice (anywhere) for the last two years. When I was a sophomore and ready to make my choice, a friend of ours who taught Home Economics at our local college told us that if I wanted to pursue dietetics as a career the best place to go was Iowa State University in Ames, Iowa. And that is where I went. There was no doubt then or now that it was the right choice of schools for dietetics. Unfortunately, at that time there were fewer career options for women and for whatever reasons it was more difficult to change one's educational course after it was begun.

I spent two and one half uneventful years at Iowa State University completing my undergraduate work, but certainly they were two and one half years of sound education and learning. When it came time to choose a dietetic internship, I applied to Peter Bent Brigham in Boston and the University of Minnesota Hospitals in Minneapolis. I was not accepted at Brigham, which was a disappointment because I had wanted to go to Boston. Instead, I set off for the University of Minnesota Hospitals, without regrets then or now about the choice. Gertrude I. Thomas was then the Director of the Department of Dietetics and the internship. It is difficult for me to describe her other than as a true character. At the time she was at least in her late sixties I am certain, or maybe in my youthful eyes she just seemed that old. She resided in the penthouse of the old nurses' dormitory, where we also stayed. She always wore a starched white uniform with a bright colored handkerchief in her breast pocket and a knitted shawl around her shoulders. We didn't see a lot of "Gertie," as we affectionately called her. The mundane activities of teaching dietetics seemed fairly unimportant to her and she left those to her many skillful staff members, who served her students well. It was rumored that she insisted the University of Minnesota male students be hired as busboys in food service so that her dietetic interns would have an opportunity to meet and date "high-caliber" men.

Every Monday morning she held an administrative seminar with us. Although the stated purpose was to discuss administrative topics, she always started the class by having us tell where we had gone and what we had seen in Minneapolis and St. Paul over the weekend. Each of us made sure to do something "cultural" because we knew that was what she wanted to hear. We rarely got to the administrative discussions. Although I enjoyed many cultural activities when I was growing up, Pocatello, Idaho—or Ames, Iowa, for that matter—had nothing to compare with Minneapolis and St. Paul. We laughed about it then, but as the years passed, I realized that Gertie saw life as far broader than one's career and her mission was to help us learn that. She taught me well and I will always be grateful to her. I kept in touch with her until she died, when she was well into her eighties.

On completing my internship, again I thought I wanted to go to Boston, but I was offered a job (sight unseen) at Butte Community Memorial Hospital in Butte, Montana. As my father was very ill by them, it seemed at the time better for me to be close to home. It proved to be a wonderful choice, providing me with both personal and professional experiences that have stayed with me all my life. Butte then was an old copper mining town and the entire economy was dependent on mining. In fact, the hospital was owned and operated by the Anaconda Copper Company. It was new, only two years old, and had all the newest equipment and a topnotch staff as well. I was hired as the "therapeutic dietitian," which also included teaching nutrition to the student nurses. The one other dietitian on the staff was designated as the Head of the Department. A staff of two dietitians for a two-hundred-bed hospital was fairly common then. My first year was a delightful experience of getting to know the friendliest group of people you could ever hope to meet. The food service employees were mostly older women from the community who treated me like a daughter, but also never lost sight of the fact that I was their "boss." The entire hospital staff was like one big happy family. During that year of teaching student nurses, I realized that my desire to teach would always have to be a part of my professional life, and it was for many years to come.

After my first year, the other dietitian, who has remained a lifetime friend, decided to leave to work on her Masters Degree in nutrition. Guess who that left as head of the department? I was scared to death. My management skills at that time were not well honed and I was only 23 years old. But I also knew that I was determined enough and that my "people skills" were good enough to see me through.

For the next year and a half I remained in Butte and was able to test my skills. I came to realize that management would always be my first love in dietetics, although learning that lesson was one of the most difficult times of my career. Incidentally, that was how most of us learned management, by being unexpectedly thrown into it in a small hospital. After eighteen months I thought I knew everything there was to know. I found out later, of course, that was not the case. But I decided to move on to bigger and better things. Also, by then my father had died and I no longer felt the need to be close to Pocatello.

This is probably a good point to tell about my two older sisters, who were certainly the finest of role models and have long supported me and my career. Joy, the eldest, is three years older than Ann, who is three years older than me. When we were youngsters and young adults they were protective of me, and I looked to them for advice and counsel. To this day we are all very close and have continued to be supportive of each other. Joy is a writer. She received her undergraduate degree in Journalism from the University of Wisconsin, and after spending some time living in the Midwest, she returned to our hometown. She is married and works for our hometown newspaper, the *Idaho State Journal*. I see her only once a year, but we still talk frequently.

My sister Ann received her undergraduate degree from the University of Michigan and her physical therapy training at the University of Wisconsin. Not long after graduation, she moved to San Francisco, knowing that the big city was for her. She never looked back. When I was ready to leave Butte, she was by then the Chief Physical Therapist at the University of California (UC) Medical Center in San Francisco. She suggested that I might want to come to San Francisco too.

So I left Butte knowing everything and nothing, to make my mark in the big city of San Francisco. After a few weeks I was hired for an administrative position by Henrietta Henderson, then Director of the Department of Dietetics at the University of California Medical Center. I might not have gotten the job had my sister Ann not put in a good word for me. In retrospect, I was not an easy student in the beginning, because I thought I knew more than I did. But Henrietta Henderson taught me well, taught me everything I know about administrative dietetics. And I mellowed some through the years that I was there. Still, I was anxious to learn as much as I could to further my career. Patience wasn't one of my virtues then and still is not. As soon as I had conquered one thing I wanted to move on to something else. Henrietta seemed to recognize this in me and allowed me many opportunities within the department that other directors might not have been so willing to do.

My love for teaching continued to be fulfilled through my work with our dietetic interns. Then and now I recognize that working with them was one of the highlights of my professional life. In fact, without that challenge I probably would have left the University of California long before I did.

Although I had developed an early interest in The American Dietetic Association (ADA) while I was an intern at the University of Minnesota Hospitals, it was not until I came to San Francisco that I became active. Henrietta Henderson encouraged this interest among her young staff members and interns. It was also during my early years at UC that I had an opportunity to attend my first ADA annual meeting in Portland, Oregon. I remember being so impressed with seeing all the women whose names I had heard and knew were important to the profession. I loved seeing them march in with their lovely gowns. Indeed, to this day I regret the discontinuance of the old ADA banquet at the annual meeting because we no longer recognize those people who made the profession what it is. I think we have taken something from our young dietitians and from our sense of history. In case you haven't guessed, I have a fierce pride about my profession and my professional association. For me dietetics is head and shoulders above most professions. Through the years I have worked with many other professional groups and most of them can't even come close to us. We may complain a lot about ourselves—maybe our complaining is what has created such high standards and our striving for excellence. This isn't to say that we have done everything right, but we really haven't given ourselves enough credit either.

In the early 1960s, then, I because actively involved in the Bay Area Dietetic Association and served as President. I met Dolores Nyhus, who was then a nutritionist with the Bureau of Nutrition, California State Department of Public Health. Dolores was active in the California Dietetic Association and was serving in the ADA House of Delegates. Dietitians in California had great personal and professional respect for Dolores and viewed her as our member who "knew the ropes" in ADA and would probably someday become ADA President. I don't know if Dolores necessarily thought that or that the presidency was one of her goals, but I never knew her when she wasn't serving on several ADA or CDA committees.

I never worked with Dolores on the job, but spent many years serving with her in the dietetic associations. Although Dolores and I were on opposite poles of the political spectrum, we did agree on association matters, and she was my mentor within the professional association. She gave me the benefit of her wisdom and guidance in association matters through my active years in CDA and ADA, until she was killed in a tragic automobile accident in 1974. So much was taken from all of us when she died. Dolores' death was very painful to all of us in California and especially to those of us for whom she had served as such a strong personal and professional role model. I knew that no one could take Dolores' place, but I had learned from the best and wanted to use that knowledge. So I decided to try to become President of the ADA if I could. It took many years for me to recover from Dolores' death, and I have never forgotten her.

After 11 years at the University of California Medical Center in San Francisco, I decided that it was time for some new challenges. It was 1967 and I was 37 years old. Little did I realize that I was about to begin another career. The passage of Medicare legislation gave those of us with entrepreneurial instincts an opportunity to try our skills. Like many others, I decided to hang out my shingle as a dietary consultant for skilled nursing facilities. I had long known that business was my major interest, and a consultant's practice seemed the perfect way to combine my education and training with what I really wanted to do.

My first account was with an organization consisting of several facilities owned by John and Marian Gellmann. They had been in the nursing home business for many years but, unlike some other old-time operators, they moved ahead and understood the need to include the new professionals in the industry. The Gellmanns had high standards and wanted to operate their facilities with a high degree of professionalism. I liked their approach and attitude—in the early years not many nursing home operators were that enlightened. And the Gellmanns liked me, and we respected each other's professional expertise. They learned a lot about dietetics and I learned a lot about the nursing home business.

Among the facilities the Gellmanns operated was a small one they had owned for many years, but were beginning to outgrow as they continued to build other facilities. One day they asked me, "How would you like to buy our Burlingame Nursing Home?" I laughed, but soon realized they were serious. I went to Ann and her husband Jim and asked them if they would like to buy it with me. In July 1968 we signed the papers.

The next few years were difficult ones as I continued to operate my consulting business while my sister Ann operated our convalescent hospital with assistance from me and some from Jim, who worked full-time as a mechanical engineer. We had strapped ourselves financially to buy the hospital and were all working sixteen hours a day. The positive side of it was that Ann, as a physical therapist, knew good hands-on patient care and rehabilitation, and I seemed to have a flair and love for the business aspects and knew food service. Jim knew building and equipment, and my sister and I both knew the health care industry. During those early years, we struggled, we worked hard and we grew with a thriving business. I loved those years because of the excitement, the uncertainty, the adventure that comes with beginning a new business. That is when I am at my best. The ordinary, day-to-day repetition, the settled, the expected were never for me.

I continued my consulting business until it had grown to the point that I could no longer handle it alone. I then had to make the choice of hiring some other dietitians to help me or giving up the practice. I chose the latter because I knew that I wanted to buy and operate other nursing homes. I guess that is when my career in dietetics ended, but not my devotion to the profession.

We went on to purchase and operate several other convalescent hospitals in the Bay Area. With each one there was always the excitement of beginning again and the thrill of seeing our accomplishments in offering good patient care and operating a stable business. I would consider myself a workaholic, although not a perfectionist, but one who takes great pride in doing well whatever I do. I have long viewed life as somewhat of an adventure and wanted to have as many experiences as I could. I have always viewed my career and my work in this way as well.

The on going upgrading of the nursing home industry under federal and state regulations brought the licensure of nursing home administrators to California. I, of course, became a licensed nursing home administrator too. Although I am proud of that credential, my greatest pride still comes from being a registered dietitian.

In the early 1970s I first became involved in ADA activities. I had served as President of the California Dietetic Association and as a delegate as well. I went on to be an Area Coordinator in the House of Delegates and served as Speaker in 1978–79. I reached my goal of being President of ADA in 1980–81. It was an experience that I would not have wanted to miss. It was a year of transition for ADA, the beginning of a new decade and turning the corner into another era for us. I like to think that we started the association on a more assertive path, if you will, although each year from ADA's early beginnings has brought progress and accomplishment and no single year has been better than another. It is the accumulation of all the years of work by all the dedicated dietitians that has brought us to a position of prominence in the health care community.

The greatest change that has occurred in the profession in my lifetime has been the emergence of so many different roles for dietitians. When I entered the profession we had two choices—be a hospital dietitian or a hospital dietitian. (That isn't quite true, but almost). Now there are so many different avenues to take. With ingenuity and perseverance, dietitians have created jobs for themselves in places that I would never have thought possible. I expect that trend to continue, and as we continue to gain public recognition, more opportunities will become available to us.

Being President of ADA was the highlight of my professional career. The professional friends and acquaintances I made during my years of being active in ADA are relationships I will always cherish. However, there are two other honors I have received that I also treasure. In 1977 I was awarded the Dolores Nyhus Memorial Award, the highest award presented by the California Dietetic Association. It is meaningful to me because one is always pleased to be recognized by one's peers and, of course, because of my association and high regard for Dolores.

The second honor came from Idaho State University, which presented me with the Distinguished Alumna Award in 1983. It was a thrill to be recognized by the university that had been such a significant part of my life since childhood.

I had always regretted that I had never taken the time to work on a Masters Degree in the earlier years of my career. Finally in 1978, I decided that I absolutely had to go back to school. I completed my work for the degree from the University of Redlands during the time I was Speaker and President-elect of ADA. It was not easy, as I was traveling a great deal, but I will never regret having done it. Believe me, though, I advise all young dietitians to get an advanced degree, the sooner the better.

In the early 1980s my sister, brother-in-law and I decided it was time for us to begin a long-range plan for "winding down." The beginning of that plan was to start selling our hospitals, keeping only one small private facility to operate in our later years. My sister and I also wanted to start another business outside the health care field, not necessarily for income, but for fun.

By 1984 we had accomplished both goals. Ann had been a doll collector since childhood, and I had become an avid collector during the last fifteen years. We had always said that when the time was right we would open a shop to sell modern collectible dolls. In October 1984 we opened our shop in our little town of Burlingame, a suburb of San Francisco.

My sister Ann and her husband Jim have played an important role in both my professional and personal life. We have been in business together for over twenty years. They have included me in their family life as well. Ann and I have always and encouraged and supported each other in every way. I was able to become actively involved in ADA because she was willing to carry the added burden of our business when I was away. It was not always easy, because Ann and Jim have an autistic daughter who has lived at home most of her life. Kylie is now 27 years old. We have all learned many lessons about life from her, and she has probably influenced our lives more than anyone else. We have shared a lot of joy and sorrow with her.

Today we continue to own and operate Belmont Convalescent Hospital and the Doll Place. I am also glad to say that the doll business is thriving and after five years has turned out to be more than just for fun. I continue to work as hard as I always have and that will probably never change. I have thought from time to time that I would like to retire, but I know I wouldn't like it. I have spent all of my adult life working hard and have achieved a moderate degree of success both professionally and in business. That has been my life. I have learned that one's success is dependent on timing and, for whatever reasons, mine has been good.

Yes, I would change a lot of things about my career and my life too, if I had it to do over again. I probably would not have been a dietitian at all and would have opted for some other career. However, dietetics gave me the background to pursue many of the things that I wanted to do, and for that I have no regrets.

Helen E. Walsh

*Helen E. Walsh, MA helped establish the
School of Public Health, University of California–Berkeley
and served as 25th President of ADA*

The distinguished career of Helen Walsh has many parallels to the development of dietetics in the United States. The ADA was only 7 years old when she entered college in 1924. It was a time when vitamins were being discovered, pellagra was being studied, and insulin had just become available for use with diabetic patients. Helen Walsh began her career in public health nutrition as a counselor in maternal and child health clinics. With the eruption of World War II, President Roosevelt proclaimed a state of national emergency and created the War Food Administration. She served as the nutrition consultant for the nine western states, Hawaii and Alaska. She was both participant and leader in many state and national dietetic association actvities, serving as ADA President in 1949 during a period of great unrest within the Association. She was also a founding member of the Society for Nutrition Education and served as its second president. Today, her top retirement priority is to briskly walk two miles a day, rain or shine. From her vantage point, the future of ADA remains bright.

HELEN E. WALSH

My career seems to parallel the development of dietetics in the United States. When I entered college The American Dietetic Association was seven years old.

Born in Des Moines, Iowa of Irish ancestry, I grew up in a loving, caring family of three brothers and a sister. After completion of St. John's Grade School, I attended and graduated from St. Joseph's Academy. Career counseling in those days was nonexistent, so selection of a college was related to factors other than a career.

For one coming from four years in a very protected environment Iowa State, the Agriculture College, in Ames, Iowa was considered an ideal choice because of its safe atmosphere with all those farm boys. I entered Iowa State in September of 1924.

If you were a woman at Iowa State you took Home Economics. The school had an outstanding and deserved reputation. When it came time to select a major, I found foods and nutrition the most interesting and challenging curriculum. McCollum and Steinbock were still discovering vitamins, Charles Glen King was working on vitamin C, and Goldberger and Sebrell were studying pellagra in white male convicts.

Dr. P. Mabel Nelson was head of the Department of Food and Nutrition. Her doctorate in physiological chemistry was from Yale. In those days chemistry was the route to nutrition. She was a most inspiring and caring person and was a great influence in my pursuing the field of nutrition as a career.

It was the dietitian at the college hospital who sparked my interest in hospital dietetics. She had just returned from a sabbatical, part of which was spent at the Cottage Hospital Metabolic Clinic in Santa Barbara, California. Insulin had become available for diabetics and Dr. Sansum, Chief of the Metabolic Clinic was among the first to allow generous amounts of carbohydrate in the diets of his patients. Her description of the activities and opportunities for participating in this new medical discovery inspired me to apply for the internship program. I was accepted and entered in September of 1928.

At the completion of the six months internship, I had decided to apply my knowledge of foods and nutrition in a different type of program than most hospitals offered at that time. Through the assistance of Dr. Sansum, I was introduced to the field of public health. His patient and close friend was the Health Officer for the Los Angeles Health Department. I spent four years there as a member of a medical team doing early diagnosis of tuberculosis in the schools. My responsibility was to interview the mother of a child who had a positive reaction to the skin test for tuberculosis. We discussed the child's health habits, physical activities and daily diet. Also, I counseled patients in the Maternal and Child Health Clinics on their daily diets. I enjoyed the preventive aspects of the programs and the interaction with patients. This experience offered, also, the opportunity to become acquainted and deeply interested in the food practices and diets of many ethnic groups.

Eager to be involved in professional activities, I joined the California Dietetic Association. Within a short time, I found myself actively participating in the work of the state and national associations. In 1935–36 I served as Secretary-Treasurer of the State Association and as Vice-President of The American Dietetic Association.

By this time the Great Depression had forced many to seek assistance from public agencies. I was asked to assist the Medical Department of the Los Angeles County Relief Administration in determining the amount to increase the food budgets of clients on special diets. It was to be a short-term assignment but it lasted four years.

It was during this assignment that I became the fifteenth president of the California Dietetic Association. It was, also, the year 1938, that The American Dietetic Association met in Los Angeles and for the first time in California for its annual meeting. I considered it one of the highlights of my early career.

Realizing that the first ten years of my career had been limited in scope because of the impact of the 1929 stock market crash and the Great Depression, I decided in 1939 to go to Columbia University in New York City to pursue a master's degree. This was the last year that Henry Sherman and Mary Schwartz Rose taught. I took advantage of their presence and attended nutrition seminars with them.

While working on my degree, I took classes in economics, professional writing and advertising research because I had decided to join many of my friends who were working in the food industry.

Just prior to my graduation, I was offered the opportunity to fill in for a professor on sabbatical at Oregon State College. My friends in the food industry encouraged me to accept the offer. They felt a year of college teaching would enhance my background for opportunities in the business field.

My dream of working in the business field never materialized. World War II erupted and a state of Unlimited National Emergency was proclaimed by President Roosevelt. He called a National Nutrition Conference for Defense on May 26, 1941 in Washington D.C. The conference presented him with 12 recommendations to serve as the basis for a national nutrition policy and as an action program that would reach every community during the current emergency.

To implement the overall recommendation of the conference, the War Food Administration was created. M. L. Wilson, Director of Federal Agriculture Extension and Dr. W. H. Sebrell, Nutrition Director for the U.S. Public Health Service were appointed as co-directors of the program. I served as the nutrition consultant for the nine western states, Hawaii and Alaska.

It was a fascinating period of time. The National Research Council had just set up a committee dealing with the biochemical and physiological side of nutrition. Its first concern was to work out recommended daily allowances for the various dietary essentials for people of different ages. The first edition of the committee's Recommended Daily Allowances was published in May of 1941, and were of calories, protein, calcium, iron, vitamin A, thiamine, riboflavin, nicotinic acid, ascorbic acid, and vitamin D.

To translate the Recommended Dietary Allowances into terms of everyday foods, the concept of the "Seven Basic Food Groups" was created. The National Advertising Council designed a poster depicting the seven food groups in a circle with the slogan

"U.S. Needs Us Strong* Eat the Basic 7 Everyday." Now it is known as the "Basic 4."

Also, at this time the enrichment program received attention. To improve the nutritive value of certain low-cost staple food products, such as flour and bread, they were enriched with the nutritive elements that had been removed from them in modern milling and refining processes. Enrichment of products was permitted only on the basis of findings of medical and nutritional experts.

During this period the workdays were long and many. The travel accommodations were rough but the opportunity to work on these programs and with such leaders as Margaret Mead, Helen A. Mitchell, Lydia J. Roberts, Agnes Fay Morgan, Mary Barber and many other leaders made it worthwhile.

As the war drew to a close, the U.S. Public Health Service established a program to study the nutritional status of certain populations groups in the United States. Lt. Col. H. R. Sandstead who had recently returned from a mission to relieve the starving and under-nourished people of the Western Netherlands was in charge. I joined the program and was commissioned as a Lt. Commander in the Coast Guard. We had four research teams. I served on the administrative staff in charge of the nutritionists and of the methodology used in collecting and processing the dietary data.

It was while I was stationed in Bethesda at the National Institute of Health that Lenna Cooper asked me to have my name placed on the 1947–48 ballot for President-elect of The American Dietetic Association. At that time, it was a single ballot for President-elect. I accepted the invitation not realizing that within six months I would be returning to California for family reasons. Subsequently, I was asked by the State Department of Health to develop a nutrition program. Also I was given an appointment to teach at the School of Public Health, University of California in Berkeley.

The following two years were perhaps the most demanding of my professional life. There was much unrest among the members of the Association. Many felt the Executive Board had too much power. The House of Delegates was concerned about its lack of authority. At the time, the President of the Association was Chairman of the House of Delegates so the House considered its primary function merely to rubber stamp action referred to it by the Executive Board.

These problems and others were addressed through a reorganization of the Association with major changes in the Constitution and By-laws. It was not an easy task and many were involved in the process, primarily Anna Boller Beach, Helen Hunscher, and Elizabeth Perry.

It was at the 1949 Annual Meeting in Denver, Colorado, where I served as President that we accomplished the adoption of the new Constitution and By-laws by the members. To me, it was the most important accomplishment of my term of office and a major turning point in the administration of Association affairs.

As I reflect on my 24 years with the California Department of Public Health and my affiliation with the University of California School of Public Health in Berkeley, I am most proud of two accomplishments.

One relates to my position in the State Department of Public Health. When I arrived there were four nutritionists assigned to the Bureau of Maternal and Child Health. Their activities were limited to the programs of the Bureau. In due time I was permitted to establish a Bureau of Nutrition which allowed for the development of a nutrition program in and of itself with a research arm and a service unit. This made it possible to participate in joint research studies with the University, the Experiment Station, State Agencies and the Federal Government. Also, it allowed for the development within the Department of the nutrition component of the programs of the Bureaus of Chronic Diseases, Hospitals, Maternal and Child Health, Cripple Children, and Food and Drug.

The second accomplishment relates to the School of Public Health. Together with Dr. Jessie Bierman, Professor of Maternal and Child Health at the University we established the public health nutrition program and recruited Dr. Ruth L. Huenemann to develop the program.

These two accomplishments provided a solid base for a strong public health nutrition program in California.

As I became more active in public health programs, I found myself accepting more and more committee assignments in public health organizations and associations. As a member of the Association of State and Territorial Nutrition Directors, I served as its president and the Chairman of the Arden House Conference to consider research in public health nutrition.

As a member of the American Public Health Association, I served as a member of the Governing Council for three terms and as Secretary, Vice-chairman and Chairman of the Food and Nutrition Section of the Association.

Recognizing the need to strengthen our efforts in nutrition education, George Briggs, Ruth Huenemann, George Stewart, Gaylord Whitlock, and myself founded the Society for Nutrition Education and I served as its second President.

At the White House Conference on Food, Nutrition and Health called by President Richard Nixon in 1969, I served as the Vice-chairman of the Panel on Community Nutrition Education.

From 1969–1972 I was a member of the Food and Nutrition Board of the National Research Council, as well as, a member of the Committee on Maternal Nutrition, the Subcommittee on Dietary Data of the Committee to Evaluate National Nutrition Survey Data, and Chairman of the Committee on Interpretation of Recommended Dietary Allowances.

In terms of honorary awards:

- Certified in 1958 by the American Board of Nutrition as a Specialist in Human Nutrition.

- Elected in 1954 to membership in Delta Omega, an honorary public health society.

- Recipient in 1971 of the Mary Rourke Memorial Awards for leaders in public health nutrition in the West.

- Special Centennial Recognition in 1971 as Distinguished Alumna–College of Home Economics, Iowa State College.

- Recipient in 1975 of the Dolores Nyhus Memorial Award, the highest honor given to an individual by the California Dietetic Association.

- First Edition in 1958 of Who's Who of American Women.

In anticipation of my retirement, I built a house in 1964 on a sand-spit in Stinson Beach, which is 25 miles from San Francisco. With the dunes and Pacific Ocean as my front yard and the Bolinas Lagoon and Mount Tamalpais to my back, I felt it was a very special place where I lived for 20 years.

Upon retirement in 1971 I became interested in the problems of the Property Owners Association and served on its Board for two years as well as on many of its committees.

The Village Association was the organization concerned with the community problems. I participated in many of its activities.

In my spare time I tried my hand at sketching and painting. Also I did considerable foreign travel. By land and by sea, I have visited 33 countries—most stimulating and educational experiences.

Five years ago I moved over the mountain to Belvedere, a quaint but modern bayside community looking over to San Francisco and accessible to the City by ferry. These days my top priority whether on land or in sea, in rain or in sunshine is a daily two mile walk at a lively pace.

As I reread this sketch and reflect on my professional career, I have no regrets. I had the opportunity to know and work with many of the leaders in my field. Nutrition research was keeping pace with advances in medicines, communications, transportation and changes in life style. The opportunities were there if one was willing to be bold and creative in approach. It has been my belief always that it is the individual who makes the job challenging and interesting or dull and routine.

Today, I would recommend the field to anyone interested in the nutritional sciences. The future looks bright. The relation of food and nutrition to health and disease is now recognized and accepted by the medical profession and the general public. This was not true in my day.

It is most encouraging to see the growth and development of The American Dietetic Association these past ten years. It has broadened its horizon and is assuming leadership as an authority in the field. This has brought the well earned professional recognition of the medical and of the allied health workers. The future is bright for The American Dietetic Association.

Donna Rising Watson

Donna R. Watson, PhD, RD
is Chairman of the Home Economics Department
at Central State University, Oklahoma.

Strong advocacy of participation in professional organizations is the byline of Dr. Donna Watson. That she puts her beliefs into action is evidenced by a long history of distinguished service to the profession of dietetics. After many active years in local and state dietetic organizations, she began national service activities in 1971 as a member of the Dietetic Internship Board. She served on the Board of Directors for 3 years, as Secretary-Treasurer, and then as 60th President of ADA in 1984. This former director of the Emory University dietetic internship program currently is Chairman of the Home Economics Department at Central State University in Oklahoma. Her doctoral studies on the British health care system sparked her interest in international health and nutrition care. This resulted in her leading nutrition excursions to China, Australia, New Zealand, and Scandinavia. Dr. Watson's early career encompassed pioneering efforts in the area of consulting dietetics. She helped develop one of the first job descriptions for consulting dietitians.

Donna R. Watson

In 1948, I thought I knew where my life was headed. Although I had recently received a BS degree in food and nutrition from Oklahoma State University and completed an internship at the Veterans' Administration Hospital in Hines, Illinois, I was prepared to walk away from my career and raise a family. I actually dropped my membership in The American Dietetic Association, thinking I would never work. In 1989, trying to picture *not* working in dietetics is nearly impossible, since I have spent the last 28 years of my life in the dietetic field.

That I chose dietetics as my profession is due, in large part, to a high school home economics teacher in Bryson, Texas, a town of 800 population, where I grew up. Although I took every course that was offered, even attending two sessions of summer school, home economics interested me most. I was one of two graduates in a class of 28 who went to college, both to become dietitians. I can't remember the name of that home economics teacher, but it can't be a coincidence that we two graduates both became dietitians.

My first two years of college were spent at Texas Women's University in Denton. There I was a member of Alpha Lambda Delta honorary society and showed an interest in creative writing. Some of my articles were published in the university's literary magazine, and I was one of a few freshmen invited to join the Writer's Club. During my second year, I was selected to be a sophomore residence hall counselor.

After my sophomore year, my parents moved to Oklahoma, and I transferred to Oklahoma State University. I received the Borden Award in Home Economics and the Oklahoma State University Award in Home Economics. I became a member of Omicron Nu and Phi Kappa Phi. Mary Leidigh was my advisor and a strong proponent of dietetics. I worked most of my way through college, in the bookstore, at theaters, and in the residence halls foodservice. However, since "all work and no play" has never been my style, I became an active member of Kappa Delta sorority and managed to find time for a well-rounded student life.

After receiving a bachelor of science degree, I went to Chicago to complete a dietetic internship at the Veterans' Administration Hospital in Hines, Illinois. Bonnie Beilfuss Miller was my internship director. She later spent many years with the American Hospital Association, writing the foodservice manual and founding the American Society for Hospital Foodservice Administrators. The Veterans' Administration dietitians and the VA system were positive professional influences which have never left me.

After my internship, I returned to Oklahoma and worked as the only dietitian in a hospital in Ponca City. Shortly thereafter, I was married and returned to Oklahoma State University to work as a dietitian in the residence halls. The following 10 years were spent being a housewife and mother of three boys, Steve, Tom, and John. I did, however, commute to Stillwater for several graduate courses at Oklahoma State University.

I returned to work out of financial necessity. When our first child started school, I started consulting part-time for a number of small hospitals and nursing homes. This was 1959. Okmulgee Memorial Hospital provided a base for my practice for eight years. With a very supportive administrator, B. Joe Gunn, I was able to develop many procedures, a set of diet instructions for use in small hospitals, and layouts for a new hospital kitchen.

In the years prior to Medicare, there were few opportunities for professional employment of dietitians in Oklahoma's small towns. However, another dietitian and I began consulting in rural hospitals and nursing homes throughout the state. In retrospect, we were true pioneers in the field of consulting dietetics. When an ADA representative came to the Oklahoma Dietetic Association meeting, she refused to talk about consulting and implied it was "not the thing to do." Any mention of comparing consulting fees brought immediate frowns and disapproval; money was not to be discussed since "dietitians provide a service." I helped develop one of the first job descriptions for the consultant dietitian. In an advisory capacity to the Oklahoma Regional Medical Program, I also pioneered in the planning of interdisciplinary continuing education programs for allied health professionals. I developed forms, policies and procedure manuals and published a set of diet instruction sheets for purchase by hospitals and physicians (to replace diet sheets distributed widely by pharmaceutical companies). One small hospital purchased one of the first Barron pumps for tube feedings, after my convincing argument. I designed kitchen layouts, assisted with the first "foodservice supervisors" workshops, and preceptored some of the first participants in a new correspondence course for foodservice supervisors.

It was during those 11 years that my deep commitment to the profession began to develop. Mary Zahasky, a former ADA president, was a leader in the Oklahoma Dietetic Association. She had a strong influence on the development of professionalism and commitment to dietetics among many Oklahoma dietitians of that time. I was one of them. I became active in the Oklahoma Dietetic Association (ODA), serving in many capacities, including those of secretary and president. As chairman of the diet therapy section, I helped publish the first Oklahoma Diet Manual.

Few persons are fortunate enough to sustain a close friendship for almost 30 years, especially when that friendship is intertwined with professional, family, and social lives. I first met Edna Langholtz at a meeting of the Executive Board of the Oklahoma Dietetic Association in 1959. An indication of our close personal and professional lives, might be that we roomed together at ODA and ADA meetings for nearly 20 years and I am godmother for one of her sons.

In 1968, I returned to OSU and received my Master's degree in human nutrition. That year I assumed the presidency of the Oklahoma Dietetic Association, as well as continuing my consulting business to support my three sons, the eldest in college. I also worked as a teaching assistant. Fortunately, I received the General Foods Fund Fellowship for graduate study and the prestigious Mary Swartz Rose Award for graduate study from The American Dietetic Association.

Armed with my degree, I moved to Atlanta to accept a rare opening as director of a dietetic internship program. My duties at Emory University included teaching in the School of Nursing besides the internship. After two years at Emory, I accepted the position of assistant professor for the Nutrition in Nursing Education Project at the Medical College of Georgia where I was part of a team developing nutrition courses for nurses. During this time I was also a private consultant to a preventive cardiology clinic, the first one in Atlanta.

I returned to Emory in 1973 and, during the next 10 years, had an unforgettable period of professional growth. I left with the title of Director, Division of Nutrition, Department of Community Health, School of Medicine. Highlights of my Emory career include developing a nationally recognized internship and graduate degree program in clinical dietetics. This came about through the incorporation of numerous innovative instructional programs including computer-managed instruction and clinical practicums in the Master's program. I also helped to establish the nutrition out-patient service at Emory Clinic as well as open a nutrition research laboratory for dietetic faculty and students.

During the Emory years, I became a consultant to the USDA Five-State Nutrition Education project with the Georgia Department of Education, managed the Georgia Nutrition Education Training program, and directed a federally-funded interdisciplinary nutrition education project in the School of Medicine.

I served as both a site visitor and a member of the review committee for the Veterans Administration Health Manpower Training grants. I published articles and conference proceedings on a wide variety of nutrition-related topics. With three other educators, I participated in the development of an instrument designed to provide a comprehensive assessment of the nutritional needs of school-age children, measuring knowledge, attitudes, and behavior components in major content areas related to nutrition. I wrote and had funded eight grants in a variety of nutrition and health care areas. I became a consultant to dietetic education programs throughout the country.

In 1983 I resigned at Emory, to return to Oklahoma because of illnesses in my family. There I assumed the position of associate professor and director of the dietetic internship in the Department of Food, Nutrition, and Institution Administration at Oklahoma State University.

A strong advocate of professional participation in association affairs, I was a charter member of the American Society for Hospital Food Service Administrators and was very active in the American Society for Allied Health Professions for a number of years. I am a member of the American Home Economics Association and the Society for Nutrition Education and The Fashion Group International Inc. For many years, I participated in district, state, and national dietetic association activities, serving as president of the Atlanta District Dietetic Association and working in several capacities with the Georgia Dietetic Association, secretary/treasurer and president of the Oklahoma Dietetic Association as well as serving on numerous committees and boards.

My volunteer contributions to The American Dietetic Association began in 1971. My first national duty was an appointment on the Dietetic Internship Board (DIB). I was in this group four years while its name changed several times to what is now the Commission on Accreditation. Poly Fitz, who became a friend and valued professional colleague, was chairman of the DIB. Other responsibilities included six years as a site evaluator for ADA program accreditation, two years on the Administrative Committee of the Council on Education Preparation, and two years as a member of the liaison committee to the American Hospital Association. I was one of the principal planners and leaders of the first Long-Range Planning Conference of The American Dietetic Association, which was held in 1981. In 1978, I was elected for a three-year term to the Board of Directors as one of the first three members-at-large, and 1981 to 1983, I served as secretary-treasurer of the Association. I was ADA President 1984–1985.

During this time I completed the course work for a doctorate at Emory University. As part of my doctoral study, I spent one summer in London reviewing the British health care system. That sparked an interest in health and nutrition care in other parts of the world, resulting in my becoming a co-leader of four nutrition and health care trips to the People's Republic of China and leader of a People-to-People Citizen Ambassador delegation of dietitians to Australia and New Zealand in the summer of 1984 and a delegation to Scandinavia and Finland in 1985. Other overseas professional trips were speaking engagements at the American European Dietetic Association (AEDA) in Lucerne and London and presenting seminars to two universities in Ariquipa, Peru.

Two recent awards I value very much are the Distinguished Dietitian of the Year in Oklahoma and a Certificate of Appreciation for Outstanding Service rendered by the Network of Blacks in Dietetics and Nutrition. Currently I serve as Chairperson in the Department of Home Economics, Central State University, in Edmond, Oklahoma. We have a Plan V and an approved preprofessional practice program (AP4) in dietetics.

It was a privilege to serve as the 60th President of The American Dietetic Association. Through this unique opportunity to serve our profession, I came to know many, many dietitians. To find such strength, commitment, and abilities among all those members of our profession is unforgettable.

Some of the highlights of 1984–85, my year as president, were implementation of the Division of Education and Research with a Ph.D. at the head; a marketing plan for ADA was developed and approved which included strong support for the ADA Ambassadors, establishment of the Recognized Dietetic Technician of the Year award. The Commission on Dietetic Registration started developing a credentialing program for dietetic technicians; state licensing was encouraged.

Perhaps the most important development during the year was the improved financial status of the Association due mostly to better accounting practices, monitoring of income and expenses, and market value increases. The reserve fund was started and the ADA Board of Directors approved an opening an office in Washington, D.C. at 1667 K Street.

ADA convened for its 68th Annual Meeting in New Orleans a city rich in history, culture, and entertainment. ADA's host at Annual Meeting in New Orleans this year, October 7 to 11, 1985, was the Louisiana Dietetic Association. The Alabama, Arkansas, and Mississippi Dietetic Associations assisted. The theme was "Directions for Action." More than 10,000 dietitians descended upon the jazz capital of the world for a week's worth of programming focused on issues of concern to dietetic professionals, including marketing, diabetes, health promotion, computers, research, education, business insights, and women's health issues.

ADA broadcast highlights of the meeting to approximately 30 sites nationwide on Saturday, October 12. Included were selected educational presentations, the exhibition, poster sessions, and other special events. Approximately 1,200 dietitians viewed the first ADA teleconference of an annual meeting.

The Board of Directors, in response to a recommendation in the *1989 Study Commission Report*, approved the establishment of an Affirmative Action Committee charged with the responsibility for developing a plan for increasing minority representation in the ADA profession.

The minority award to a school that has implemented an innovative or significant minority recruitment and retention program was increased. One thousand dollars per year will be contributed by ADA to the ADA Foundation to establish a permanent minority award.

The American Dietetic Association Foundation ended its 1984–85 fiscal year with preliminary fund balances totaling more than $1.45 million. This represents a greater than 30 percent growth over the previous year's audited fund balance.

The Foundation's scholarship funds increased; the scholarships continued to provide support to deserving dietetic students at graduate, undergraduate, and intern levels. More than $112,000 in scholarships were awarded to 133 students for the 1985–86 school year.

On Friday, December 14, 1984, representatives of Chicago, Dallas, and St. Louis made proposals to the Board of Directors for locating the National Center in these cities. After considering the proposals and a review of all major population centers by the consulting firm of Ernst & Whinney, the Board voted to locate the Center in metropolitan Chicago. Also, the ad hoc Committee on Programmatic Development for the National Center for Nutrition and Dietetics was appointed by the ADA Board of Directors in October 1984 to refine a proposed program document. The Center building committee chaired by Loyal Horton, implemented its charge to review space needs and organization as well as Center needs and to screen possible buildings.

The first joint meeting of the ADA and ADA Foundation Boards of Directors took place on May 2, 1985, when I was ADA president and Edna Langholtz was ADAF president. Joint meetings of the boards have continued.

This 1984–85 year brought both the rigorous demands and the gratification that come with the office of president. As I reviewed the year, I recognized that many outstanding committee members, leaders, headquarters staff, advisers, and friends contributed immeasurably to the successful solution of problems and the achievement of ambitious goals. Also, it is quite obvious that many strongly committed people, sometimes unrecognized, are the Association. I realized more than ever before that we are talented people with a unique commitment to the wellbeing and future of the Association, to the profession of dietetics, and to the health of the U.S. population.

Times change rapidly. We are well into the technological age. Our Association is proving to be flexible, resilient, and powerful. We are capable of responding, of conforming, to changing, or new, situations; of being able to recover, to adjust, to withstand stress. We are gaining prestige and influence, and we are becoming the leaders in the field of nutrition and dietetics. I believe in what we do and that we can only go on to achieve greater recognition for our profession and for our Association.

Nancy S. Wellman

*Nancy S. Wellman, PhD, RD is Chair
and Associate Professor, Department of Dietetics and
Nutrition, Florida International University, Miami, FL*

From questioning "whether I *wanted to* belong" to an organization she was told was a must, to eventually serving proudly as its 65th President, Nancy S. Wellman offers us a glimpse into the influence of her personal life on her professional career. Along her career path she was acknowledged as Florida's Recognized Young Dietitian of the Year and later recognized as Outstanding Dietitian of Florida. She describes her own "minority" struggle in terms of working in a medical school where non-physicians were generally considered second class. She candidly describes her beginning negative acquaintance with the Association which quickly changed to admiration and respect. In describing her philosophy, she says she tries to focus on doing the right things rather than doing things perfectly right; advising us to aim for excellence, not perfection. She notes that she has been a risk taker at key points in her life. She does not see her activities and energies ending with her Presidency, as there are "miles and miles to go for dietitians and for the Association." No doubt Nancy Wellman will continue to be a leader, even when her formal duties are through.

Nancy S. Wellman

Career Decisions . . . In Retrospect

It's surprising how many key decisions in life happen almost by chance. My decision to major in Home Economics Education at the State University College at Buffalo in 1960 was approved by my father who said at the time "You can always use that kind of information." Looking back, the actual depth of that decision had more to do with the challenge of using leftovers creatively, because I doubt I had a career in mind then. I didn't want to risk being bored for years at home, and knew I'd need an "outlet" later in life.

After I earned a bachelor's degree, I taught part time for one year while taking science prerequisites for a new interest, nutritional biochemistry. That led to my decision to pursue a master's degree at Columbia University—another significant step. This was followed by one year's work in a cancer research laboratory where I made an important discovery—that I enjoyed working with people much more than with mice. About that time I married Keith and moved to Miami where I looked for positions in public health or clinical nutrition. It was my first realization that perhaps I had a marketable degree. Having had few role models regarding a career in nutrition, an awareness about career paths, raises, promotions, etc., was just beginning.

I was surprised to find that many jobs required membership in The American Dietetic Association (which was unfamiliar to me as there were no dietitian professors in Home Ec Education). Upon hearing of ADA, I was intrigued that a group existed in which members were likely to be interested in nutrition as I was. Yet I do recall another reaction—that of being told I *had to* belong to an organization making me question whether I *wanted to* belong—a typical '60's reaction.

Qualifications for membership then (1969) required one year of supervised work experience. I had accepted a position as a staff nutritionist at the University of Miami Child Development Center. Levina Phillips, Director of Nutrition at Dade County Health Department, agreed to be my year long "supervisor—on paper" since my job was a quasi-public health position. At Levina's encouragement, I went ahead with the lengthy process of filling out application forms for ADA and assembling supporting information.

After acquiring the year's experience, I was surprised to learn my full membership was approved. Thus, I came into the Association through a non-traditional route. I was grandfathered in as a registered dietitian since I did not have to take the national examination, which was being offered for the first time in 1969. Levina's mentoring was one in a series of important influences in my career that appeared on the scene at exactly the right moment.

Mentors

I was ten when my mother died of cancer of the breast after a lingering three year illness at home. At a crucial time in my development I did not have a strong or consistent female role model, though a series of aunts and a grandmother filled in as best they could. I realized early I had to grow up fast to "fill my mother's shoes" in this all-male household.

I actually found the role of surrogate "lady of the house" with my dad and two brothers natural and comfortable, but my mother's absence created a lack of cohesiveness and nurturing. My independence was fostered prematurely in this fairly undemonstrative environment. I learned not to expect much praise or approval. This may explain my later ability to cope in unsupportive environments like the medical school, and why I set high standards for myself and others. Speaking of standards, mine were directly influenced by my father, who encouraged me to do things well. I recall when sewing clothes, he once noted that they "didn't have to look homemade," thus establishing high expectations even in everyday household tasks.

My father sent me to a Catholic girls high school because he thought I needed the nurturing of nuns, as mother substitutes. In fact the nuns were sweet, but aloof and impersonal and another importance influence in my developing sense of independence and ability to cope with being left alone.

I was fortunate to have had several mentors along the way whom I respect a great deal. The first was Muriel Wagner at the Merrill-Palmer Institute in Detroit. The second was Levina Phillips in Miami, and the third Carol Shear, a pediatrician in Miami. I enjoy the comraderie of working with bright women like these because I can learn from them and gain from their creativity and encouragement.

Another mentor was my husband, Keith, whose maturity being eight years my senior and whose perseverance and fortitude build a solid foundation for us both.

Serendipitous life events and mentors seem to be intertwined. I hadn't gone away to college for economic reasons, but had always wanted to try a taste of residential college life. My opportunity came along during my junior year when I learned that one or two seniors were chosen by the faculty to attend the Merrill-Palmer Institute in Detroit for one semester. I was selected to spend fall semester of my senior year at the Institute in what would be the first of many significant career markers.

Muriel Wagner's "Developmental Nutrition" course was thought provoking and exciting. Her interest in nutritional biochemistry encouraged my interest. I remember conversations with her and a photographer named Donna after class in her office. I enjoyed those talks immensely, perhaps because I was encouraged to think about my future and to realize that I might shape it.

When I looked into the requirements for becoming a nutritional biochemist, I found I needed many more basic science courses. So after my Home Ec Education degree, I took a part-time job teaching junior high school and enrolled at the University of Buffalo, taking mostly chemistry prerequisites. That's where I met Keith, who was my Organic Chemistry teacher. But more about that later.

Admitting I knew little about biochemistry, I investigated graduate programs and found the one year master's program in nutrition at Columbia University included several biochemistry courses. My father encouraged my pursuits saying "you can never get too much education."

I realized I would have to pay for my graduate education myself and had inquired about expanding it over two years so I could work. I was fortunate to be offered a U.S. Public Health traineeship and I enrolled at Columbia. Again, a crucial career choice at another important junction. Had the traineeship not come along, I might have become an airline stewardess. The allure of travel and glamour was really tempting.

I dated Keith over the summer following two semesters in his class, and we kept in touch while I was in graduate school in New York city. I returned to Buffalo to check out that relationship, after a summer of doing field work in Haiti for my M.S. degree. It was then I worked in cancer research at Roswell Park Memorial Hospital in Buffalo, but didn't find that professionally or personally satisfying. As mentioned earlier, I liked people more than laboratory animals, and didn't like the thought of spending a large portion of my waking hours in the lab.

Keith and I married in December, 1967. The next fall Keith took a job at the University of Miami, and we were off on a new adventure. When I was job hunting there, I was surprised to find I was one of only two people in Miami with a master's degree in nutrition, giving me my pick of several jobs. It was during job interviewing that I met Levina Phillips and we kept in close touch during my years at the Child Development Center as our offices were nearby. Levina would call frequently to tell me ten things to do. And though I might tackle only two or three, she always gave a little extra push in the right direction. She deliberately picked out those she believed had potential, to focus her attention on. She was very directive, but tempered her "you shoulds" with many strokes.

I took the job at the Child Development Center because it was a team approach to helping families and children with mental retardation and developmental disabilities. I was intrigued by children with inborn errors in metabolism, and this seemed to be an important role for nutrition. But I was an inexperienced dietitian/nutritionist, knowing only that PKU children needed a diet low in phenylalanine. As the Center was situated in the Department of Pediatrics and the School of Medicine, I had many opportunities to learn.

I worked directly for Dr. Carol Shear, a conscientious pediatrician, who helped me develop my writing skills. She was bright, quite a perfectionist and generous with her time. As she and I became more confident of my developing skills, a partnership evolved, and we worked as an effective team helping many children and families. I liked to train the mothers of PKU patients to become independent of me. There was no reason to keep the calculations a mystery and by teaching parents how to do them, I could be an enabler.

I stayed at the Child Developmental Center for 13 years. The teaching environment fostered new skills and new perspectives. Because of the multidisciplinary nature of the Child Developmental Center, I learned not only about clinical nutrition, but also about interpersonal dynamics and the special skills of people from many health disciplines.

"Minority" struggles for me included, as mentioned, my working for a long time in a medical school where all non-physicians were generally considered second class. The preponderance of males in administration throughout my work experience has frequently been a challenge, as had finding willing mentors in this group of males. Fortunately, Keith has been more than a good mentor in many, many ways. Particularly in my current academic position, he understands the job demands and is supportive of the unique aspects of academia. These are related to the academic life not being a 9–5 job (odd hours, weekend work, etc.); pressures to publish; grantsmanship; university politics ("pettiness at a sophisticated level"); expectations to stretch academically; and low pay (of course traded for independence). I frequently try out strategies with him prior to discussing them with supervisors, and his advice has been invaluable.

Milestones

It became obvious that, not being an M.D., not being a male, and not being a Ph.D. were definite handicaps working in a medical school. Although several people had encouraged me to get my doctorate, it was easier to put off that decision. I wish someone had nudged me just a little harder, just a little earlier. I finally went back to school ten years after my master's degree and completed my Ph.D. at age 39. The decision was also pragmatic in that I recognized having a Ph.D. itself was more important than the actual major at that stage in my life.

I continued to work full-time while pursuing graduate course work in Early Childhood Education. I recall pushing pretty hard for about three years taking two or more courses each semester in the evening to satisfy a host of requirements. I choose early childhood education because the faculty seemed to be very mutually supportive. This sharply contrasted with some of the less friendly interactions in the medical school setting.

Another significant life event in looking back was the year that Keith, Scott (my stepson) and I spent in Brazil. Keith took a visiting professorship at a university in San Paulo. Although I did not succeed in finding paid work in nutrition, I did teach English part-time. I played the non-working wife role to the hilt, enrolling in every leisure time activity or course I could find. I had such a good time, at the end of that year I remember being quite amazed to find that I was qualified to be paid for some professional competence. My one year of unemployment shook my confidence regarding my marketable skills. I missed the challenges of working, the stimulating interactions with people, the feeling that what I did made a difference, and the tangible paycheck acknowledgement of my value.

Being away for a year provided some perspective on both personal and professional goals. Coming back to Miami helped me focus on the decision about doctoral programs. I also decided I needed some hobbies. I had tried yoga, ballet, crocheting, needlepoint, etc. while in Sao Paulo and had enjoyed the new challenges. I decided to take up tennis, mainly because Keith and Scott seemed to be having fun on weekends playing tennis. I found my athletic ability had been pretty well untested, and that although I wasn't a klutz, I had little awareness of coordinating the movements of my own body parts.

I enjoyed the social and competitive aspects of tennis. I saw tennis as a skill to be mastered, and following Keith's example of perseverance, decided to put in the time to get better at it. As my snow skiing had improved gradually over the years, I was optimistic that my tennis, too, would improve. All of these personal pursuits bought a balance to a demanding work schedule and built confidence that carried over to my professional life. As RDs, we tend to like structure and to fit ourselves into preconceived molds, worrying unduly about the *"shoulds."* In our zeal of control our environment and to be perfectionists, some of us need to work at not being too one-sided.

As my biological time clock was also ticking, I thought about adding biologic motherhood to stepmotherhood. Scott had come to live with us at age 12, five years earlier, and we were all still adjusting to one another. Fate, via genetics, ultimately made the biologic decision for us, although I had been struggling with the decision before it became a foregone conclusion. I had grown up quickly at age ten when my mother died prematurely, and perhaps I had done enough mothering of my own brothers.

Professional Accomplishments

In the meantime, I had been busy with the Miami Dietetic Association first, and then almost immediately with the Florida Dietetic Association, due to Levina Phillips' encouragement. At ADA's first legislative workshop I met ADA president Isabelle Hallahan. Because we had gone to the same undergraduate university in Buffalo, she recalled me later when making appointments to various ADA committees. She appointed me to the Association membership committee. I was quite interested in learning from my roommate, Barbara Benoit, during the first committee meeting, how one could continue this type of committee work with ADA. Barbara seemed on target when she said it would happen almost automatically as long as you were conscientious and did a good job.

My experience as a Delegate from Florida for two three-year terms, and my subsequent stint as an Area Coordinator prepared me well to be Speaker of the ADA House of Delegates. Through those elected offices I learned about the intricacies and operations of a large organization. I'm particularly indebted to Judy Dodd when she was Speaker-elect. She and I had mutually supportive yet quite different styles.

It is special to get recognition from one's peers, and I have been fortunate in that way. I was the Florida Recognized Young Dietitian of the Year and Outstanding Dietitian. At the midpoint of my career with about 20 years behind me and probably another 20 ahead, I am most proud to be elected to represent the 59,000 members in The American Dietetic Association. It's a weighty responsibility, but I have seen our Association and profession progress so far that I am equally optimistic about the future.

Looking back, a significant event was the keynote address I gave in Tampa for the Florida Dietetic Association in 1980, entitled "Selling the Dietitian." To prepare I read widely in areas quite new to me. Several psychologists at the Mailman Child Development Center directed me to literature regarding professional appearances, body language, professional style, and so on. Preparing for that talk helped me realize dietitians were often not playing the game in the business world that everyone else was playing. I discovered if dietitians could become more attuned to their work environment, they could easily be much more successful.

Subsequent to that talk (Selling the Dietitian), I expanded and polished the speech, changed its name to "First Impressions and Winning Images" and presented the new version at many state and district dietetic associations. The audience response was so positive I knew I was on target with a theme that had great potential to rally dietitians. I recall two quotes from the speech, in particular, struck a chord with the audience:

> "Dietitians are up to the challenge of recognizing that impression management is one of the games being played. We can catch up and play the game very well."

> "You can make changes to bring yourself closer to the professional you want others to see in you. As we know from our nutritional counseling, first we must see that change is a possibility, then we need to decide to make the change, and lastly recognize that we can learn from others who have gone before us."

That keynote address at the Florida Dietetic Association was the reason I was offered the position of department chairperson at Florida International University (FIU). Although still working on my doctoral degree, I was invited to apply for the position. It was one of the few job opportunities in Miami that interested me. It would have been easier to stay at the Mailman Center while completing my dissertation, but this was another one of those career junctions when timing was critical.

During the ADA presidency of Anita Owen, I chaired the Marketing and Public Relations Committee. It was an exciting time, because the Association had formed a new Marketing and Public Relations Division. Ann Cole, the first director of that division, and I, along with the committee, had a very productive and energizing year. It was a year of innovations as there was no blueprint to follow. Most notable among the accomplishments was the production of the *Competitive Edge*, popularly called the "Marketing Manual" for dietitians. The Association whole-heartedly embraced the need for helping each dietitian to become her own personal marketing agent. Knowing how much good is going on in and because of the Association, I find it hard to understand how dietitians can keep up with new knowledge without maintaining their membership in ADA.

Professional Perks

Aspects of the profession that have served as motivators include the independence and flexible time of an academic position. My former job at the Mailman Center also allowed considerable indulgence in areas of focused interest.

I believe there are also many advantages to a career in dietetics in general. I believe the nutrition profession is exciting and holds considerable potential, particularly for those who are creative and adventuresome. A favorite quote is Helen Keller's "life is either a daring adventure or nothing at all." I would personally add to my list of adventures the partnerships I've enjoyed with other health professionals. In teaming up with these professionals to help retarded youngsters, I could demonstrate the unique worth of our discipline to other staff members in helping clients and reassuring parents. It's interesting that in partnerships like these staffings, RDs can shine without fear of being swallowed up. It's just the opposite. One need not have autonomy or full control to demonstrate competence. If you do your homework and set high standards for the quality of your work, you can confidently take your place on the team.

I've always held a strong belief in the importance of food choices and hence nutrition in terms of one's health and well-being. I also believe that traditionally many women have expressed their creativity in the kitchen. Food preparation and even food purchasing, allow one considerable freedom of expression. Did I really just say that? Perhaps Judith Chicago's "The Dinner Party" is the ultimate example of creativity at the table! The central role of food in the profession as a vehicle for nurturing is tied to the female and probably has much to do with the profession's continued dominance by females.

I enjoy working with other committed dietitians, another professional perk. All along I have found dietitians involved in the district, state or national association have been bright, enthusiastic and stimulating. As the status of dietitians has risen in the eyes of the public, so has our pride in our profession. The indispensability of the registered dietitian should no longer be a well kept secret, known only to those who have passed the registration exam!

I chose my early career focus in pediatrics because of the natural link between nutrition and infancy and childhood. People speak of the "glamour" area of nutrition in metabolic disorders. For me glamour was not the point. I liked working with inherited conditions because diet could make a dramatic difference in those children's lives.

Another career focus I have found to be beneficial began in 1981 when I was selected to be among the first group of ADA Ambassadors, or media spokespersons. In seeking Ambassadors and State Media Reps, the ADA and the states are looking for dietitians with a broad perspective of the field who project an air of authority, come across convincingly, show genuine concern and who do their homework as part of a commitment to getting out an accurate message. I had always been annoyed that so much misinformation was being conveyed to the public via radio and television talk shows. Yet I felt I had little right to be openly critical unless I was willing to do something about it. ADA Ambassadorship provided this unique opportunity. The media training gave me the skills and the confidence to work in print and broadcast. Success in media relations comes if you put in the *preparation time* and have a genuine interest in conveying solid, accurate information to your audience.

Being an Ambassador really increased my self-confidence. The credibility bestowed on the speaker by the public and fellow RD's through mere media appearance is quite interesting because the media's shallowness is readily apparent to those involved.

The adage seems true—in the media business, the amateur thinks of the topic and the pro thinks of the audience. Whatever the reporter skims off the top to print or to broadcast, if you hit the target and speak to the needs of your audience, your message (albeit superficial) will be received and understood.

Professional Style/Philosophy

The list of suggested questions to answer in preparing this material included: "What led you to conceive or develop your professional style?" Whatever that style is, I doubt I created it intentionally. But I'm certain my sense of humor has played a role. I'm convinced we take ourselves much too seriously, and stick by our own rules too rigorously. We dietitians should be more flexible in interpreting our own rules and be willing to admit that as times change, rules must also be changed. Our rigidity makes us take ourselves much too seriously. Also, our fear of peer criticism (when we should be each other's best supporters) needs to be addressed to improve our professional status. Seeing humor in situations would help us be better team players, more willing to bend.

One of my goals has always been to aim for excellence, not perfection. As noted, my father had always encouraged my brothers and me to do things well and not to settle for just O.K. I find at times I must fight my perfectionist tendencies. I'm quite conscientious and very thorough. One way to temper this tendency is to concentrate on the BIGGER PICTURE and not allow yourself to become mired down in petty detail. Also, more recently, I have tried to focus on doing the right things, instead of just doing things so perfectly right. The book *Perfection Salad*, by Laura Shapiro, is a case in point in it's espousal of the theory that there's a scientific way to approach every problem, even the most mundane task of housekeeping. In our compulsion to be in control, we often channel too much energy into doing everything "the right way."

I've worked hard at developing my sense of security. Discovering that all people are insecure at different times and with different degrees of intensity at those different times, has been somewhat comforting. I found that *acting* secure makes one *feel* more secure. Also because of my high standards and conscientiousness (maybe that's just another word for compulsivity) I read a bit about stress management. I like the two-rule approach to handling stress described in a June '83 *TIME* magazine cover story on stress. The first rule is "don't sweat the small stuff," and the second rule is "it's *all* small stuff." Maybe I'm getting too philosophical, but these seemingly simple tenets have helped me keep my perspective, and my sense of humor and sense of values intact!

I enjoy books by female authors. Regrettably I don't have much time for non-nutrition reading. Favorite authors include Margaret Atwood, Margaret Drabble, Ann Taylor, Beryl Markum, Gail Godwin, Doris Lessing. I enjoy the depth of the characters that women writers seem better able to develop, and that strength of characters can often be a source of inspiration or a type of role model. I also enjoy biographies about successful people. One can learn much from successful women, in particular because one can easily identify with them. Similarly, one can learn much from reading about successful men, and at the same time gain insights into the male mindset. That's pretty important because it's still a man's world.

In looking back, while there was no Grand Plan or Blueprint, it wasn't a haphazard series of coincidences either. I *did recognize* opportunities when they presented themselves and was not afraid to take risks at key choice points. Being open-minded and focusing on the BIG PICTURE also contributed to prudent decisions at significant career junctions. And I believe the undercurrent or driving force throughout the decision-making process was the search for ways to MAKE A DIFFERENCE.

Career Perspectives

As with many young woman in the 1960's, I never truly believed I had a real career until at least 10 years into dietetics. When I began in the field, I was not really aware that women worked outside the home. I certainly didn't think of myself as a career person, or even having a "career" until I heard other dietitians talk of *my* career as a beacon for theirs. By then I was enjoying my job and was ready to acknowledge my serious commitment to my chosen field.

Risk-taking seems to be difficult for many women. We internalize failure as evidence of our own personal shortcomings. Mistakes aren't bad as long as we don't repeat them. But men are better able to project their failures onto others. In my early days I never thought about my sometimes unorthodox approaches as risk-taking. But I've always been fairly comfortable doing what I believed was right, even when it was not the popular course. I try to remember that it's easier to get forgiveness for taking a chance and making the wrong choice, than to ask permission.

If I knew then what I know now, I would encourage others to get advanced degrees, especially doctorates, sooner. Doctoral degrees today for dietitians are equivalent to master's degrees twenty years ago. A Ph.D. is essential for an RD who aspires to be acknowledged for research contributions in an academic setting. More applied nutrition research is needed and dietitians are uniquely qualified to do it. Understanding food preferences and eating habits are key to motivating people to eat healthier. Population studies will help define the role of diet in chronic diseases. Much investigation remains to be done regarding interrelationships among food, diet and health.

I would also encourage dietitians to see applied research possibilities in everyday job activities. Today's need for cost benefit data—because no firm third party reimbursement system for nutrition services is in place—is a consequence of a naive, fairly female, do-gooder philosophy. We should always have been collecting data and documenting our cost effectiveness and the importance of nutrition services in the health outcomes of Americans—our patients and clients.

Dietitians have many opportunities to conduct and publish applied research projects. I wish I had learned earlier to focus on tangible outcomes, specifically publications, because they're so important to one's academic career and to the profession.

308

Changes in the Dietetic Profession

Changes in the profession that I have observed over time are quite interesting. I can personalize . . . calling myself a nutritionist was more comfortable for at least the first fifteen years of my career. However, I have come to the conclusion that it's not so important whether I am called a dietitian or a nutritionist, just that I'm *called*—by the media, by colleagues, by students, by patients, etc. To quote from an item I wrote in 1986:

> "A large number of us are preoccupied with what to call ourselves. The protected title 'Registered Dietitian' or 'RD' is indeed a powerful baseline professional credential and a distinct marketing advantage. If you've earned it, flaunt it! *Always* include the initials after your professional name so you can be easily identified as a bona fide nutrition expert.
>
> From a marketing standpoint, the more generic term "nutritionist" may seem to carry certain advantages in some situations. We all know that all RDs are nutritionists, but not all nutritionists are RDs. This fact doesn't, however, negate the use of the term nutritionist. Rightfully, RDs more than anyone else should capitalize on the interest in nutrition and the positive image "nutritionist" conveys in the minds of many (the media, health care professionals, wellness entrepreneurs, etc.) but *always* coupled with the RD initials. The fact that not all nutritionists are RDs should be kept uppermost in our own minds. RD is the only designation that is uniquely ours and sets us apart from other real or self-proclaimed nutritionists."*

Increased visibility of dietitians was greatly affected by Project IMAGE, the media spokesperson program which Susan Finn had the foresight to initiate. Project IMAGE gave all dietitians, not just Ambassadors, permission to be more visible and outspoken. The ready success of the Ambassadors encouraged many dietitians to appear in public and on radio and television, to write more articles for the print media and professional journals, and above all, to *have opinions*.

The media had a great deal to do with changing the negative image of dietitians in the eyes of physicians. Dietitians have always had to vie for approval in the "hospital battlefield." This struggle simply does not exist with the media who are receptive to dietitians and unequivocally accept our expert opinions in matters of nutrition. In this way, the media have significantly advanced our cause in the patient/client area.

Other changes I've observed in the profession are the enthusiasm and commitment to the profession by young members. There is an increased variety of settings in which dietitians are being recognized for their valuable contributions. It's heartening to see more and more dietitians pursuing and completing advanced degrees. Continuing education requirements of registration have had a positive impact on the profession in that more dietitians keep up to date. Simultaneously, the public, now more nutritional savvy, expects dietitians to know more than ever before. Public interest in nutrition continues to be high, providing greater visibility for dietitians. The entrepreneurial dietitian, in

*Excerpted from *The Competitive Edge: Marketing Strategies for the Registered Dietitian*, by Kathy King Helm and James C. Rose, The American Dietetic Association, 1986.

particular, has almost unlimited potential for creative, satisfying, and personally rewarding professional ventures.

The Next Twenty Years

Reflecting on the past has given me an interesting perspective on the future. For me, being the ADA President is another beginning. I can't just retire to the tennis courts and say, "I've done it."

There are "miles and miles to go" for dietitians and the Association, and I'm intrigued about what the future holds. As I see it, the mile markers will include spearheading the national initiative toward food labeling, strengthening our industry relations programs, capitalizing on the liaison potential for our Association, developing creative recruitment strategies for youngsters in the elementary school and junior high, tracking nutrition issues and consumer interest so that we can be more proactive rather than reactive with the media, and the unlimited and exciting opportunities that lie ahead as our Association establishes the National Center for Nutrition and Dietetics.

Our future is dependent on those that we recruit into the profession today. Most people agree that female-dominated professions are experiencing unique challenges in the competitive marketing environment that will continue to dominate the '90's. After we increase salaries, we must continue to recruit the best and the brightest by turning them on to the vast potential that exists in the nutrition field. Today's dietitians must keep up-to-date by striving for excellence, reading the current scientific literature, and by being assertive and taking a stand on issues. Armed with confidence we must *act*, knowing that dietitians *can make a difference*—on a health care team, as motivators to improving food choices, or managing personnel, and above all as supporters of other risk-taking dietitians.

My personal goals at my career midpoint are to continue to learn and be involved, build coalitions with industry around important issues for dietitians, remain active in the media, serve as a mentor to more young dietitians, learn how to fly . . . and take a little more time to savor life.

Esther A. Winterfeldt

Esther Winterfeldt, PhD, RD is Interim Department Head
Department of Nutrition and Foods
Auburn (AL) University

A Great Plains farm upbringing and 10 years of 4-H involvement formed the early backdrop of a career in dietetics for Dr. Esther Winterfeldt. Her professional positions have covered the spectrum in the field—clinical, foodservice management, administration and academics—including department chair and associate dean at Oklahoma State University. Her keen interest in public policy was nurtured by two positions in Washington, D.C., with USDA; one in research and the other as administrator of the Human Nutrition Information Service. Dr. Winterfeldt has served ADA as Secretary, Speaker of the House of Delegates, and President in 1979 when membership was growing at a pace of 4000 members per year. She also served as President of the ADA Foundation. Among her reminiscences are the days when pernicious anemia was treated with prodigious amounts of liver, the starting salary of a dietitian was $360/month, and all food for hospitalized diabetes was carefully weighed on gram scales!

Esther A. Winterfeldt

I had what is probably the ideal background for a career in dietetics. Growing up in southeast Oklahoma, I learned early about the work ethic and a healthy lifestyle. There was no other choice and besides, those were the values learned through the influence of hardworking parents of modest means. High school home economics and science classes (all the school had to offer) as well as ten years of 4-H involvement formed the backdrop for my later career. So it was a logical step choosing a major in college that would somehow combine early interests in science and foods, in other words, dietetics. A high school home economics teacher whetted interest in nutrition by assigning a three day dietary intake record to be modified for ideal weight and activity and meet RDA's. Looking back, it was an assignment now routine in college classes accomplished with the use of computer programs. I didn't realize until much later, it was early exposure, too, to competency based, applied learning. I graduated as valedictorian of my relatively small high school class of 30, decreased in number because several classmates had already joined the World War II Armed Services.

A dietitian in a residence hall at Oklahoma State University gave me my first job at college and I soon knew I had found a profession. It was the first I knew about dietetics. Hattie Bentley was a real role model, as hardworking and dedicated a dietitian as any I have ever known. She encouraged a farm girl from a small high school to learn everything about food service and over the next three years I did just that. I gained further experience as a counselor in the dorms. The university was a training center for WAVES (Navy women) and Navy officers and my dining hall was occupied by the WAVES. It was also the era of sugar coupons and food shortages of all kinds as well as rationed shoes and tires. Halfway through school, the war ended and the Navy departed.

I had marvelous old school teachers who were experts in quality food preparation and application of scientific principles to foods. There is no way I will ever forget the fat-gluten principles in making pie crust and egg-sugar complexes in angel food cake. Whatever the combination of diligence and scholarship, I was honored in being named to Mortar Board, Phi Kappa Phi, Omicron Nu, Who's Who in Colleges and Universities and later, Sigma Xi and Phi Upsilon Omicron.

The next step was a dietetic internship at the University of Michigan Hospitals, one of the best at that time. Fifteen of us for 12 months received excellent training, $50.00 a month (not including board) and a week vacation. I used part of the week to go to Niagara Falls which in January was mostly fog. As interns, we worked at all meal times and had classes during afternoon breaks. Weekends off were rare. Some aspects of diet therapy were quite different; for instance, ulcer patients received Sippy and Meulengracht diets. Pernicious anemia patients were treated with prodigious amount of liver in all forms and combinations and there was a special hospital for these patients. Vitamin B12 was known but not how it related to anemia. The diabetic diet food lists were complicated and used very precisely. All food was carefully weighed out on gram scales. Before the year was over, the first set of Exchange Lists was issued and we immediately began the conversion to the newer plan.

We worked under the direction of a staff of 25 dietitians who were excellent role models. Later, we appreciated fully what we received there because we were, in fact, ready for almost anything in dietetics or so we felt. We were also ready to try our own wings.

Other degrees came later. I went back to Oklahoma State in Stillwater when Dr. Ruth Leverton extended an offer of an assistantship to help on a project for analysis of the nutritional content of meats. It was the flagship study on meats for almost 20 years. Funded in part by the National Livestock and Meat Board for the purpose of establishing data on the major nutrients for several of the major meats and meat cuts, it was published and quoted widely. Dr. Leverton left for the U.S. Department of Agriculture before my degree was finished but the mails and telephone worked fine and the master's degree was accomplished. I then went back to dietetics several more years before entering Ohio State University for the doctorate. I was by then already at Ohio State and moved over from the University Hospitals to the College of Home Economics for the degree. The faculty included Levelle Wood, Virginia Harger, Eva Wilson, and my advisor, Virginia Vivian. Co-students during some of the time were Roy Maize, Sue Finn, Eleanor Pao. I was the older returning student by that time; they were the younger. My research was at Children's Hospital right next to George Owen's labs where his technicians kindly ran the plasma vitamin C samples for my study with children who had osteogenesis imperfecta. It was a center for treatment of this particular congenital bone disease and children came from all over the state. I completed the degree in 1970.

Positions in Dietetics

The first approximate 20 years of my career were in hospital dietary departments which provided exceedingly rich experience. It was constant continuing education as my responsibilities increased. From the first position as only dietitian in a 50 bed Children's Hospital to director of a large university hospital department, the full spectrum of dietetic practice was covered. Everything I knew and yet more was needed. In Louisville, Kentucky, where an internship friend and I took our first positions, the small hospital was a microcosom of everything happening in dietetics and like in every first experience, a quick study in personnel management. The well run University of Michigan Hospitals, with a large staff of specialized dietitians and compartmentalized experiences never necessitated one person putting it all together in one. Learning to deal with people in all their variations and motivations; employees, hospital staff, administrators, salesmen etc., is formidable at best and overwhelming at first. Suddenly, a whole new array of responsibilities descends which cannot be delayed or avoided. When the administrator says casually, "we're building a new hospital soon and need your approval of the already completed plans for the dietary department," one learns fast.

In contrast, my next position at the University of Chicago Hospitals was again in a comprehensive medical center with a large staff. As the administrative dietitian for food production in a decentralized system, I found further new challenges such as dealing with unionized employees with militant union stewards and fast turnover of employees who came primarily from surrounding unstable Chicago neighborhoods. During that time, too, Michael Reese Hospital in Chicago turned over foodservices to a management company and had to immediately relinquish their internship. It was very similar to what had happened at Johns Hopkins Hospital some five years earlier. In the 1950's, such events created great shock waves in dietetics.

After I had completed the master's degree, I returned to the University of Chicago as Internship Director and associate director of the department. The internship was soon to be closed and another opportunity for me came not long afterward. There were marvelous role models in dietetics at that time such as Ella M. Eck, my boss, one of the early lay leaders in ADA and a true genius in organization and facilities planning. Beulah Hunzicker and Merme Bonnell were at the University of Illinois. Henriette Gebert, Vivian Laird, Ruth Kahn and Marion Perkins and many others were influential in my life and remained friends.

From Chicago, I went to the Ohio State University Hospitals as Director of the Dietary Department. Martha N. Lewis was in the process of starting the first Coordinated Dietetic Program in the School of Allied Health and the hospital was the clinical training center. This became the model program for all those that followed throughout the country. Mrs. Lewis was later awarded the Copher Award in recognition of this and her other accomplishments as a leader in dietetics. In the department, Joan Sharp, Rachel Hubbard and Virginia Millholland were a triumvirate responsible for specific areas of the department. When I later entered the University for the doctorate, Jo Sharp became the director and remained in the position until recently.

In the hospital, one of the greatest challenges was maintaining a staff. Starting salaries for dietitians were $360 per month. They did begin rising, thanks in part to pressures nurses brought through strikes and salary demands at that time. Nursing had the force of numbers and since administrators could not allow salaries for any one group of allied health professionals to get too far out of line, dietitians also benefitted. I well remember, too, the feeling of accomplishment when my own salary reached the lofty $10,000 per year mark.

In the late 1960's, student riots over the Vietnam War were at their peak. The University was literally under siege. It was an unsettling experience to be caught in the middle of a riot between students and state police while innocently on the way to the library. On one particular day, the tear gas was so thick over the entire campus that businesses and a grade school close to the campus had to vacate. Shortly thereafter, the University was closed for over a month until the school year was over and by that time demonstrations themselves were almost over.

The Ohio Dietetic Association (ODA) has always been an active association with many dedicated members. Perhaps as a consequence, many ADA leaders have been as-

314

sociated with or had a connection with Ohio. The several metropolitan centers in Ohio meant there were many health care institutions and as a result, a large association membership. I served in several capacities in both the Columbus and Ohio Associations and as president of ODA in 1967–68. At almost the same time, one of the first Dial-A-Dietitian programs was successfully launched in Columbus. Peg Hinkle and Pat McKnight were responsible for this; anything the pair worked on always turned out a success and there were many such projects.

My academic career actually began during graduate school at Ohio State when I taught the Diet Therapy class and also one for student nurses at Capital University in Columbus. I have always enjoyed teaching and have taught one or more courses every semester along with other responsibilities since being in a university. The Dean of Home Economics, Dr. Lela O'Toole, called as I was finishing the PhD and talked about the need for a department head of Food, Nutrition and Institution Administration at Oklahoma State and had, in fact, been looking for a while. I was not at all sure I wanted to go back into administration just yet but she was persuasive and the offer was good. I therefore went back to Oklahoma State and was the department head until 1985, when I became Associate Dean for Research in the College until 1988. After this, I took advantage of an early retirement program and went to Auburn University as the interim department head of the Department of Nutrition and Foods, my present location.

I am proud of the number of dietitians who were prepared for careers at Oklahoma State and the dietitians who received updating of their course work and "retreading" for return to dietetics after being inactive for periods of time. In the early 1970's, dietitians were needed in nursing homes and hospitals receiving Medicare funds due to the new regulations mandating dietetic consultation. Elizabeth Hensler, the Director of the Nutrition Division of the State Health Department, was responsible for finding qualified staff so we formed a partnership and offered any number of concentrated one day a month courses updating dietitian's knowledge and practice skills. As a result, by far the majority of nursing homes in Oklahoma were staffed with qualified dietitians. Any dietitian wanting a position could find one or more. At about the same time, the Oklahoma Dietetic Association started a Peer Review Committee for which I was named the chairman. I believe this may have been among the first in the country. The federal Professional Standards Review regulations had come into being shortly before that and both movements were the forerunner of the PSR movement in ADA which later became Quality Assurance. I was then appointed chairman of the ADA Professional Standards Review Committee by President Isabelle Hallahan who saw the need for ADA to be aligned with this national movement.

At Oklahoma State, a futuristic department head and dietetics leader, Dr. Daisy I. Purdy, began an administrative dietetic internship and later, the Hotel and Administration program in the 1930's and 1940's. Many outstanding administrative dietitians went through the internship starting in the 1930's. Much later, many also went through the master's degree plus experience program as well as a statewide traineeship program organized at Oklahoma State. All these experience programs have now given way to others as circumstances and ADA requirements changed.

I am proud of the 42 masters and doctoral graduates from Food, Nutrition and Institution Administration I advised. Almost every one is now active in dietetics in education.

My career was further enhanced by two stints in Washington, D.C., on leave from the university. These experiences not only contributed to my ongoing education but also gave me a continuing interest in public policy as well as many Washington contacts. This was important later in ADA legislative matters in which I was involved. Both positions in Washington, three years apart, were with the U.S. Department of Agriculture. The first was in the Cooperative State Research Service agency which reviews research in Colleges and Universities receiving federal funds. My leader and mentor in this agency was Dr. Elizabeth Davis, a friend and colleague then and ever since. The second was as Administrator of the Human Nutrition Information Service, the agency which conducts the National Food Consumption Surveys and issues Handbook 8, the Bible of nutrition values. The Food Consumption surveys, which have been conducted at intervals for a long time, are also a vital component of the current National Nutrition Monitoring Bill. For various reasons, the USDA does not support the present bill although it has been and would continue to be responsible for this part of the data gathering. I worked with many outstanding professionals such as Betty Peterkin, Cathy Wotecki, Eleanor Pao, and Bob Rizek in USDA as well as Grace Ostenso in Congress, Donna Porter in the Library of Congress, Lenora Moragne in Health and Human Services and Evelyn Johnson in Extension Service. During this same period I was a representative from ADA to the National Nutrition Consortium where Kristen McNutt was the Executive Director.

Washington experiences formed the basis for teaching a course in public policy several summers as well as a close continuing interest in the Washington scene. They were exciting and challenging experiences but it personally was a relief for me to return to the university each time.

Experiences in Dietetics

I started in local and state associations, having always felt it was important to participate in associations at all levels. Along the way, I served as president of the Chicago Dietetic Association and the Ohio Dietetic Association as well as a member of committees. I enjoyed these experiences totally and, from my standpoint, gained more than I gave. I "went national" when ADA President Isabelle Hallahan first appointed me to the Journal Board which was a demanding but thoroughly enjoyable experience. About a year later, I was asked to be on the ballot and was elected ADA Secretary, thus becoming a member of the Executive Board. The Secretary was also chairman of the Membership Committee which was a very active position in the early 1970's when membership categories and requirements were undergoing change. The committee worked closely with Dorothy Bates and her staff and met several times in Chicago to work through the new categories. Dietetic technicians had just become eligible as members and the Associate category had been created without any precise definition as to who would be eligible. The three year experience as a qualifying route to membership was also allowed—a plan which has come and gone more than once and now of course no longer exists.

Elsie Haff was ADA President when I joined the Executive Board, followed by Annie Galbraith and then Jean Sturdevant. It was also the period during which the separation of membership and Registration was approved. This was a concept not fully understood at the time but which in fact is one that has functioned exactly as intended and planned ever since. It was feared membership would drop as members realized they could remain fully qualified to practice by simply retaining the R.D. That this did not happen and still has not is a credit to the leadership. ADA has been able to continue to hold and increase members when that has not happened in many other associations. This may well have been due, at least in part, to the foresight of very early leaders who tied eligibility to practice to association affiliation and positions the Association itself as the standard setting and monitoring body. The Association has of course continued to grow steadily and without fragmentation.

I was then elected Speaker of the House of Delegates while Maxine Wilson was Speaker. The new Bylaws were in the final stages of preparation by a committee who had worked diligently on them several years. The Bylaws were accompanied by a plan for a new organizational structure. This was a fairly radical change whereby the Council on Practice, the Council on Education and, for a while, the Commission on Operations were all created. The Board was also enlarged by three Members-at-large. The Bylaws also gave more power to the House of Delegates, such as in passing the Association budget, setting membership standards and others. Changes in the Association governance could further be made by the House through revision of the Bylaws without an all-member vote. The campaign to sell the new Bylaws and structure was fought hard and, in some instances in which I was uncomfortably involved, by negative campaigning against a "too powerful Board of Directors." The plan had many merits going for it on its own and I wondered then and often since why it was felt necessary to attack in order to sell. In any event, it did pass and became a well organized and functional structure with much broader input by more groups. It was also the initiation of Practice Groups which was probably one of the most timely and important steps taken in the Association.

In 1978–79, I became President-elect and then President the following year. This was just after initiation of the new structure with a larger Board and many players in new roles. As an Association, we were growing fast, adding some 4000 new members per year and moving in many important directions. Yet, it became very obvious that leadership in the headquarters office was not keeping pace; people were not being utilized in the best ways; decisions that should—or should not—have been made were not handled well or in timely ways. The Board regretfully arrived at the decision in a major change in leadership must occur. It was beyond question a turning point in the Association about which there were mostly positive reactions from the membership. However, some personal relationships which I had prized were fatally wounded and remain so to this day as a result of this action. However, a standing ovation at the Annual Meeting in Atlanta that fall convinced me that members were in accord with the directions the Board had taken and that they were supportive and ready to move ahead.

One of the activities presidents are often called on to do is testify before Congressional committees and I did my share of this also. For the most part these occasions went well and ADA's position was respectfully received although not always heeded. Perhaps the best example was the frequent attempt at legislation establishing third party payment for dietetic services. Isabelle Hallahan and Betty Blouin worked as hard on this year after year as anything that came along and, of course, it is still not a reality. One of these testifying experiences stands out for being almost ludicrous although it was deflating at the time. Senators Metzenbaum and Schweiker were having a hearing on Nutrition Education and we were asked to testify. As it turned out, they were mostly interested in nutrition in the medical school curriculum. When it was suggested that a major boost from Congress such as declaration of a nutrition emphasis week or even a day would lend visibility and credibility, there was an instant reaction from Senator Metzenbaum. Drawing up his full impressive importance, he informed us they already recognized every cause that came along and could not be expected to consider such a thing. It did seem ironic that the subject it was felt important enough to hold national hearings on was not important enough to award Congressional recognition.

The International Congress of Dietetics convened in Sao Paulo, Brazil, that year and I went with a group of about 40 dietitians and families as the official U.S. representative. It was a tremendous experience seeing Rio de Janeiro and the beach and large statue there as well as Sao Paulo, the industrial city and capital of the country. I soon found out however that being the U.S. delegate accorded no special attention. It was a fascinating experience which could almost serve as a textbook study on international maneuvering. Even the topic I was asked to speak on appeared in the program as a completely different subject. I am sure the representatives who heard it there still wonder about that speech.

How to describe what its like to be president of this leading professional association? The responsibility for influencing policies that affect the profession, that literally set direction and impact on the livelihood of thousands of dedicated professional dietitians is awesome. It is humbling in realizing that members expect much from their leaders but also accord them a certain adulation, deserved or not. It is also stressful and demanding because presidents serve as volunteers; usually continuing on with their own positions back home, hopefully with superiors who understand the tremendous time and travel commitment required. The true pleasure comes in meeting and interacting with people everywhere—people both within and outside the profession who have influence and impact. The prestige of the office opens doors to experiences never available otherwise. In short, there's nothing quite like it.

I was pleased to be asked to become a member of the ADA Foundation Board after my year as President was over. The Foundation was also at a turning point after a long period of mostly funding scholarships and developing contacts with industry and it was poised to become much more active. Incredibly dedicated members such as Katherine Manchester, Lee Horton, Dee Downey, Margaret Klink, Audrey Wright, and Edna Langholz conducted the business while dreaming of much bigger things yet for the Association. I didn't realize just how big the dreams were at first or what would be involved but it soon became clear. First, the Board was enlarged by addition of key members of the ADA Board of Directors for policy decisions in concert with the Association. Then the plan unfolded: by an ambitious fund raising undertaking, a building housing the Association headquarters would be brought which would also be the site of the newly created National Center for Nutrition and Dietetics. When I became President of the Foundation in 1986–87, much activity was centered around trying to find the right building, however this did not become a reality until 1988. The Association now is happily settled into the Jackson Boulevard Building. The National Center is still evolving but when fully operational, should be the most important nutrition information center in the country. Already there is a link to the National Agriculture Library in Beltsville with access to food and nutrition literature throughout the world. I count my several years on the Foundation Board as a time when exciting, important things were happening in the Association.

Reflections

There have been manpower studies over the years predicting growth in various areas of dietetic practice and decline in others. Regardless, the number of members continues to grow and the career opportunities remain broad and varied. Dietitians are now in positions and areas of practice which did not exist earlier. The public's interest in health and fitness has created entire new industries in which dietitians are also becoming entrepreneurs in their own businesses. It seems to be the outlook for dietetics is almost unlimited.

The major changes I have observed in the profession are increasing sophistication of members, more leadership and more risk taking. Dietitians are becoming more visible in the mainstream of professional and public life. The increasing emphasis on outcomes of education is a trend hoped for by educators in dietetics programs. The missing link of measuring outcomes through later performance on the job is ideal but at present can be done only informally at best and by persons themselves or by employers. Requirements for the experience component for membership are more closely circumscribed than ever before and the R.D. exam has evolved into an instrument driving education.

In the Association, there has been continual development of programs in response to the increasing educational levels and specialization among members. The growth and success of Practice Groups and the number of quality of continuing education events recognize the broad range of interests and needs among members. The initiation of research through the Council on Research and the phenomenally successful research abstracts and sessions at the Annual Meeting, the high quality journal and the Annual Meeting itself are all tangible evidence of the care and attention given to professionals and their needs. Of course, fees and dues increase. I well remember the registration for the first Annual Meeting I attended was $5.00. In present times, I firmly believe value received far exceeds the cost.

I am now into traveling. As educational tour leader for two trips to Russia and one to Australia and New Zealand, there have been fascinating opportunities to see wonderful sights as well as visit health care institutions and meet other professionals in those countries. I will go to China this fall which is another long awaited wish.

My chosen profession has truly been a fortuitous choice. If I have given some, I have gained much more and would do it all over again.

Audrey C. Wright

Audrey C. Wright, MS, RD is Administrator,
Father Walter Center for Handicapped Children,
Montgomery, AL

Although Audrey Wright works as a health care administrator, she has always maintained her strong dietetics identity. She has demonstrated her ability to combine family life and career, making the best of every opportunity which presented itself as her husband's career necessitated a move. In the recount of her decision to leave her beloved Barnes Medical Center (St. Louis, MO) where the foundation of her professional career began, her professional philosophy comes through. "There was an accountability measure in my practice required to myself, as well as the recipient of my services." Her commitment to the profession has been exemplified in long-term activities with ADA/ADA Foundation and has led to much-deserved recognition including Outstanding Dietitian* of Alabama and the ADA Medallion Award. No doubt she receives professional and personal pride in her daughter's decision to become a registered dietitian and active member of the Association.

Audrey C. Wright

As I reflect on the past 37 years of membership in The American Dietetic Association, and my commitment to the profession, I realize my interest in dietetics began in high school. The sister of a family friend was a dietitian at Lutheran General Hospital, Chicago, Illinois and mentioned this as a career to pursue. The biological sciences were already a keen interest for me. With added encouragement and support from my mother, Margaret Clever Hoefling, I searched for information related to career opportunities in dietetics, as well as the educational requirements.

I was a senior in El Dorado High School in 1947, when I wrote for information from The American Dietetic Association, 620 North Michigan Avenue, Chicago, Illinois. From the pamphlets sent to me that listed the academic requirements in college, the necessity, at that time, for completing a dietetic internship at an approved hospital, and the career opportunities that lay ahead, I knew that this was my chosen field. Realizing at that time, that the field of dietetics was geared to hospital, community service or possibly the Army Medical Corps, I began planning my college selection to those institutions that offered this curriculum. I found out very quickly that in 1947, and in Arkansas, only the University of Arkansas could afford me this opportunity.

I entered the University of Arkansas, Fayetteville, Arkansas in September, 1947. Since I had chosen dietetics, I was assigned to the College of Agriculture. My advisor, Vera McNair, Ph.D., an active member of The American Dietetic Association, was very pleased to have four young women assigned to her. I was very frightened of her at first, as this was the most knowledgeable person in the field of nutrition that I had ever met. She was businesslike and plotted my four year course of study, perfectly. I remember being able to select only one course my freshman year, none my sophomore and junior years and two courses my senior year.

As I began the core curriculum that was required by the Home Economics Department, I realized that we were certainly in the minority, since most of the students were studying to be Home Economics teachers or Home Economists. Dr. McNair was our champion and was constantly justifying the need for courses in food and nutrition. Never did she let her students realize that we were the "step-children" of the department. She was insistent that we attend the state dietetic meetings in Little Rock, which I am sure that even though we traveled in a University car, she paid for the gas and other expenses from her own pocket.

In 1949, my sophomore year, I won a trip to St. Louis as part of the Danforth Award, sponsored by Ralston Purina. This was a very prestigious Home Economics Department award, not often achieved by a foods and nutrition major. Part of the trip was a visit to Barnes Hospital, the clinical facility for Washington University School of Medicine. Immediately, I felt a kinship with the dietitians and dietetic interns there.

It was, also, in the summer of that same year that my father, George Martin Clever, was transferred to Shreveport, Louisiana. He was a tremendous support in my career pursuit. I was not happy over thoughts of leaving the University of Arkansas. My family wanted me to stay on my planned course, so I continued my studies. For visits, it took me a day and a half by train from Fayetteville to Shreveport, which was about 400 miles away.

On May 13, 1950, about two weeks away from finals, my father died of a heart attack at forty-seven. Not only was he a wonderful father, but also a beloved friend and supporter. This was a devastating time for me. My mother was very courageous, now left with a nineteen-year-old and a twelve-year-old and widowed at forty-two. She decided to move back to El Dorado. When I look at what confronted her, I marvel at how she took hold and became a motivating force in my life.

That fall in 1950, I began looking at dietetic internships. There were few in the southeast. I wanted to stay close to home, but again Dr. McNair influenced my choice. She insisted that I apply for only one internship at Barnes Hospital in St. Louis, Missouri. Since she had been a guiding force, during college days, I trusted her judgment and applied. To my relief, my appointment came in the spring of 1951. I had wondered what I would do if I did not get that internship. Dr. McNair said to me, "Henrietta Becker knows me and knows that I would never let anyone apply for her internship that she would want to reject!" I was happy she was so confident, because I was not, at that time. My mother and my sister Mary Ann were caught up in the excitement of getting ready for my internship, during the summer of 1951.

In September of that year, I boarded the train bound for St. Louis full of enthusiasm. Arriving at Barnes Hospital and receiving my room assignment and roommate, I was both scared and excited. My roommate, Adele Heumann Lang, who was from St. Louis, was there and we, immediately, became dear friends. There were 12 of us who, for the next 12 months shared experiences with our work and lives. Through this sharing, we developed a bond of friendship that has lasted through the years.

The new charges were treated well by department director, Henrietta Becker. She believed in the dietetic profession and in her presentation, I knew I was on the right course in my chosen field. In those twelve months, I grew from a green college graduate to a person who felt comfortable and somewhat knowledgeable in the practice of dietetics. Miss Becker was a leader and a mentor to me and I feel her guidance and leadership fueled my interest and desire to achieve excellence in the field of dietetics. She paved the way for each of us to take our places as co-professionals and team members with hospital administration, nursing and the physician. During my internship, I always felt I was a viable participant in the health and welfare of the patient, in every setting from food service administration to the clinical setting.

Upon completion of my internship, August, 1951, and joining The American Dietetic Association, Miss Becker offered me the position of Clinic Dietitian for Washington University Clinic. I was honored, as this was a prestigious position for a new graduate. I was considered a department head in the Clinics, and it was an honor to practice at the Barnes Medical Center. Also, that year Dr. Frank Bradley, Administrator of Barnes Hospital, and current President of the American Hospital Association, initiated a residency program in Dietetics that would enable us to take classes with master's program students in Hospital Administration. Miss Becker felt that was a great opportunity for her staff and allowed us to participate. I was awarded a certificate for completion of this program in the spring of 1953.

In the summer of 1953 the ST. LOUIS POST DISPATCH did a two-page story in the Sunday supplement on "Three Career Girls in St. Louis." This story, with pictures, depicted the professional lives, as well as outside activities of myself and my two roommates, Carolyn Kavanaugh (Rogers), clinical dietitian, St. Louis Children's Hospital and Kathryn Phillippi, clinical dietitian for the surgical floors of Barnes Hospital. The three of us had become such good friends during our internship that we decided to stay in St. Louis and share apartment living. There are many fond memories of those days and the publicity was a very exciting event in our lives.

I worked for two rewarding years as a Clinic Dietitian for Washington University Clinics, but I felt I wanted to move on in my career and since my mother had moved to New Orleans, Louisiana, I interviewed at the hospitals in that vicinity. It was truly a difficult decision to think about leaving the Barnes Medical Center, as truly I felt this Center was the ultimate in health care. I knew the foundation for my professional life began there at Barnes, because of the outstanding role models, not only in dietetics, but also in hospital administration and medicine. I learned that as I advanced up the ladder of professional life, there was an accountability measure in my practice required to myself, as well as the recipient of my services. I found, also, that humility was a virtue to attain in any successful venture. I have always been proud to say that I was a product of Barnes Hospital, as I had the privilege of knowing Dr. Glover Copher, husband of the late Marjorie Hulsizer Copher; Dr. Barry Wood, Dean of Washington University School of Medicine; Dr. Robert Shank, a leader in the establishment of the Recommended Dietary Allowances; Dr. Carl Moore, noted hematologist; Mary de Garmo Bryan, who with her husband was a frequent visitor to the Washington University; Dr. Frank Bradley, Past-President of the American Hospital Association and a leader in the field of Hospital Administration, just to mention a few.

My trip to New Orleans, in August of 1954, proved to be successful as I was offered the position of Educational Director of the Dietetic Internship Program at Charity Hospital in that city. I, reluctantly, closed the chapter of my wonderful three years in St. Louis and moved to New Orleans in mid-September. I was about to meet my husband-to-be that August, when my mother had some young people in for a gathering to meet her daughter. Rex Wright was one of them.

My adjustment to Charity Hospital was difficult in that I had left a private hospital that offered food service served on china with an exciting selective menu to a state hospital that served the indigent population of south Louisiana. Sister Theresa Cain, Daughter of Charity, was the director of the department. Sister Theresa was "old school" and insisted the dietetic interns be handled in the same manner as if they were in a girl's school, with rigid restrictions. Sister Theresa became a good friend and I soon became the buffer between the interns who were not much younger than I. In time, I won Sister over to the fact that these girls were college graduates and very capable of handling their personal lives, and that we were there to help them develop their clinical skills and professional confidence.

Charity Hospital was a mammoth institution to me, as we had patients on eight floors, with a census of around 200 per floor, in a 19 story building. There were five surrounding buildings; three that housed tuberculosis patients, one that had only polio patients and one that housed contagious diseases that were prevalent in the south. Charity was the clinical facility for two school of medicine, Tulane University School of Medicine and Louisiana State University School of Medicine, as well as affiliations for about 20 Schools of Nursing in the Charity Hospital School of Nursing. A wealth of information was within this mammoth institution. Also, there was an affiliation with the new Oschner Foundation Hospital and their excellent dietetic department, under the leadership of Sally Cloud Oster and Sara Crumley.

During this time, I was being courted by Rex, so this was an exciting period in my life. I attended my first meeting of The American Dietetic Association that October, 1954, in Philadelphia, Pennsylvania and roomed with my former director and mentor, Henrietta Becker. I attended the educational sessions at the beginning of the meeting and audited the House of Delegates. Miss Becker saw that I met many of our leaders, Dr. Bessie Brooks West, Dr. Helen Mitchell, Mrs. Grace Shugart, and many more. It was a thrilling experience for me and I believe the event strengthened my allegiance to The American Dietetic Association.

I became engaged in January, 1955. Our wedding was May 28, 1955. The dietetic interns were as much a part of the exciting parties and events of this period as were my social friends. In less than a year, Rex was advanced to manager of the Farm Chemical Division of Armour & Company in Havana, Cuba.

Rex left New Orleans in February, 1956 and I joined him the next month in March, expecting our first child to arrive in June. This was a traumatic time for me, as I could not continue my career and I was about to have my first child in a foreign country. Rex was assured by his company that if necessary I could come back to the states to have my baby, but my doctor in New Orleans felt that was not necessary. He said, ''Most of the Cuban doctors trained in the states and women had been having babies in Cuba for years!''

Rex William Wright arrived June 10, 1956 in Havana, Cuba. Our lives there turned out to be both exciting and eventful. I was immediately asked to be on the Board of Directors for the Anglo-American Hospital, which was an honor and a challenge. I was to be a regular patient in this hospital as Margaret Ann Wright arrived November 13, 1957 and Karen Louise Wright on March 25, 1959. During this time, I remained an active member of The American Dietetic Association and received my ADA Journals, monthly. In October of 1958, The American Dietetic Association Annual Meeting was held in Miami, Florida, and my dear friend, Henrietta Becker, extended her trip to include a visit with us in Havana. She brought me up-to-date on many of the happenings in the profession and I realized how much I missed having contact with other dietetic practitioners.

At the same time, Fidel Castro and his "Barbudos" were initiating the overthrow of the Batista regime. We lived through the revolution, which began December 31, 1958 and witnessed the downfall of the government that January 1, 1959. We loved Cuba and were distressed to see the destruction of a way of life to be replaced by communism. It was not blaringly evident at first, but the presence of the eastern bloc countries, immediately, in Cuba was an indication of what was to come. We lived for one and a half years under Fidel Castro and witnessed many sad events befall our Cuban friends.

On July 4, 1960, Rex took the children and myself out of Cuba to his mother's home in Tuscumbia, Alabama. He returned to Havana and in two weeks the government took over Armour & Company and told Rex he could leave the country. Believe it or not I heard him being interviewed the day it happened, by NBC newsman Richard Valariani. We could only take with us what we could get into suitcases, which was very limiting, and choices had to be made as to what was irreplaceable.

This was a chaotic episode in our lives and, luckily, we were transferred to Birmingham, Alabama. With three small children, my hands were full, but we were able to sponsor and to help our housekeeper, Louisa Stewart, to leave Cuba and to join us in December, 1960. Adjusting to life in the United States was pleasant for the family and soon the happenings in Cuba seemed like a bad dream. The next September 20, 1961, we were blessed with the arrival of Susan Marie Wright.

While in St. Vincent's Hospital, having the baby, the Administrator, Sister Mary Carlos visited me. She had just arrived in Birmingham, after spending 20 years in New Orleans at Charity Hospital and Hotel Dieu. She had been Administrator at Hotel Dieu, the oldest hospital in New Orleans, for the last ten years and was thrilled to have someone to talk New Orleans with her. In fact, we knew many of the same people, since Hotel Dieu was a field experience for the Charity dietetic interns, and we quickly became friends.

Sister Carlos called me many times in the next few months, as she was having problems with the dietary department. In January, 1962, she asked if I could come to her office, as she wanted to offer me a part-time position. Sister Carlos was an outstanding administrator and a leader in her profession. I accepted a position as Director of the Department of Dietetics on a part-time basis, and I was thrilled to return to my professional career as St. Vincent's, which was one of the most respected hospitals in Birmingham.

The next four and a half years at St. Vincent's were productive and satisfying. Sister Carlos soon became another mentor and together we initiated innovative changes in the food service delivery of that hospital. The medical staff was very supportive and the department was recognized as a viable participant in the health and welfare of the patients.

In that fall of 1961, I made contact with University Hospital, in Birmingham, and met Janet Mastin, the Director of the Dietetics Department. Janet was in the process of establishing a dietetic internship and was very active in the state association activities. Before I knew it, I was involved myself, as I was appointed Public Relations Chairman,

1964; Program Chairman, 1965 and elected President-elect of the state association in 1966. I soon formed friendships with my fellow professionals in the state that lasted throughout the years. The year I was Program Chairman we were fortunate to have past ADA Presidents, Dr. Neige Todhunter and Anna Mae Tracy and Mary Zahasky, the President-elect. This was an exciting meeting and I observed the professionalism of the Alabama dietitians.

My husband was transferred to Montgomery, Alabama in the fall of 1965. It is the capital city, located 95 miles from Birmingham, and we moved there in July, 1966.

Arriving in Montgomery, I was soon involved in the local dietetic association. Since I was to take office as President in October, 1966, I already knew many of the dietitians in this city. Emma Clinkscales, Director of Nutrition Services for the Department of Health was out-going President and I enjoyed her as a dear friend. I traveled with Emma throughout the state and soon became acquainted with dietitians in all the major cities.

In the fall of 1967, I was elected as a Delegate from Alabama to finish the unexpired term of Ernestine Jackson, who had been elected to the Council of the House of Delegates. I served as both President and Delegate for 1966–67. It was, also, the fiftieth anniversary year of The American Dietetic Association and the national meeting was held in Chicago, Illinois at the Hilton Hotel, with Mary Zahasky as President. In March, 1969, I received one of my most treasured honors by being selected as Alabama's "Outstanding Dietitian." I served as Delegate to the House until 1972, when I was elected as Delegate from the House of Delegates and a member of the Coordinating Cabinet to serve until 1974.

During my tenure in the House, I was fortunate to chair the Code of Ethics Committee, the first attempt to have an accepted code of professional practice; the Membership Categories Committee that recommended expanding membership in the Association; and serve on the Committee to Study, Evaluate and Make Recommendations for Implementation of the Study Commission Report, "The Profession of Dietetics," with Dr. Charlotte Young as Chair.

It was, also, during this period that I entered graduate school at Auburn University. Mildred Van de Mark, head of the department, was my advisor and having received my B.S. degree 20 years before, this was truly a tremendous undertaking for me. Needless to say, without the help and support of my husband and four children, ages 15, 13, 12, and 10 years, I would never had succeeded in this venture. It was an outstanding experience and I was honored to have my research article published in the Journal of The American Dietetic Association, November 1972, entitled, "Hemoglobin and Folate Levels of Pregnant Teen-agers." During graduate school, I was invited to join Omicron Nu, National Honor Society in Home Economics.

After completing my Master's Degree, I was encouraged by the Administrator, Sister Mary Bernadine of Father Walter Memorial Child Care Center, a skilled care nursing home for mentally and physically handicapped children, to complete a licensure course in Nursing Home Administration at the University of Alabama in Birmingham.

After completion, I took the exam and received my license as a nursing home administrator. Beginning in 1972, I, not only, was the consultant at Father Walter's, but also acted as administrative assistant, on a part-time basis.

My move to Montgomery had been truly rewarding, since upon my arrival, nursing homes were desperate for consultant dietitians. I acted as preceptor for several dietary managers to finish correspondence courses to enable them to be eligible to manage food service in their respective nursing homes. In fact, Prenttella Rudolph, the dietary manager at Father Walter's, became President of their state association known as the Hospital Institutional and Educational Food Service Society (HIEFSS). HIEFSS received its' charter as an affiliate with the national association, during my tenure as President of the Alabama Dietetic Association and, during this period, dietitians were advisors to HIEFSS.

The 1970's were very eventful in my professional growth, especially, when I was elected as a Delegate-at-Large, a member of the Coordinating Cabinet 1974–1983. I served on the Committee to Study Registration Independent of Membership 1972–74; House of Delegates Committee to Implement Membership Categories 1974; Finance Committee of The American Dietetic Association 1974–1976; the first Appeals Committee of ADA 1977–1980; Chairman, Continuing Education Advisory Committee 1979–1980; and the Conceptual Framework Committee 1979–1980.

My election to the Foundation Board of Directors in 1977 was particularly exciting, as Loyal Horton was President and I served under the presidency of Colonel Katherine Manchester, who has been a spectacular leader in the profession. I was elected President of the Foundation for the two consecutive years, 1981–1983, as I had previously served as Secretary, Treasurer, and Vice-President.

The Foundation's assets were limited and I was privileged to be a part of the outstanding growth in its scholarship program and nutrition education for public programs. It was during my tenure as President that the ADA/ADAF Building Fund Task Force launched the project for a National Center for Nutrition and Dietetics. Thanks to past presidents Edna Langholz, Colonel Katherine Manchester, and Dr. Kathleen Zolber, the campaign was a success. The membership of ADA was receptive to the concept, since nutrition education for the public has always been the primary mission of the Association. This period saw corporate advisors included in Foundation planning and fund-raising activities that enabled growth. Robert Knight—Hobart Manufacturing Company, Charlie Boyce—Diamond Crystal Corporation, Ted Reiple—Diversey Wyndotte Corporation, and Jane Young Wallace—Restaurants and Institutions Magazine were some of the first advisors. These and others continue to support Foundation and Association activities as well as Mead-Johnson and their long-standing support of the scholarship program.

The 1980's have been significant as my older daughter Margaret Ann Wright graduated from the University of Alabama in May as a dietitian. In August of that year, I was about to finish my year as Chairman of the Council on Practice, when tragedy touched my life. My daughter Karen Louise Wright died from cardiac arrest. That year she would have been a senior in dietetics at the University of Alabama. Needless to say, this was the most traumatic event in my life and only through faith and prayers were my family and myself sustained. Donations came in from our many treasured friends throughout the Association and the Karen L. Wright Lecture Fund was established in the Foundation, which affords a lecture given at the Alabama Dietetic Association Annual Meeting. That same August, I had just accepted and embarked on the challenge as Administrator of Father Walter Memorial Child Care Center.

At the October, 1981 meeting of The American Dietetic Association in Philadelphia, Pennsylvania, I was honored to receive the Association's Medallion Award, under the presidency of Mary Lou South. I continued to be active in Association and Foundation affairs, as I was a Site Visitor for the accreditation process for ADA and took the helm as Chairman of the ADA/ADAF Building Fund Task Force for the National Center for Dietetics, for the period 1983–1987. This was an exciting project and the realization of raising two million dollars from membership solicitation was achieved. Also, the major fund-raising project of publishing *FOOD FAVORITES COOKBOOK*, proved to be a tremendous success. On a personal note, my oldest daughter, Margaret Ann Wright, was married in 1982 and my youngest daughter, Susan Marie Wright, was graduated from the University of Alabama in December, 1983. My son, Rex William Wright, finished his Master's Degree in Civil Engineering from Georgia Tech and married in the fall of 1985.

In the spring of 1987, I was elected Secretary/Treasurer of The American Dietetic Association. This office proved to be very exciting and stimulating, since the Association was able to reach the financial reserve goal set in 1983 and yet continue to advance programs in legislation and public policy, dietetic practice, research for the profession, and marketing and communication. I also served as Chairman of the Fiscal Affairs Committee, a committee of the Board, which monitors the financial affairs of the Association.

In the span of a nine-year period, I was very involved in seeking licensure for Alabama dietitians, which was achieved in May, 1989. My activities with the Alabama Nursing Home Administration are many. I am a licensed nursing home administrator in my position with Father Walter Memorial Center for Handicapped Children. I served as chairman of the Peer Review Committee and served on the Board of Directors as a Region Vice-President 1981–1986. I served as President of the Alabama chapter of the American College of Health Care Administrators 1981–1982. Another eventful happening was my appointment by the Governor of Alabama Guy Hunt, to serve as a Board member for the Alcoholic Beverage Control Board of Alabama 1987–1991. This was the second time in 50 years that a woman had been appointed to the Board.

As the 1980's close, I look forward to continued participation in the affairs of The American Dietetic Association and its Foundation. I was honored to have my name placed in nomination for the office of President-elect of the Association. This election will be decided in April, 1990. My past 37 years have proven to be eventful, stimulating, challenging and meaningful in my career as a dietetic professional.

Kathleen Keen Zolber

Kathleen K. Zolber, PhD, RD is Professor
and Nutrition Chairman, Loma Linda University

Those who know Dr. Kathleen Zolber well have summarized her career in two words—dedicated excellence. From her first teaching job as part-time instructor at Walla Walla College to her current position as full Professor and Chairman of the Nutrition Department and Director of the Approved Preprofessional Practice Program at Loma Linda University, her interest in and commitment to students have been guiding forces in her career. She has admirably blended the dual roles of administrator and educator approaching each with equal vigor and thoroughness. She served as Chairman of the Commission of Evaluation of Dietetic Education (Commission on Accreditation) and the ADA Representative to the National Nutrition Consortium. Dr. Zolber became the 58th President of ADA in 1982. She was also invited to be a member to the National Task Force on Education for the Veterans Administration. Although at one point she considered a career change to consumer law, she decided to remain with dietetics, the challenging and rewarding profession she has enjoyed for over 48 years.

Kathleen K. Zolber

Walla Walla, Washington is where I was born, attended elementary school, three years of high school and college. The senior year of high school was taken at Yakima Valley Academy in Granger, Washington. It was a church-related academy which provided the opportunity to live in a dormitory environment. In September, 1935, I enrolled as a freshman at Walla Walla College. Since I was financially on my own and responsible for college tuition and related expenses as well as dormitory living expenses, it was necessary for me to be a student employee half time and attend classes on a half time schedule. During the freshman year I was employed in the college bakery 2 a.m.–8 a.m., attended classes between 8 a.m.–2 p.m. as scheduled, then slept and studied . . . . , but mostly studied. By the beginning of the sophomore year I had changed student employment and began a four year employment schedule in the cafeteria food service department.

My mother had always hoped I would become a registered nurse but since I was too young my freshman year to enter the nursing program I decided to major in food and nutrition in the Home Economics Department. This worked well with my employment in the college cafeteria. Combining the academic coursework with the practicum experience over a four year period worked out to be a valuable asset as I began my professional career following graduation from college.

While I was a student in college my concept of leadership began to develop, influenced by the writing of Mary Parker Follett, born in Boston in 1868. She studied at Radcliffe College and her work there and later accomplishments gave her a place among the college's fifty most distinguished graduates. As early as 1930 she wrote that some are beginning to conceive of the leader, not as the man in the group who is able to assert his individual will and get others to follow him, but as the one who knows how to relate these different wills so that they have a driving force. He must know how to create a group power rather to express a personal power. He must make the team. The leader is regarded as the man who can energize his group, who knows how to encourage initiative, how to draw from all what each has to give. . . . The ablest administrator has a vision of the future. The person who influences me most, she wrote, is not he who does great deeds but he who makes me feel that I can do great deeds (1). If this were true of men, could it be true of women as well?

Extracurricular activities of a college program held special interest for me as I enjoyed being involved in group activities and it was an opportunity to achieve predetermined goals. During my five years in college I was elected to fill different offices in student association affairs. Working on the college newspaper initiated my desire to develop skills needed in writing for publication. Serving as the director for student association social activities was a very valuable experience in developing leadership and public relation skills relevant to organizational activities.

During my junior year in college I met an architectural engineering student, Melvin Zolber. Dating continued and we were married a year later. Fortunately for me he has been very supportive of my continuing advanced education program as well as my involvement in professional association activities. As our busy schedules permit we enjoy traveling, attending cultural as well as sports events, and for Melvin a high priority is playing golf at the Country Club.

Upon completion of the B.S. degree I was invited to become Director of Food Service and an Instructor in Foods and Nutrition at Walla Walla College. This position was very exciting to me as it afforded the opportunity to work closely with college students as they pursued their own educational and professional goals. Many students who were student employees in the cafeteria were enrolled in pre-medicine, pre-dentistry, pre-nursing, elementary or secondary education, etc., and after they completed professional training our paths continued to cross and they would keep me updated on their achievements. To me this is an important reward which accrues from working with college/university students.

After teaching several years I enrolled in the master's degree program in food and nutrition at Washington State University (Pullman). To my good fortune my academic and research project advisor was Marion Jacobson, Ph.D. In addition to being an advisor she became my mentor and role model for the kind of teacher I hoped to become as I returned to teaching and advising college students. Some years later I was indeed humbled to read comments made by Dr. Jacobson relevant to her reflections on my time spent as a graduate student under her guidance in the master's degree program:

> "Two words describe Kathleen Zolber's career—dedicated excellence. From her actions, one senses that her dedication to service and warm concern for people stem from a deep religious faith. The excellence has developed from intelligence and abundant energy. Kathleen's motto might well be, 'It can be done.' Further, she goes about doing more than her share to see that it will be done" (2).

When my master's degree was completed I returned to full-time teaching as an Assistant Professor in Foods and Nutrition at Walla Walla College and remained in that role for three years.

In 1964 my husband accepted a position in California and we moved to Loma Linda. At that time I joined the School of Nutrition and Dietetics faculty to teach graduate courses in the Dietetics Internship as well as in the Master of Science degree program. The following year the University sponsored me in beginning a doctoral program in Food Administration at the University of Wisconsin–Madison. I will never cease being thankful for having the guidance of Beatrice Donaldson David, Ph.D., R.D., well known and respected nationally for her excellence in teaching, research, publications and as a management consultant. Her published research has focused primarily on the study of productivity and labor time analysis in food service systems. She not only served as advisor for my doctoral program but she also became an outstanding mentor providing the environment which promotes a student to be highly motivated to achieve predetermined goals. I think often of the continuing contribution which Dr. David is making as the many master degree and doctoral degree graduates from the program she directed in food service administration are filling leadership positions in teaching, research and management. In 1983 The American Dietetic Association presented her the Marjorie Hulsizer Copher Memorial Award. Financial support for my pursuing a doctoral program includes the Mead Johnson Graduate Study Award given through The American Dietetic Association in 1965–66 and 1966–67.

Dr. David's comments relevant to my activities as a doctoral student were:

"A member of Kathleen's doctoral committee asked the director of her graduate study and research program for the Ph.D. in Food Administration how she motivated a graduate student to take on such an extensive study and research program, complete it within a designated time, and do it so well. The answer was that Kathleen Zolber does not need to be motivated: she *is* motivated. Kathleen's enthusiasm and philosophy for living and working are contagious, but she gives those with whom she has contact, particularly professionals, much of the credit for her special achievements."

In 1967 the School of Nutrition and Dietetics (which had been organized in 1922 as the School of Dietetics) became the Nutrition Department in the new School of Public Health. I returned to Loma Linda University in June, 1967, to teach in the Master of Science in Food Systems Management Program in the Graduate School and became Director of the Dietetic Internship in the School of Public Health. I was awarded the Ph.D. degree in Food Administration by the University of Wisconsin in June, 1968.

Dietetics education was changing and a new concept implemented at Ohio State University was the Coordinated Undergraduate Program (CUP) in Dietetics which I found very intriguing. For several years I had questioned why it needed to take four years of college coursework plus a one year dietetic internship to become a dietitian when nursing students could enroll in a four year baccalaureate nursing degree program and become eligible to become a registered nurse in that period of time. As our nutrition and dietetics faculty explored the possibility of developing the CUP in Dietetics program it seemed that it was an appropriate time to move in that direction. We learned that several other colleges and universities had followed Ohio State University's model and implemented this new type of coordinated program. Since the new 564 bed Loma Linda University Medical Center had become a reality in 1967, the decision was made in 1970 to phase out the one year dietetic internship and replace it with the CUP. Approval by The American Dietetic Association to offer this new program was given to the School of Allied Health Professions in 1972. Five students were accepted that first year. Soon it was possible to accept up to 26 junior students a year. As CUP program director I also became Director of Nutritional Services Department at the University Medical Center, a dual role which worked out to be an ideal situation for providing quality preprofessional practice for both the junior and senior students in both clinical dietetics and administrative dietetics. This program has enjoyed continuous accreditation status by The American Dietetic Association and over 266 students have graduated from one of the two emphases offered. The dietetic internship was phased out in 1974 from which 203 dietetic students had graduated. Alumni from this internship program as well as from the CUP are serving in different places in the U.S. and many are serving in other countries.

Filling the dual role of CUP Director in Dietetics, School of Allied Health Professions, and Director of Nutritional Services at the University Medical Center continued to be very exciting and stimulating as it gave me the opportunity to be involved in teaching, research and management practice. Seeing graduates of the dietetics program be successful in performing at a high level of competency and advancing the profession of dietetics is a most valued reward. A major activity to which I gave considerable attention was the implementation of a computer-assisted management information system for the Nutrition Services Department. The project was started in 1972, when Part I of the system became operational. Part II was to add a program directed primarily toward patient nutritional assessment and care plan.

When I had completed the doctoral program, I participated more actively in state as well as national affairs of the ADA. There have been numerous opportunities to serve at the national level including being Chairman, Commission on Evaluation of Dietetic Education (Commission on Accreditation), 1975–77; a Site Visitor for Accreditation, 1975–78, 80–81, 1984–88; Board of Directors, Member-at-Large, 1978–80, President-elect and President 1981–83; ADA Representative, National Nutrition Consortium (Washington, D.C.), 1979–83; Committee to Advise Implementation of Study Commission Recommendations for the ADA, 1984–85; Evaluation for Pilot Testing the Standards of Education, ADA, 1985–87. The rewards of serving the Association in various roles far outweigh the time involved. Hopefully colleagues and students with whom I am currently or have been associated will become active in their respective district, state and national association activities.

An outstanding educational opportunity for me was to serve as a member of the Task Force on Education, Veterans Administration Central Office, Washington, D.C., 1974–76. In 1978–79 I was invited to be a member of the Task Force on Productivity in Hospital Dietary Departments, Veteran Administration Central Office, Washington, D.C. Never before did I realize how effectively Registered Dietitians serve the U.S. veteran population who are hospitalized or are receiving nutritional care on an outpatient basis.

During my year as ADA President many short-term objectives and long-range goals were achieved as addressed in The President's Annual Report, 1982–83 (3). The history and traditions of the profession and of the ADA have been built on a goal of excellence. We have learned much from the past; we recognize the achievements of our predecessors; yet there is the continuing challenge for the future, with change being the only constant. In reflecting on the events of that year as President I believe the endorsement by the ADA Board of Directors of The American Dietetic Association Foundation's (ADAF) establishment of a building-fund program was the exciting highlight. This endorsement paved the way for the ADAF to actively pursue acquisition of a building, which would have two major benefits:

It would provide rental space for ADA Headquarters and would give the Foundation a permanent source of income for funding projects. As the concept of a national resource center for nutrition and dietetics evolved, a fund-raising program was initiated at the Annual Meeting in Anaheim, 1983. The success of that endeavor yielded more than $200,000 in donations and pledges from charter members of the Founders Club for the Let's Build Our Future Campaign.

In 1988 the ADAF announced the partnership acquisition of a permanent headquarters facility, The American Dietetic Association Building, to which all units moved in August. The National Center for Nutrition and Dietetics became a reality, thanks to the support of the ADA membership. Corporate contributions will add to the building fund and support of the programs provided through the Center.

Research became a major priority for me after I completed my doctoral research project and dissertation on Distribution of Work Functions in Hospital Food Systems. Focus of the research was on the innovative assembly-serve food system implemented by Kaiser Foundation Hospitals in California. Reports of the research were published in the Journal of The American Dietetic Association in 1970 Vol. 56 and in Hospitals, Journal of the American Hospital Association in 1971 Vol. 45. A Master of Science degree program in Food Systems Management was offered at Loma Linda University through the Graduate School between 1967 and 1984. Sixteen graduate students completed the program which included a research project and a thesis or publishable paper in a peer reviewed journal. Areas of research included a) performance of task functions by dietetic technicians, b) work measurement in hospital dietary departments, or c) computer-assisted information systems for food service systems.

In January, 1984, I informed the School of Public Health Dean, the School of Allied Health Professions Dean and the University Medical Center Administrator that I planned to retire in June of that year. Retirement benefits were available and I decided it was time to use them. The Associate Director of the Nutrition and Dietetics CUP who was also Associate Director for Nutritional Services at the University Medical Center was Bert Connell, Ph.D., R.D. He had carried the major responsibility for both positions while I had been so heavily involved with ADA activities and his performance was outstanding. He could fill both positions extremely well. Soon after I told the School of Public Health Dean about my plans for retirement he made an appointment to talk with me about returning after my retirement in June to assume the position of Nutrition Department Chairman. The current chairman had requested that he be permitted to return to full time teaching and research and be relieved of the administrative responsibilities. After several weeks of deliberation I accepted the invitation to return to the School of Public Health.

In July and August 1984 my husband and I had a wonderful trip to the Scandinavian countries plus Scotland and England. We joined a group of our friends from our college days for the excursion which made the experience especially enjoyable. When we returned from that vacation I assumed responsibility for serving as Nutrition Department Chairman, School of Public Health, effective September 1984. Though I had been a member of the Nutrition department in Public Health since 1964, my major responsibilities changed in 1972 when I became Director of the CUP in Dietetics organizationally housed in the School of Allied Health Professions. Returning full time to the School of Public Health in September, 1984, changed the focus of my direction. The primary responsibility was to direct the master's degree program offered in public health nutrition.

For a number of years nutrition faculty had talked about exploring the possibility of offering a Dr.P.H. degree in Nutrition with the emphasis in Community Nutrition. Before any plans could be laid we had to evaluate the resources available, conduct a needs assessment for such a program, develop an appropriate curriculum, and appoint an advisory council. The outcome of that effort was that nutrition faculty collectively developed the program proposal, submitted it to the University Academic Council for review and hopefully approval. Action by the Council was approval and the proposal was submitted to the University Board of Trustees. Their approval was granted in May, 1986. It was approved by the Board of Higher Education in 1987. The first doctoral student in the Dr.P.H. Nutrition program in the School of Public Health enrolled in 1987. Currently there are four students pursuing that degree in 1989.

Since 1978 the Nutrition Department had sponsored graduate students who completed the Master of Public Health in Nutrition degree or the Master of Science in Nutrition degree for six months' qualifying experience in dietetics to establish eligibility to write the Registration Examination of The American Dietetic Association to become a Registered Dietitian. In 1986 we were advised that the Commission on Dietetic Registration had voted to amend the registration eligibility schedule for dietitians. October 1, 1988 was the last postmark date to submit an application for prior approval of a qualifying experience with an advanced degree. Since a high percentage of the students in the master's degree programs wished to become a Registered Dietitian, the nutrition faculty voted to develop a Self Study for a Proposed AP4 Preprofessional Practice Program in Dietetics to replace the Qualifying Experience route for registration eligibility. The Self Study was submitted to the ADA on November 25, 1987, and approval was granted by ADA in May, 1988. Currently the Nutrition Department has accepted 24 graduate students into the AP4 Program since it was approved.

From the research in which I have been actively involved to date fifteen articles have been published in refereed journals including the Journal of The American Dietetic Association, Journal of Home Economics, School Food Service Research Review, and Hospitals: Journal of the American Hospital Association. From 1985–88 I was a member of the Editorial Panel, School Food Service Research Review, American School Food Service Association. Since 1985 I have served on the Editorial Board, Topics in Clinical Nutrition, Aspen System Corporation.

ADA members can be proud of the progress made to date by current Association leadership in defining the vision of where we want to be in the 21st century. The Strategic Plan, adopted at the 1988 House of Delegates meeting in San Fransisco, is designed to guide the Association, its Foundation, and the National Center for Nutrition and Dietetics.

Collectively, Association leadership has been responsible for the success in legislation and public policy which has been viewed as related to dietetics visibility. Legislative issues include licensure. In 1987–88 six states passed laws bringing the total, to date, to 23 states with licensure, title or registration acts.

Dietetic educators are being trained by the Council on Education on the new Standards of Education and the new accreditation/approval processes.

Many dietitians are becoming successful entrepreneurs and establishing private practices in clinical dietetics or food systems management. Others are employed in sales or serve as nutrition educators for the food industry or pharmaceutical organizations. Some are innovators as consultants for layout and design of foodservice operations. I have watched with interest the success some dietitians have achieved in enhancing visibility for the Registered Dietitian by the leadership they have demonstrated in print and TV media.

As I reflect on the Board of Directors activities during my term as ADA President (1982–83), one of the major challenges was to select the new editor for the Journal of The American Dietetic Association (JADA). Dorothea Turner had been an outstanding editor since June 1946 and had submitted her resignation to enjoy the benefits and lifestyle of retirement. It took seven months to complete the recruitment and selection process to finalize on selection of a new editor. Questions had been raised relevant to selecting an editor who was not on-site at the Headquarters Office. When the decision by the Selection Committee was made that an off-site editor could function successfully, Elaine Monsen, Ph.D., R.D., School of Medicine, University of Washington, was employed as full-time editor. Dr. Monsen has made ADA membership proud of the quality of the Journal under her leadership. The timeliness of the content the Journal brings to the membership is deeply appreciated.

Serving the Association at the district, state, and national level has brought reward of recognition for which I do not take credit. Rather the recognition should go to the many nutrition and dietetic professionals with whom I have been privileged to be associated.

AWARDS:

Delta Omega Society National Merit Award for Outstanding Achievement in Public Health, 1988

International Woman of the Year/Work-Professional Life Award, Associate of Adventist Women and General Conference of Human Relations, 1985

Distinguished Faculty Service Award, Loma Linda University, 1984

Management Service Award, Loma Linda University Medical Center, 1984

Distinguished Faculty Lecturer, Loma Linda University, 1979

Dolores Nyhus Award, California Dietetic Association, 1978

Distinguished Home Economics Alumnus Award, Washington State University, 1978

Alumnus of the Year, Walla Walla College, 1977

American Men and Women in Science, 1977

Delta Omega Award, Public Health Honor Society, 1972

Who's Who in California, 1970

Who's Who in American Women, 1969

In a high-performance organization, every member is expected to make a personal contribution to accomplish the stated goals. Participation by networking, working through common problems, and developing strategies for solutions, by being aware of the changing practices and technologies that may transform our role, by exploring and working together professional is imperative.

My professional life as a registered dietitian, a teacher, an administrator and researcher has been challenging and extremely rewarding. Several years ago it was suggested that based on my experience and background that I pursue a career in consumer law relevant to food and nutrition. As I explored a change in career decision I weighed the possible outcome against the advantages of my teaching role at this point in time. The final decision was to continue what I have enjoyed immensely for over 40 years.

References

1. Metcalf, H.C. and L. Urwick. Dynamic Administration: The Collected Papers of Mary Parker Follet, p. 247–285. Harper and Row Publishers, 1940.
2. Matthews, M.E. Kathleen Zolber, Ph.D., R.D., President, 1982–83, The American Dietetic Association. J. Am. Diet. A. 1982; 81(5):592.
3. Zolber, K. The President's Annual Report, 1982–83. J. Am. Diet. A. 1984; 84(1):80.

About the Authors

Connie E. Vickery received a B.S. degree in home economics from the University of Alabama and completed a dietetic internship at Massachusetts General Hospital. She earned her M.S. degree in nutrition science from Syracuse (NY) University and her doctorate in human nutrition and foods from Virginia Polytechnic Institute and State University. She has held positions in clinical dietetics and currently holds the rank of Associate Professor in the Department of Nutrition and Dietetics at the University of Delaware. She is co-author of *Effective Counseling for Dietary Management.*

Nancy Cotugna is Assistant Professor in the Department of Nutrition and Dietetics at the University of Delaware. At the time of this publication she will be on leave from that position to serve as a post-doctoral fellow at the National Cancer Institute. Dr. Cogugna received an undergraduate degree in home economics from the University of California, Santa Barbara, a master's degree in nutrition from Rutgers University and a doctorate in public health from Loma Linda University. She completed a dietetic internship at the Massachusetts General Hospital. In addition to her teaching experience, she has held positions in clinical dietetics, inservice education, and consulting.